Concise Textbook of Large Animal Handling

This concise instructional guide condenses the most important aspects of large animal handling. It provides a portable, durable, beside-the-animal means of learning, as well as a convenient way to refresh on how to strive for safety and efficacy in animal handling techniques. It is ideal for use during veterinary placements in all settings from farm to laboratory, to riding school. The text covers:

- Handler safety
- Animal safety
- Sanitation
- Approach and capture
- Routine handling and release procedures
- Handling for medical procedures
- Use and supply sources of restraint equipment

Important reading for undergraduate veterinary students on EMS rotations, as well as practicing veterinarians, technicians, and assistants, the book covers species encountered in farm, equine, and laboratory settings.

A Companion Website provides additional self-assessment questions and answers to aid learning.

Concise Textbook of Large Animal Handling

A Practical Handbook

C. B. Chastain
Emeritus/Adjunct Professor
College of Veterinary Medicine
University of Missouri, Columbia, MO

Line Drawings by Lynn Vellios

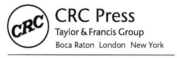

CRC Press
Taylor & Francis Group
Boca Raton London New York

CRC Press is an imprint of the
Taylor & Francis Group, an **informa** business

First edition published 2023
by CRC Press
6000 Broken Sound Parkway NW, Suite 300, Boca Raton, FL 33487–2742

and by CRC Press
4 Park Square, Milton Park, Abingdon, Oxon, OX14 4RN

CRC Press is an imprint of Taylor & Francis Group, LLC

ISBN: 978-0-367-62812-3 (hbk)
ISBN: 978-0-367-62809-3 (pbk)
ISBN: 978-1-003-11091-0 (ebk)

DOI: 10.1201/9781003110910

Typeset in Minion
by Apex CoVantage, LLC

Access the Companion Website: www.routledge.com/9780367628123

CONTENTS

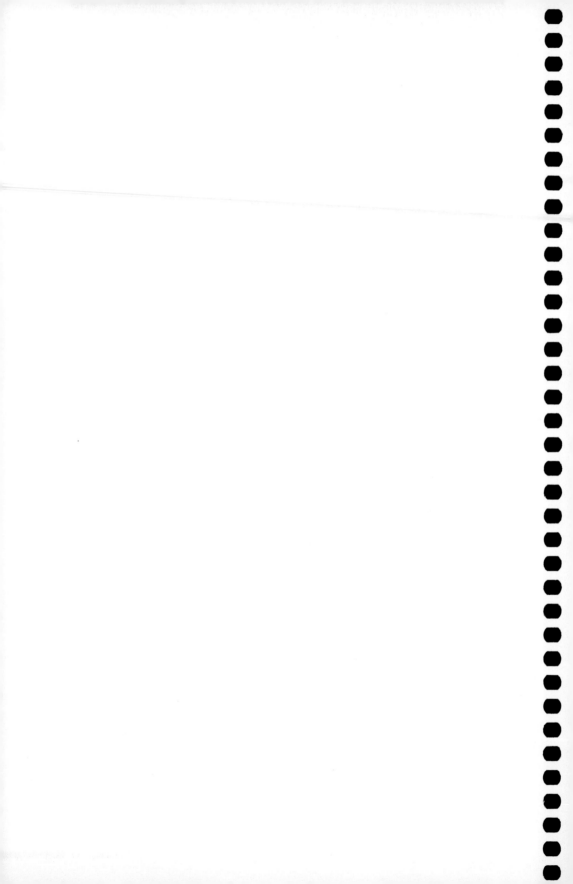

PREFACE

Proper handling and restraint are essential to the welfare of captive animals. Animals that are properly handled and restrained can be examined, groomed, and treated in ways that contribute to their optimum quantity and quality of life.

Veterinary medicine is both art and science. Teaching the science of animal handling is relatively easy. Learning the art is more difficult as it requires much experience, continual practice, and an open mind to new challenges. Each animal is an individual and each handling environment provides its own advantages and disadvantages.

The most basic part of the art of veterinary medicine is the safe handling of animals. The needs of pre-veterinary and veterinary students to become knowledgeable in safe, humane animal handling was the impetus to write the textbook *Animal Handling and Physical Restraint*, which is the predecessor to this handbook.

The goals of this handbook are to assist future veterinarians; veterinary technologists, technicians, and assistants; and others who deal with animals to be able to handle animals more safely and humanely. It is for quick reference and use next to animals. No handling or restraint of animals is without risk, but proper animal handling and restraint aid in reducing the chance of the handler or animal experiencing physical injury or infectious diseases that can be transmitted between species.

Means of confinement (fences, gates, pens, and stalls) can affect animal handling, but they are not covered in this handbook. For more information on confinements, the history of domestication of various species, or horseback riding safety, see the textbook *Animal Handling and Physical Restraint*, published by CRC Press.

Each time a handler handles or restrains an animal the handler is training it how to accept the next time it is handled. Ideally, the response to the next time it is handled is better than the last.

Self-assessment questions and answers based on the information provided in the book are available to book buyers on a Companion Website at https://routledgetextbooks.com/textbooks/9780367628093

The greatness of a nation and its moral progress can be judged by the way its animals are treated. Mahatma Gandhi, 1869–1948.

ACKNOWLEDGMENTS

I owe many thanks to my mentors on large animal handling, including veterinarians Leonard E. Palmer, Ed Ebert, Toney Reynolds, Joe McGinity, Tom Eagle, Jim English, and Art Dobson. Other large animal handlers I worked with and to whom I owe gratitude are Bill Donaldson, Jerry Stone, and Bill and Fannie Robinson.

Ultimately, the greatest instructors I have had are the animals I have handled and restrained, who taught me more about safe, humane, and efficient animal handling each time I had the privilege of working with them.

Special thanks go to Lynn Vellios, whose line drawings have permitted non-distracting backgrounds and emphasis on key visual aspects of animal handling. In addition, thanks to Alice Oven, Senior Editor Life Sciences & Veterinary Medicine at CRC Press, Taylor & Francis Group, who has always been encouraging and immensely helpful in the creation of this handbook. The proofreading efforts of Kaitlin Sulkowski were also of great help.

The encouragement of my wife, Joyce, and daughters, Andrea and Danielle, and my daughters' families as well as their willingness to forgive my obsession with better animal handling has been essential and much appreciated.

C. B. Chastain
September 2022

CAUTION

No handling nor restraint of animals is without risk, but proper animal handling and restraint aids in reducing the chance of the handler or animal experiencing physical injury or mutual infectious diseases.

Learning, acquiring, and maintaining the skill of animal handling and restraint is a methodical progression of stages to (1) learn, (2) see, (3) practice, (4) do, and (5) maintain. To translate knowledge of the art of animal handling into practical skills requires long practice of proper procedures. Early training, life-long practice, and an open mind to acquiring better techniques are the keys to successful animal handling. Practice yields improvement but not perfection. Each animal is an individual and each handling environment provides its own advantages and disadvantages.

Serious injury or death can result from handling and restraining some animals. Safe and effective handling and restraint requires experience and continual practice. Acquisition of the needed skills should be under the supervision of an experienced animal handler.

AUTHOR BIOGRAPHY

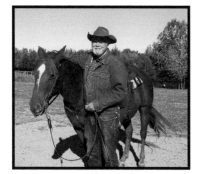 **C. B. Chastain** is a professor emeritus and adjunct professor of veterinary medicine and former Section Head of Small Animal Medicine and Associate Dean for Academic Affairs at the University of Missouri. He also has been on faculty at Iowa State University and Louisiana State University. In addition to being a Diplomate of the American College of Veterinary Internal Medicine, he has authored journal articles, book chapters in veterinary medical and allied publications, and textbooks on clinical endocrinology and animal handling and physical restraint.

Prior to entering academic veterinary medicine, he was a horse wrangler for a horseback-riding stable and a licensed guide in Rocky Mountain National Park, Colorado; worked in mixed animal veterinary medical practices in Missouri, Illinois, and New Mexico; and a captain in the U.S. Air Force Veterinary Corps. He has handled, restrained, and trained a variety of animals in differing environments and taught aspects of animal handling for more than 40 years at the undergraduate and professional school levels. Currently, he is a professor and consultant for Veterinary Online Programs at the University of Missouri.

1

SAFER ANIMAL HANDLING AND PHYSICAL RESTRAINT

DOI: 10.1201/9781003110910-1

The reasons to handle or restrain individual animals include physical examination; prophylactic, medical, or surgical treatments; grooming; training; recreation; and companionship. The single action that veterinary medical personnel do for each and every patient is the application of handling techniques.

HANDLING AND ANIMAL WELFARE

Handlers should become familiar with animals in their care, including their normal habits of eating, drinking, sleeping, urinating, defecating, and exercising so that problems can be identified early and corrected when possible.

GOOD HANDLING NEEDS TRANSPARENCY

Handling animals in seclusion without public visibility by employees or agents of owners fosters an environment that allows the attrition of good animal handling (Table 1.1).

Table 1.1	Examples of Contributors* to the Attrition of Good Animal Handling
•	Animal trainers who require appointments for owners to see training practices
•	Closed confinement of livestock and poultry that prohibits public observation
•	State laws that prohibit photographs of animals in confinement
•	Veterinary practices that prohibit observation of their handling of patients.

* These situations do not innately cause poor animal handling but they permit and protect environments without transparency to the public that can harbor poor animal handling.

- **Evidence of the Quality of Handling:** The best, and only meaningful, source of evidence for good animal handling, restraint, or confinement is what the animal reveals by their behavior when the handling and restraint are repeated or persist.
- **Stereotypic Behaviors:** If the behavior is unnatural (stereotypic or exaggerated fear), poor handling or restraint methods have taken place. Stereotypic behaviors include pacing, weaving, chewing cages or stalls, or self-mutilation, among others. Unnatural behavior as a result of poor handling, restraint, or confinement should be among the primary means of assessing the need for improved management of animals, along with the number of animals demonstrating excessive lameness, external injuries, and vocalizations.

DEFINITION OF ANIMAL WELFARE

The American Veterinary Medical Association has defined animal welfare as "when an animal is healthy, comfortable, well nourished, safe, able to express innate behavior, and not suffering from unpleasant states such as pain, fear, and distress." The basic needs of animals are referred to as freedoms (Table 1.2).

Table 1.2	Five Basic Needs (Freedoms) of Domesticated Animals
•	A suitable environment
•	A suitable diet
•	The ability to exhibit normal behavior
•	The need for an animal to be housed with, or apart from, other animals
•	Protection from pain, suffering, injury, and disease.

THE MORE EFFECTIVE HANDLER: THE ART OF FIRM KINDNESS

Proper animal handling for husbandry, treatment, and safety is quiet, methodical, and should allow the animal to be easier to handle the next time. Guidelines for physical restraint of animals are contained in the American Veterinary Medical Association's position statement on the "Physical Restraint of Animals." The essentials of the AVMA's position statement are listed in Table 1.3.

Table 1.3 Essentials of Proper Animal Restraint	
•	The least restraint required to allow the procedure to be performed properly
•	Protection of both the animal and personnel from harm
•	To plan, formulate, and communicate restraint prior to its application
•	The use of chemical restraint when physical restraint presents excessive risk of injury to the animal or its handlers.

AFFECTION FOR THE ANIMALS

- **Empathy:** Lack of empathy is the hallmark of a poor animal handler. Handlers may be empathetic toward one species and effective with that species but dislike other species and be ineffective with them. Use of derogatory terms toward animals such as "dumb," "stupid," "mean," etc. affect handler attitude and actions and should disqualify that person from handling the animals to whom the terms were directed.
- **Affection:** A good animal handler has to like the type of animal that will be handled.
    - **Danger of Food Rewards:** Using petting, scratching, grooming, or verbal praises are beneficial under the correct circumstances. However, larger prey animals seeking food can endanger people if they invade human personal space.
    - **Avoid Food Association with Hands:** Food treats should only be offered to horses and livestock in pans or buckets. They should not be taught to associate hands or pockets as a source of food. Seeking food directly from a handler can lead to dangerous invasion of the handler's personal space.

PROPER ATTITUDE

Good animal handlers are calm, deliberate, patient, organized, and determined, and they attempt to prepare animals to better tolerate future animal handling experiences.

- **Calm, Deliberate, and Patient:** Extroverted behavior (i.e., direct stares, exaggerated facial expressions, frequent hand and arm movements, and loud or spiking speech patterns) can attract the attention of humans and may engender a good first impression, but these mannerisms do not gain or maintain trust from animals. Animal handlers should move and act calmly, deliberately, and patiently.
- **Organized Approach:** Being organized and having a plan before handling or restraining animals is important for success for each handling event and all future handling events with the animals handled.
- **Determination:** Determination is an essential quality of a good handler. A handler must be confident and determined that the plan to handle or restrain an animal will be successful.
- **Controlled Release:** The release must be as quiet and calm as possible and it must be under control of the handler, not the animal. Each handling, and especially restraint experience, is a lesson learned by the animal, and their release is most remembered.

ALLOCATION OF SUFFICIENT TIME: POWER OF PATIENCE

Sufficient time to observe the animal or animals to be handled is important in determining the best approach to handling and to allow the animal or animals to adapt to handler presence.

- **Disadvantage of Being in a Rush:** Once a plan of handling is determined, sufficient time must be allocated to perform the handling with minimal stress to the handler and the animals.
- **More Time for Special Cases:** Longer times need to be allocated particularly for handling young or new animals. The luxury of adequate time is always subject to weather conditions.

USE OF VOICE, TOUCH, AND BODY LANGUAGE

Restraint begins with the handler's voice or body language.

- **Voice:** Animals like to hear a handler's voice if it is soothing and has rhythmic tones.
- **Body Language:**
  - **Primary Means of Communication:** Large animals use body language to a greater extent than any other means of communications.
  - **Perception of Human Body Language That Is Imperceptible to Humans:** Some animals are especially sensitive to human facial expressions and other body language.
    - ○ **Clever Hans:** An Orlov Trotter horse in Germany, named Clever Hans, was famous for this in the early 1900s. He appeared able to perform arithmetic and other mental tasks by reading subtle human body language.
    - ○ **Clever Hans Effect:** In recognition of his abilities, the observer-effect is also referred to as the *Clever Hans Effect*.
- **Preferred Body Language of Handlers:**
  - **Lowered Posture:** Non-threatening body language includes keeping the arms down and close to the body, with palms toward the thighs. Raising the arms is threatening, but can be used to drive large animals in a desired direction. An erect posture is less threatening than slumped shoulders or rounded back which simulates a pouncing and threatening posture.
  - **Avoid a Direct Stare:** A glancing gaze or indirect stare is less threatening than a direct stare. Staring at an animal's eyes is threatening to prey animals.
  - **Rhythmic Movement:** Moderately rapid, rhythmic normal movements are less threatening than rapid, jerky, or slow, creeping actions.
- **Touch:** Touch can readily convey handler confidence and intentions to an animal being handled.
  - **Touch Pressure:** Excessively light touch or stroking does this poorly causing signs of apprehension in most animals. Moderately firm, deliberate gentle touch conveys more confidence and is less threatening than very light touch or stroking.
  - **Hand Position:** Touching should be done with fingers together and applied with either the palm side or the back of the hand. Touching with the tips of the fingers while the fingers are spread or with the end of the thumb is less well tolerated. Using spread finger tips or the end of the thumb can be a much more useful means of moving a horse in a desired direction than pushing with a flat hand.
  - **Patting or Slaps:** Very firm, pushy, or slapping-type touches may be perceived as a challenge to social position in the herd or a reprimand for misbehavior. However, it can be beneficial for handlers to desensitize horses to moderate slaps to prevent flight reactions if tack or clothing accidently slaps them while mounting or riding or if the handler or rider needs to slap a biting fly, especially horseflies.

- **Better Tolerated Locations:** The shoulders are not densely innervated by touch receptors and this is not a location that fatal injuries can be inflicted. As a result, animals tolerate touch on the shoulders more easily than touch around the more vulnerable areas such as the eyes, ears, throat, belly, or legs.

ALWAYS ON GUARD: SAFETY FIRST

Animals should always be handled with precautions against injury. The safest animals may be safe 99% of the time, but handlers should always be prepared for the 1% chance that the usually safe animal will become unsafe due to pain, perceived territorial threats, illness, or a myriad of other situations unlike those in the past. Handlers must be constantly aware of the risks of injury to themselves, other people, or the animal being handled.

- **Individual Animal Reactions Vary:** Each species has its inherent species behavior, and within a species, each individual has a unique temperament and behavior. Factors which affect an individual animal's reactions to handling are familial tendencies; prior handling and training; trust, or the lack of it, in the handler; and stressful events preceding or during the handling. As a result, the assumption that all domestic species or animals within a species are the same can lead to serious injury.
- **Overconfident and Ill-Prepared:** Most handler injuries from animals are caused by the handler being overconfident and under-competent. Animal handlers must always position themselves to eliminate or minimize the chance of injury to all involved.
- **Special Risks to Veterinary Staff:**
  - **High Risk:** Many animals that veterinary personnel must treat have not been socialized to humans or previously handled. In addition, sick or injured animals may act atypically because of pain or fear.
  - **Under-Appreciation of Risk:** Sick or injured animals often hide their disease or injury until a handler disturbs them. Some owners do not appreciate the risk of handling sick or injured animals or animals being handled by new people whom the animal has not yet established a bond of trust. The need for precautionary measures may have to be explained to owners.

DISTRACTION VERSUS PAIN FOR RESTRAINT

Distractions are the basis for most humane and effective animal handling techniques and are not painful when correctly used.

- **Pain:** Pain is a message sent to the brain that body tissue is being injured. Painful procedures leave a physical or psychological mark on the animal.
  - **Signs of Pain:** In addition to evidence of tissue damage, other signs of pain in animals can be present (Table 1.4). Animals, particularly prey animals, may mask some signs of pain if in unfamiliar surroundings or otherwise feeling threatened.

Table 1.4	Signs of Pain in Large Animals
•	Decreased appetite
•	Failure to groom
•	Lack of effort to nest
•	Hunched posture
•	Grinding of teeth
•	Glazed stare
•	Elevated heart rate and/or respiratory rate
•	Thrashing movements.

- **Fear That Mimics Pain:** Some animals will react to distraction in fear as if the distraction was painful. When this occurs, chemical restraint may be needed if there is a reasonable possibility that fear will be intensified and hinder future efforts to handle the animal.

- **Distraction:** Distraction is applying a non-painful stimulus that supersedes competing stimuli.
- **Avoid Painful Distractions:** When a distraction technique is applied severely or incorrectly, it can inflict pain. For example, when a nose twitch, a pinching distraction technique most often used on the upper lip of horses, is applied correctly there is no tissue injured and therefore no pain. If used inappropriately and the twitch causes pain, there is evidence of tissue damage (i.e., soreness persisting after releasing the twitch, loss of function of the upper lip, or a change in the appearance of the tissue such as swelling, cuts, or bruising).

RESPECT FOR HANDLERS
- **Gaining Respect:** Animals should be respectful, not fearful, of human handlers. Respect is gained by their knowledge that either pleasure (e.g., praise, petting, undisturbed rest, food treats) or discomfort, not pain (e.g., requirement to move, distraction techniques), will consistently occur with certain behaviors.
  - **Control of Movement and Access to Resources:** Leaders of animals establish their social position by the control of movement and access to resources. Effective handlers do the same.
  - **Danger of Food Rewards:** In the case of large animals such as horses, the use of food rewards can be impractical or dangerous due to the risk of the animal invading the handler's personal space.
  - **Proper Rewards for Large Animals:**
    - **Livestock Wish to Be Left Alone:** Requiring large animals to respond to a stimulus and then removing that stimulus so that they are again undisturbed is a great reward. Rather than using food rewards, large animal respect for human personal space is more safely established by simply staring at the animal or moving a hand away from the handler's body. The stimulus, such as staring or raised hands, is immediately removed after a desired response from the animal.
    - **If Food Is Used:** Additional positive reinforcement with food rewards may be desirable in some cases, but the large animal's access to the food should never be associated with being close to the handler, particularly their hands or pockets.
- **Avoiding Fear:** Fear can result from the expectation of pain. If fear is from instinct, it can be moderated. If it is from having experienced pain, it is often permanent.
- **Danger of Lack of Respect:** Animals that are either fearful of handlers or have no respect for humans are the most dangerous to handle. Bulls and stallions are often raised in relative isolation of their own species. That, plus an excessive exposure to humans, often leads to dangerous habits which result from the lack of respect for humans.

ADAPTATION TO SPECIAL CIRCUMSTANCES
Animal handling is not a set recipe that fits all situations. An effective animal handler must adapt techniques to the species, the surroundings, and the individual.

- **Surroundings:** Each animal handled should first be observed to assess its current attitude and physical condition.
- **Current Attitude and Condition:** Young, elderly, and pregnant animals need special handling. How immature animals are handled can ingrain their responses to handling for the rest of their life.

- **Need for Special Handling:**
  - **Young Animals:** Young animals may be more easily injured due to the risk of injuring growth plates in bones and because of their uncoordinated attempts to resist handling.
  - **Elderly Animals:** Elderly animals may have a lifetime accumulation of good or bad experiences with being handled and a greater probability of failing organ function and arthritis.
  - **Pregnant Animals:** Pregnant animals may be more fearful from the instinct of knowing that their escape, if needed, will be more difficult.

APPROPRIATE ATTIRE, GROOMING, AND PERSONAL HABITS

Proper handler attire for the type of animal handling to be done is important for handlers and animals.

- **Clothing:** Inappropriate attire can be dangerous (Table 1.5 and Figure 1.1).

Table 1.5	Inappropriate Attire and Grooming for Large Animal Handlers
•	Loose clothes
•	Loose long hair
•	Dangling jewelry (earrings, bracelets, necklaces)
•	Bulky rings
•	Hoods or other head gear that obstructs peripheral vision
•	Boots with slick soles.

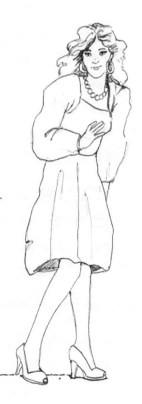

Figure 1.1   Inappropriate large animal handling attire.

- **Shirts, Coats, Trousers, and Coveralls:** Clothing should be reasonably clean and untorn. Short sleeves or rolled up long sleeves are needed to keep arms from being easily caught on fences, gates, and handling equipment. Coveralls or thick trousers in muted green or khaki color are appropriate for routine handling of livestock or poultry (Figure 1.2).

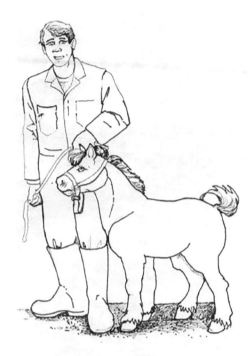

Figure 1.2 Appropriate large animal handling attire.

- **Belts and Leggings:** A strong belt can be used as a temporary lead rope around the animal's neck or a flag to direct animal movement. Leather leggings are advisable if handling ratites to protect legs from forward strikes.
- **Footwear:** Boots should be loose fitting, water impermeable, with non-skid soles. Metal toe caps may be advisable when working with cattle, small ruminants, or ratites.
- **Worn at Appropriate Time:** Attire for animal handling should be worn only when handling or restraining animals and then changed to reduce the risk of transmitting disease among other animals and to humans.
- **Fingernails:** Fingernails should not extend beyond the end of the finger to reduce the risk of injury to other handlers or to animals being handled and because longer fingernails are more capable of entrapping disease agents.
- **Identification Badges:** If ID badges are needed, they should either be attached to the clothing or worn using a safety, breakaway lanyard around the neck.
- **Cuts and Abrasions:** Handler cuts or abrasions should be treated and covered before handling animals.
- **Food and Tobacco Products:** Smoking or consuming food or drink while working with animals or in animal handling areas should be strictly avoided due to the danger of introducing infectious organisms to the handler's mouth.

- **Personal Protective Equipment:**
  - **Waterproof Apron:** Waterproof aprons should be worn when bathing animals.
  - **Eye Protection:** Safety glasses or goggles should be worn if handling animals that may sling body secretions or bath water or when dust is prevalent. Goggles should be used if working with horses or cattle in wet/muddy conditions. Temporary blindness, particularly around livestock and horses, can be dangerous.
  - **Ear Protection:** Ear plugs should be worn if noise from animals, particularly swine, or their handling equipment prevents conversation in a normal voice.
  - **Face Protection:** Nose and mouth masks (N95 or N100) are needed in circumstances that could involve infectious diseases or dusty environments, particularly in total confinement poultry environments.
  - **Gloves:** Latex rubber or nitrile gloves should be worn if hands have cuts or cracks.
  - **Hats:** Hats for handlers of livestock or poultry aid to protect from overexposure to sunlight and head injury.
    - **Brimmed Hats:** Ball caps are popular, but a simple brimmed hat will also help protect against sun on the ears and back of the neck. When working in tight quarters, brimmed hats give the handler an early warning of the possibility of hitting his or her head on structure beams or handling equipment. They also help keep spider webs in barns out of the face and hair.
    - **Hoods:** Hoods, other head gear, or long hair styles that obstruct peripheral vision or might become snagged and entrap the head should not be worn when working with livestock, particularly cattle, horses, or swine.
- **Adherence to Standard Farm and Ranch Rules:** If working on a farm or ranch, trust and respect from owners of animals are gained by adhering to common farm and ranch rules (Table 1.6).

Table 1.6 Common Courtesies When Working on Farms or Ranches	
•	If you open it, close it
•	If it was open, leave it open
•	If you unlock it, lock it
•	If you move it, put it back
•	If you make a mess, clean it up
•	Do not climb on fences or gates without permission
•	Do not leave an animal in a dirty stall, clean it as often as you find it dirty
•	Unless certain of probable safety or animal welfare risks, do not tell an owner how to handle their animal without being asked.

CONDITIONS FOR HANDLING AND RESTRAINT

Outcomes of handling and restraint of animals can be affected by health of the animal, the time of day, lighting, ambient temperature, setting and facilities, personnel, and duration.

PRE-HANDLING CONSIDERATIONS

An unhealthy animal can have an altered temperament requiring special handling techniques or elevated risk of injury from being handled due to illness or previous injury. Before handling any animal, it and its surroundings should be visually inspected (Table 1.7).

Table 1.7 Pre-Handling Evaluation of the Animal and Its Surroundings

•	Check for signs of injury or disease
•	Be alert for abnormal vocalizations
•	Ascertain current appetite, thirst, and quantity and appearance of eliminations
•	Observe for signs of abnormal attitude
•	Assess signs of mobility
•	Watch for abnormal depth or rate of respirations
•	Evaluate the safety of the animal's containment area.

PRE-RESTRAINT CONSIDERATIONS

Restraint, if needed, must be applied effectively on first attempt or the animal will learn to escape the restraint in the future.

- **Formulate a Plan:**
  - **Plan with Contingencies:** Pre-restraint considerations are to formulate a plan, consider the effects on the animals, and what safety precautions are appropriate. Although a plan for restraint should be designed to be successful on first attempt, a contingency plan should be formulated in case circumstances are unexpected and inappropriate for the initial plan.
  - **Check Equipment:** A plan needs to first include a check of equipment.
  - **Capable Assistance:** If others will assist, everyone must be physically capable and trained to handle animals, and they must know the current plan thoroughly.
- **Determine What Safety Precautions Are Appropriate:**
  - **Escape Plans:** When dealing with large or otherwise dangerous or potentially aggressive animals, an escape should be planned in advance in case it becomes needed.
  - **Chemical Restraint Option:** Chemical restraint should be ready for some animals in advance of attempted physical restraint so that if chemical restraint becomes necessary, it can be administered without delay.

EFFECTS ON ANIMALS

The effects of handling and restraint on animal safety should be considered.

- **Current and Future Effects:** What lesson will be learned by the animal? To yield the best lesson that might be learned by the animal, a handler should use the minimum needed restraint, maintain a calm environment, and carefully manage the final release to be perceived that the release was the handler's choice, not the animal's.
- **Impact of Past Experiences:** If adverse effects occur when handling or restraining an animal, the animal will associate events, people, and objects that immediately preceded the handling and occurred during the animal's handling. They may respond with signs of stress or fear when exposed to similar handler clothing, locations (cage, pens, etc.), and other sounds on re-exposure. This displayed distress may seem inexplicable to a new handler.
- **Poor Handling Aftereffects:** See Table 1.8.

Table 1.8 Effects of Poor Handling of Large Animals

•	Lack of trust in handlers and trustworthiness in horses
•	Lack of weight gain and/or lameness in beef cattle
•	Reduced milk production and/or lameness in dairy cattle
•	Diminished lambings, impaired growth, and/or poor wool production in sheep
•	Small litters, decreased rate of growth, lameness, and/or delayed age of first estrus in sows.

SURROUNDINGS AND CONDITIONS

The time of day or amount of light can affect animal handling.

- **Ambient Lighting:**
  - **Nocturnal vs. Diurnal Animals' Reactions:** Nocturnal (night active) animals are more docile when handled in bright light. Diurnal (daytime active) animals are more docile when handled in subdued light.
  - **Shadows:** Livestock and horses (prey animals) avoid shadows and darkened areas and will move more willingly to well-lit areas, but not if the light is glaring, impairing vision.
- **Ambient Temperature:**
  - **Livestock:** Pigs and sheep are particularly susceptible to heat stress and should be handled early in the cooler part of the day. Fans and water spray on legs and lower abdomen should be applied, when needed.
  - **Horses:** Cool, brisk temperature enlivens horses, making handling more difficult. Hot weather makes them more tractable.
- **Reduce Risk of Injury or Escape:** Before working cattle in chutes, a check of all chutes, alleyways, and stalls should be conducted. Stalls and stocks should be inspected for potential hazards to horses before their use. Areas for casting a large animal (laying an animal down) should be checked for hazards where the animal could get its legs caught underneath a nearby structure.

PERSONNEL

If an assistant is present to help a primary handler, it is the primary handler's responsibility to make sure that the assistant is knowledgeable in proper animal handling and is fully aware of the handling or restraint plan.

- **Qualified Assistants:** An assistant should be behaviorally mature and physically strong enough to carry out the needed assistance. Otherwise, if the assistant or the animal is injured, the primary handler can be liable for damages.
- **Unqualified Assistant Liability:** In the case of veterinarians or veterinary technicians being primary handlers, animal owners should not assist with handling and restraint of their own animal. In less than ideal circumstances, when no one else is available to assist, an owner may insist on helping in a desire to ensure proper care of their animal or to prevent injury to it or the veterinarian. If assistance from an owner is the only means to provide reasonable safety for the animal or people present, the owner must not be allowed to assist without first being instructed in the proper technique, the risks involved, and a stated willingness to defer to the veterinarian's directions during the procedure, preferably in writing.

DURATION

The duration of animal handling or restraint should be as short as possible to complete the task. Longer durations cause unnecessary stress to the animal and exhaust their patience to tolerate the handling. Pre-handling preparation is absolutely essential to minimize the duration of handling and restraint.

RISKS OF INJURY

GENERAL RISKS

Few domestic animals are naturally aggressive toward humans. When fearful or stressed, most animals' first reaction is to attempt to flee. When fleeing is not an option, they will resort to their means of offense or defense, which may involve teeth that bite; hooves that kick, stomp, or strike; heads that butt or crush; or horns that gore.

- **Risks by Species:** One of six farm injuries are animal related, due to bites, kicks, and crushing. Male and elderly handlers are demographically at highest risk. Cattle, especially bulls, are responsible for 40% of deaths, horses for 27%, and hogs for 1%.
- **Injuries and Deaths from Cattle:**
  - **Deaths:** Cattle cause deaths in humans by mauling, charging, goring, kicking, or knocking people down. Most deaths are the result of attacks by bulls or cows with newborn calves.
  - **Beef Cattle:** Beef breeds of cattle are handled less than dairy cattle and are more inherently dangerous than dairy breeds.
  - **Dairy Cattle:** As a result of how they are typically raised in isolation, dairy bulls are considered the most dangerous of all domesticated animals. Dairy handlers are most often injured by cows during the milking process or treating mastitis, sustaining leg or facial injuries.
- **Injuries and Deaths from Horses:**
  - **Deaths:** Most horse-related human deaths are associated with riding, such as falling off or being thrown off. Other people are killed by being crushed, trampled on, or kicked (particularly in the head) by horses.
  - **Injuries:** Brain and craniofacial injuries from animals are most often caused by horses. More than 100,000 people are admitted to an emergency room in the U.S. from horses each year. Approximately two-thirds of horse-related injuries are from riding, and more than 12,000 injured people have head injuries.
- **Animal Injuries to Humans:** Large animal-related physical injuries to humans can be intentional from the animal involving butting, goring, bites, and kicks resulting from aggression or fear. In other cases, injury to the handler may be unintentional such as crushing from falls, stepping on feet, and blows to the body while the animal struggles to get free. Most causes of animal to human injuries are preventable (Table 1.9).

Table 1.9	Causes of Handler Injury
•	Lack of animal handling knowledge
•	Overconfidence or under-confidence
•	Being rushed
•	Becoming angered
•	Error by an assistant
•	Pain experienced by the animal
•	Equipment failure.

- **Human Injuries to Animals:** Human-related physical injuries to animals can be intentional from the inappropriate release of anger or from sadistic injuries. Unintentional injuries to animals can occur to those that are handled or restrained inappropriately. Many unintentional injuries of animals involve horses and are caused by handlers without adequate training on the proper handling of horses.

RISKS TO VETERINARY PERSONNEL

Based on most reported epidemiologic studies of animal-related injuries to veterinary personnel, more than half of all veterinarians will be seriously injured by animals some time in their careers. The U.S. Bureau of Labor Statistics lists veterinary medicine among the top 10 most dangerous jobs.

- **Types of Injuries:** The most common large animal-related injury is being kicked, followed by crushing (both occur more often from cattle than horses). The injuries from species received in large animal practice from highest to lowest are: dairy, cow-calf, and equine. The number of veterinarian or veterinary technician injuries from horses are less than the injuries to nonprofessional handlers and equestrians due to the latter's lesser training and the greater danger involved in riding.
- **Species Involved:** In private practices, the species inflicting injury are most commonly cattle and then horses. In contrast to private veterinary practices, Veterinary Teaching Hospitals where cattle are handled in carefully designed stanchions and chutes while horses are handled with less restraint devices, the risk of injury from horses is 4 times the risk from cattle per 1,000 animals handled. Rams, bucks, and swine can also inflict serious, even lethal injuries.
- **Rates of Veterinarians' Injuries:** Large animal veterinarians are injured at 1.75 times the rate of injuries to small animal veterinarians.
- **Preventive Measures:**
    - **Assistants Should Be Present:**
        ○ **Handling Sick Large Animals:** An assistant should always be present when a sick, large animal is being examined to provide a diversion for the examiner.
        ○ **Handling Mature Male Large Animals:** Mature bulls, stallions, rams, bucks, and boars are always unpredictable. Handlers should never lose sight of their presence and attitude.
        ○ **Handling Mothers with Young:** Cows, mares, and sows with nursing young can also be unpredictable and dangerous.
    - **Pre-Plan an Emergency Exit:** Whenever handling mature male or nursing female livestock or horses, handlers should always have a planned emergency exit.

RISKS OF DISEASE TO HANDLERS AND OTHER ANIMALS

ZOONOSES: TRANSMISSION OF DISEASE FROM ANIMALS TO HUMANS

A zoonosis is any infectious disease of animals that can be transmitted to humans under natural conditions.

- **Incidence:** Of the more than 1,400 known infectious diseases of humans, 60% are zoonotic. Most are associated with the gastrointestinal tract and transmission is fecal-oral.
    - **In the U.S.:** More than 50 zoonotic diseases are known to be present in the U.S.
    - **U.S. Zoonotic Disease Examples:** Examples include rabies, salmonellosis, cryptosporidiosis, plague, sporotrichosis, psittacosis, and ringworm.
- **Means of Transmission:**
    - **Direct Transmission:** Means of exposure to zoonoses are varied. Direct transmission can be contact with animal saliva, blood, urine, or feces with handler eyes, nose, or mouth which can occur from splashing of body fluids or eating, smoking, or touching the face. Contamination of a skin cut, scratch, or crack with animal saliva, blood, urine, or feces are also forms of direct transmission.
    - **Indirect Transmission:** Indirect transmission can include inhalation of contaminated dust. Vector-borne indirect transmission can be the bite of a fly, mosquito, tick, or flea carrying a zoonotic organism.

- **Risks:**
  - **Realistic Perspective:** Every animal can carry some diseases that humans could acquire. However, handling apparently healthy domestic animals using basic sanitary practices such as keeping hands away from eyes, nose, and mouth, keeping skin cuts covered, and washing hands after handling animals carries very little risk of acquiring zoonotic diseases.
  - **Higher Risk Situations:**
    - **Age-Related:** Children 5 years old or younger should have supervised exposure to animals due to immature immune systems and a tendency to put unwashed hands in their mouths. Animal handlers that are more than 70 years old may have increased risk of zoonoses from declining immune responses. Young children and immunosuppressed adults should especially avoid nursing calves, all reptiles, and baby chicks and ducklings.
    - **Stress-Related:** Systemic diseases in handlers such as HIV, congenital immunodeficiencies, diabetes mellitus, chronic renal failure, alcoholism, liver cirrhosis, malnutrition, and certain cancers can depress immunity. Pregnancy may also reduce the nonpregnant immune response. Treatments for cancer, organ or bone marrow transplants, and autoimmune diseases can also depress immunity.
    - **Type of Animal-Related:** High-risk animals for transmitting zoonoses are the young, females giving birth, and unvaccinated, stray, and all reptiles and wild or exotic species. Others include those fed raw meat diets, kept in crowded conditions, and with internal or external parasites.
- **Prevention of Transmission:** Special precautions are needed if working with animals with diarrhea, or skin or mouth sores.
  - **Maintain Health:** Keeping animals healthy can also lower the risk of zoonosis and transmission to humans. Routine veterinary care, vaccinations, and parasite screenings should be maintained. High-quality food is advisable.
  - **Sanitation and Avoiding Exposure:**
    - **Hand Washing:** Hand washing is essential to controlling the transmission of disease (Procedural Steps 1.1). All animal handling locations should have a means for handlers to wash hands. Animal handlers should keep their fingernails short and, if necessary, use moisturizers to keep the skin from cracking and creating portals of disease entry.

Procedural Steps 1.1	Hand Washing Procedure
1.	Clean fingernails and remove rings.
2.	Wet hands.
3.	Apply an olive-size amount of liquid soap to a palm.
4.	Scrub both hands while counting to 20, slowly.
5.	Rinse thoroughly and dry with paper towels.

- - - **Hand Sanitizers:** Alcohol-based rubs are effective against most disease-producing agents if the hands are not visibly soiled with organic material.
    - **Wound Care:** If the skin is broken by cuts or pointed penetrations, the wound should be thoroughly cleaned with soapy water. Compression should be applied, and if bleeding persists, a physician should be consulted.

- **Special Precautions during Pregnancy:** Pregnant women should not handle cat litter or ewes in the process of lambing.
- **Vaccination Protection:**
  - **Tetanus:** All animal handlers should be vaccinated against tetanus every ten years, as recommended by the U.S. Centers for Disease Control. Horse handlers are particularly at risk.
  - **Influenza:** Handlers of hogs or poultry should be vaccinated with the current human influenza virus vaccine.
  - **Rabies:** Veterinary personnel are also advised to receive pre-exposure vaccination against rabies and have serum titers checked every two years.
- **Control of Disease Vectors:**
  - **Ectoparasite Disease Vectors:** Some animal-related diseases are transmitted to humans indirectly via ectoparasite vectors, such as mosquitoes (encephalitis viruses) and ticks (Rocky Mountain Spotted Fever and many others). The animal carrying the ectoparasite may or may not become ill.
  - **Control of Ectoparasites on Animals:** Livestock are protected from ectoparasites by using dusters, dust bags, back rubbers and oilers, pour-ons, impregnated ear tags, feed-through larvicides, or boluses of insect growth regulators.
  - **Premise Control of Ectoparasites:** Premise control may include sprays, traps, and baits. Yards need to be mowed frequently enough to keep grass height short. Pastures and pens should be either cleaned of manure or harrowed on a weekly basis, and manure piles and other compost should be turned weekly.
  - **Rodents and Birds:** These vectors are controlled by eliminating entry to animal dwellings and hiding places. Access to food sources should be eliminated by maintaining food storage in rodent-proof sealed containers and proper disposal of garbage.
- **Increased Risks for Veterinary Personnel:**
  - **Food Animals:** The greatest zoonotic risks to food animal and mixed practice veterinarians are *Campylobacter*, ringworm, and rabies.
  - **Equine:** Equine veterinarian zoonotic risks have recently been greatest for West Nile virus (acquired from mosquitoes).
- **Personal Protective Equipment:** Personal protective equipment (PPE) should be considered in possible zoonotic risk situations.
  - **Eyes and Face:** PPE can include protection of the eyes with properly fitted goggles or ANSI-approved face masks.
  - **Ears:** Ears should be protected from excessive noise with earmuffs or molded ear plugs (cotton plugs are insufficient).
  - **Torso:** Protection for the torso can be lab coats, coveralls, gowns, or aprons.
  - **Arms and Hands:** Long sleeves protect against scratches and splashes. Hands are typically protected with rubber or nitrile gloves.
  - **Scalp:** The scalp can be partially protected from exposure to cuts, splashes of infectious liquids, and ringworm with a hat.
  - **Feet:** Feet may be protected with closed-toe, slip resistant, water impermeable shoes or boots.
- **Summary of Recommendations to Prevent Transmission of Zoonotic Disease:**
  - **Essential Preventive Measures:** Essential recommendations for the prevention of large animal zoonotic disease are listed in Table 1.10.

Table 1.10	Recommendations to Prevent Large Animal Zoonotic Diseases
•	Thoroughly wash your hands after feeding or touching animals or moving their waste; do not dry hands on clothing
•	Do not eat or drink in animal handling areas
•	Wear appropriate clothing when handling animals
•	Do not kiss animals
•	Wash cuts thoroughly
•	Keep animals from where human food is prepared or handled
•	Deworm animals on regular basis and provide reasonable control of flies, ticks, and mosquitoes
•	Vaccinate animals against zoonotic diseases and maintain tetanus vaccinations in all animal handlers and rabies vaccinations in high-risk animal handlers
•	Use proper low-stress handling techniques and containment practices and facilities to reduce stress-induced shedding of zoonotic diseases
•	Routinely train animal handlers on the prevention of zoonotic disease and animal handling safety measures.

- **Additional Information for Veterinary Personnel:** Precautions for veterinary personnel handling overtly sick animals are beyond the scope of this book. For these circumstances, consult the current *Compendium of Veterinary Standard Precautions for Zoonotic Disease Prevention in Veterinary Personnel*, published annually in the *Journal of the American Veterinary Medical Association* and *Veterinary Standard Precautions* at www.nasphv.org/.

TRANSMISSION OF DISEASE AMONG ANIMALS BY THEIR HANDLERS

Handlers can easily carry diseases from one animal to another.

- **Sanitation and Disinfection:** Sanitation (reduction of possible disease agents) or disinfection (complete or nearly complete elimination of disease agents) techniques are needed to reduce the chance of inanimate objects (clothing, handling equipment, confinement structures) from becoming inanimate transmitters of disease (*fomites*). The degree of sanitation needed varies with the risk of transmission.
  - **Cleansing:** In low disease transmission risk situations, simple washing of handling equipment and hands may be sufficient. Higher risk cases require disinfection of equipment as practically possible.
  - **Careful Preparation of Disinfection:**
    o **Dilution:** Disinfection should be preceded by cleaning of all organic matter (feces, blood, saliva, dust, urine, and hair) before using the disinfectant. Disinfectants can be sanitizers which reduce the number of microorganisms, antiseptics which kill or stop the growth of a few specific microorganisms, or sterilants that kill all microorganisms. The manufacturer's directions for dilution and use of the disinfectant should be closely followed.
    o **Practical Disinfection:** A common, effective, and inexpensive disinfectant (sterilant) is household bleach diluted to 1:32 (one cup bleach per gallon of water). NOTE: Bleach (sodium hypochlorite) must never be mixed with an acid or ammonia which will result in the release of toxic gases.
- **Risk of Transmission:** See Procedural Steps 1.2.

Procedural Steps 1.2	Order of Handling to Prevent Disease Transmission
1.	**First:** Handle young apparently healthy animals
2.	**Second:** Handle apparently healthy adult animals
3.	**Finally:** Handle isolated or sick animals.

- **Closed Group:** The risk of transmission of disease is low if all animals appear healthy and belong to the same household, farm, or ranch. When animals drink from the same water source, eat from the same ground or containers, touch noses, and have other frequent physical contacts and appear healthy, the risk of handling procedures spreading disease is mild to nonexistent.
- **Segregated Age Groups:** The risk is lowered further if animals of different age groups are segregated. Older animals are more likely to be disease carriers without signs and capable of transmitting disease to younger animals.
- **Separation of Sick Animals:** Sick animals should always be segregated and handled separately after disinfection or change of handling tools, boots, and clothing. When handling animals from different sources (households, farms, ranches), disinfection of handling tools, boots, and clothing should take place between handling the different groups of animals.
- **Containment:**
  - **Wash Hands:** To prevent the transmission of disease, handlers should always wash their hands after handling animals.
  - **Proper Foot Covering:** Water impermeable boots should be worn if walking on surfaces on which urine or feces may have been present, and boots disinfected before moving to another animal holding area.
  - **Clean Clothes:** Clothes worn during handling of animals that may have been ill should be washed near handling areas with commercial equipment.
  - **Clean Containment:** Animal confinement areas should be properly cleaned before introducing new animals.
  - **Quarantine New Animals:** New animals being introduced to an established group of animals should be held in quarantine until the effects of transport stress and the typical incubation period for infectious diseases have passed (usually ten days).

ANTHROPONOSIS: TRANSMISSION OF DISEASE FROM HANDLERS TO ANIMALS

In rare cases, diseased handlers can transmit their infection, such as tuberculosis, to animals. This is referred to as reverse zoonoses or *anthroponosis*. Animal handlers should not handle animals while sick, due to the risk of reverse zoonosis, as well as the added risk of physical injury from impaired judgment and delayed reactions.

ETHICAL CONCERNS

Ethics are based in part on social mores and therefore not static. Past methods of animal handling, restraint, and discipline once considered acceptable may not be tolerated by society today. Certain actions are considered inappropriate for handling, restraining, or disciplining large animals (Table 1.11).

Table 1.11	Unacceptable Handling, Restraining, or Disciplining Animals
•	Use of force beyond that needed for self-defense or protection of others
•	Use of force as punishment
•	Punishment delivered in anger or to inflict pain
•	Striking an animal on the head or other sensitive or injured body parts
•	Choking an animal
•	Shaking an animal violently
•	Striking an animal with a rigid object, if not to avert a dangerous attack
•	Unnecessary use of chemical restraint.

USE OF FORCE

Force is considered permissible if handlers are in full control of their emotions at the time and only the minimum amount of force needed is used to protect the safety of the humans, the animal being handled, or other animals. Force must be used with consideration of the animal's nature and with empathy for the animal. An example of necessary force is being charged by a bull or boar and using a stout stick to strike it on the nose to escape the attack.

RESPONSIBILITY FOR THE ACTIONS OF ASSISTANT HANDLERS

Handlers who are also supervisors of other animal handlers bear the responsibility to ensure that the other handlers are appropriately trained and supervised.

- **Written Guidelines:** Written guidelines, although they may only deal with extremes, should be provided along with a no tolerance policy on cases of animal abuse.
- **Penalties for Abuse:** Immediate termination of employment should be written and understood by all employees handling animals as a consequence to unequivocal animal abuse. It is well established that there is a link between willful abuse of animals and eventual domestic violence against humans.
- **Legal Gray Areas:** The designation of what is proper handling, restraint, and discipline is often murky. There are no universally accepted guidelines. Because of this, state statues on animal abuse usually prohibit forms of handling in vague extremes, such as overworking, overloading, and inflicting unnecessary cruelty upon animals.

LEGAL CONSIDERATIONS

Most states have laws that require animal handlers to exercise adequate control over animals to prevent them from harming themselves, other animals, people, or property.

LIABILITY

- **Waivers:** Liability waivers, signed by people involved in animal handling other than the primary handler may help win a legal case for a defendant, but they do not prevent lawsuits and the cost of defense. Waivers of responsibility also do not absolve handlers of liability in an injury or death that is due to their negligence or incompetence.
- **Negligence Versus Incompetence:**
  - **Incompetence:** Incompetence is simply not having the knowledge or ability to control an animal. It is important to ascertain that any assistant animal handler is mature enough, strong enough, and trained sufficiently for each task to be performed.

- **Negligence:** Failing to properly contain or control an animal that causes injury to a human is negligence. Knowing that an animal is potentially dangerous and not taking extra efforts to protect others is also considered negligence. Inadequately training assistants can be considered negligence on the part of the primary handler (supervisor).
- **Indirect Injuries:** Injury received in an attempt to flee from an animal demonstrating threatening behavior can be owner or agent negligence.
- **Insurance:** It is prudent to have adequate liability insurance that covers activities of an animal handler.
- **Role of Assistants:** A handler assumes responsibility for the safety of the animal and that of the people who may become injured by the animal being handled. This responsibility includes adequate supervision during animal handling. If all safety precautions are taken and cautions given to others, an injury to people or to the animal(s) may be attributed to inherent danger and an assumption of personal responsibility.

INHERENTLY DANGEROUS ANIMALS

Inherently dangerous animals should only be handled by specially trained and experienced personnel.

- **Adult Male Large Animals:** Stallions, bulls, rams, boars, and ratite cocks are inherently dangerous after puberty and especially during breeding seasons.
- **Mothers with Nursing Young:** Mares, cows, ewes, sows, and ratite hens inherently dangerous if they perceive their babies to be in danger.
- **Wild and Exotic Animals:** Ratites, deer, elk, and bison are examples of wild and/or exotic large animals that are inherently dangerous.

ANIMAL ABUSE REGULATIONS

Domestic animals have traditionally been viewed legally as property. Still, there are laws to protect the inhumane care of animals.

- **Felony Potential:** In more than 30 states, at least one form of animal cruelty constitutes a felony. The Federal Bureau of Investigation (FBI) reclassified crimes against animals in 2016 as a Group A offense and included cases in the FBI's National Incident Based Reporting System.
- **Veterinary Professionals:** If the handler is a veterinary medical professional, there is risk of malpractice charges that could lead to disciplinary action under the state veterinary practice act.
- **Stepping Stone to Abuse of Humans:** A history of willful abuse of animals is known to be associated with domestic violence, child abuse, and other violent crimes toward people.

ROLES OF CHEMICAL AND PHYSICAL RESTRAINT

PROPER USE OF CHEMICAL RESTRAINT

Chemical restraint should only be used when physical restraint techniques are substantially less safe for the animal or the handler, not just for convenience, to supplement income, or as a substitute for good handling and physical restraint methods. In addition, when chemical restraint must be used, it should be supplemented by sufficient humane physical restraint to optimize the animal and handler safety during administration, induction, and recovery from the drug's effects.

ADVANTAGES AND DISADVANTAGES OF CHEMICAL RESTRAINT

- **Potential Advantages of Appropriately Used Chemical Restraint:**
  - **Safety:** Recent innovations in chemical restraint (sedation and anesthesia) have been highly beneficial to animals, owners, and veterinarian personnel in alleviating animal stress and possible physical injury.
  - **Convenience:** The convenience of chemical restraint can lead to decreased risk to the handler and shorter handling time.
- **Potential Disadvantages of Unnecessary Chemical Restraint:**
  - **Altered Vital Signs of the Physical Exam:** Chemical restraint can also interfere with a physical exam by altering vital signs (heart rate, respiratory rate, and body temperature).
  - **Adverse Health Effects:** All sedatives and anesthetics have potentials to cause adverse health effects (Table 1.12).

Table 1.12 Potential Adverse Health Effects of Chemical Restraint
• Respiratory or cardiac arrest
• Physical injuries to animals or handlers during the chemical administration, induction, or recovery
• Organ damage from over dosage, individual variation in response, drug interactions, or idiosyncratic reactions.

  - **Fostering Fear:** Chemical alteration of consciousness may alleviate some of the fear and resistance to restraint in animals. Although in some cases, memory of the loss of full control of their body during induction or recovery may instill fear in other animals.

DRUGS TO FACILITATE HANDLING OF LARGE ANIMALS

Prescription drugs administered for the purpose of facilitating handling of large animals are primarily used in horses.

- **Tranquilizers:** Tranquilizers are supposed to produce relaxation and decrease aggressiveness with mild sedation. They are prescription medications.
  - **Acepromazine:** Acepromazine is a relatively short-acting tranquilizer that can cause protrusion of the third eyelid, hypotension, and protrusion of the penis.
  - **Reserpine:** Reserpine is a relatively longer-acting tranquilizer that can cause colic, hypotension, protrusion of the third eyelid, protrusion of the penis, mild diarrhea that may last for days, and sweating over the back and hind legs.
- **Alpha-2 Agonist Sedatives:** Alpha-2 agonists are prescription medications for sedation and analgesia. Adverse effects may be reversed with yohimbine.
  - **Xylazine:** Xylazine is a moderate-term sedative (1 to 2 hours) with muscle relaxant effects and brief analgesia. Hypotension, arrhythmia, incoordination, and sweating may occur.
  - **Detomidine:** Detomidine is administered intravenously or as a sublingual gel for moderate to deep sedation and analgesia in horses for up to an hour. It can cause cardiac arrhythmia, hypotension, sweating, ataxia, and muscle tremors.
  - **Romifidine:** Romifidine is similar to detomidine but with a longer duration of effects (1 to 1.5 hours).
- **Benzodiazepines:** Benzodiazepines are Schedule IV, controlled prescription sedative hypnotic anti-anxiety drugs used off-label in horses. Learning and memory can be suppressed by benzodiazepines which inhibits effective training.
  - **Diazepam:** Diazepam causes sedation and muscular relaxation. It can cause muscle twitching, weakness, and ataxia at dosages sufficient to cause sedation.
  - **Alprazolam:** Alprazolam is similar in effect to diazepam with a shorter duration of action.

CHEMICAL RESTRAINT FOR DEEP SEDATION OR GENERAL ANESTHESIA

Drugs that cause deep sedation or general anesthesia may be used for the temporary control of dangerous large animals, but these replace handling techniques and do not facilitate handling of large animals after they regain consciousness.

KEYS TO GOOD HANDLING OF LARGE ANIMALS

Good handling of any type of domestic or tame non-domestic animal involves proper preparation (Procedural Steps 1.3) and ten basic keys (Table 1.13).

Procedural Steps 1.3	Proper Preparation to Be an Animal Handler
1.	Read about animal handling.
2.	Observe normal animal behavior.
3.	Gain guidance from a good handler.
4.	Observe a good handler with animals.
5.	Practice under a good handler's supervision.

Table 1.13 Keys to Good Animal Handling
• Frequently, but briefly and gently handle young animals during their critical socialization period to reduce their natural fear of humans while being mindful not to eliminate their inherent respect for humans.
• Quietly handle healthy adults frequently for short periods to habituate the animals for handling without an association with fearful, painful events to follow.
• Confine animals in environments as similar to their ancestors' natural habitat as reasonably possible (e.g., pastures as ancestral steppes for horses).
• Provide environmental enrichments that will prevent or reduce boredom and stereotypic behaviors.
• Confine animals with as much personal space as needed to prevent or minimize stereotypic behaviors.
• Maintain social like-species support for animals by keeping prey and flock animals in groups with numbers appropriate for the species.
• Minimally handle elderly, neonatal, or sick animals to prevent their exhaustion or pain.
• Handle animals with confidence, using smooth rhythmic movements along with a calm low-pitched voice.
• Be able to recognize abnormal behavior for the species and the individual, including fear or signs of health problems.
• Use correct timing and type of responses to favorable or unfavorable animal conduct to beneficially shape their future behavior to handling.

IDEALS AND REALITIES

IDEALS CAN BE ELUSIVE

Large animal handlers should always be advocates for ideal animal handling conditions and scheduling. However, in the reality of day-to-day animal handling, animals often must be handled in less than ideal conditions and during less than ideal times due to medical or hazard emergencies or because of owners who are unwilling or incapable of providing ideal conditions.

BEST INTERESTS OF THE ANIMAL

There are situations when delay of handling is in the best interests of the animal, while other situations may mandate doing the best handling possible under less than ideal conditions to act in the timely best interests of the animal.

FLEXIBILITY ADVANTAGE IN HANDLING METHODS

Unless a handler is comfortable with leaving animals in danger or being handled by less competent personnel, it is advisable for a handler to become familiar with, and skilled in, a variety of means of handling animals, some of which may not be needed in ideal conditions or at ideal times. For example, using a rope on a stick for capture, steel tube panels for traps, casting a cow with ropes, and using a detached tubular gate as an emergency glide are not needed in ideal conditions, but these can be the best, or only, methods to successfully handle animals in some handling conditions.

LESS THAN IDEAL SITUATIONS SHOULD NOT DEFAULT TO NO CARE

To provide no assistance in handling animals whose welfare is in danger because conditions are less than ideal is a form of handler negligence. A good animal handler provides the best assistance for the animals in danger with the tools and techniques that are available at the time, as long as there is reasonable expectation of safety for the animals and the handlers.

BIBLIOGRAPHY

1. Austin HE, Hyams JH, Abbott KA. Training in animal handling for veterinary students at Charles Sturt University, Australia. J Vet Med Ed 2007;34:566–575.
2. Bender JB, Shulman SA. Reports of zoonotic disease outbreaks associated with animal exhibits and availability of recommendations for preventing zoonotic disease transmission from animals to people in such settings. J Am Vet Med Assoc 2004;224:1105–1109.
3. Busch HM, Cogbill TH, Landercasper J, et al. Blunt bovine and equine trauma. J Trauma 1986;26:559–560.
4. Cawdell-Smith AJ, Pym RAE, Verrall RG, et al. Animal handling as an integrated component of animal and veterinary science programs at the University of Queensland. J Vet Med Ed 2007;34:542–549.
5. Centers for Disease Control and Prevention Morbidity and Mortality Weekly Report: Compendium of Measures to Prevent Disease Associated with animals in public settings, 2011;60(RR04):1–24.
6. Chapman HM, Taylor EG, Buddle JR, et al. Student training in large-animal handling at the School of Veterinary and Biomedical Sciences, Murdoch University, Australia. J Vet Med Ed 2007;34:576–582.
7. Cockram MS, Aitchison K, Collie DDS, et al. Animal-handling teaching at the Royal (Dick) School of Veterinary Studies, University of Edinburgh. J Vet Med Ed 2007;34:554–560.
8. Cogbill TH, Strutt PJ, Landercasper J, et al. Injuries from horses and cows. Complic Orthop 1989;120:112–114.
9. Epp T, Waldner C. Occupational health hazards in veterinary medicine: Zoonosis and other biological hazards. Can Vet J 2012;53:144–150.
10. Epp T, Waldner C. Occupational health hazards in veterinary medicine: Physical, psychological, and chemical hazards. Can Vet J 2012;53:151–157.

11. Esch KJ, Petersen CA. Transmission and epidemiology of zoonotic protozoal diseases of companion animals. Clin Microbiol Rev 2013;26:58–85.
12. Farm and Ranch Safety and Health Association. A health and safety guide for handling farm animals and poultry. www.farscha.bc.ca. Accessed 11/20/2015.
13. Frechette D. Liability law: Reality check. Equus 2008;374:45–49.
14. Hanlon A, Gath V, Mulligan F. Practical animal-handling classes at University College Dublin. J Vet Med Ed 2007;34:561–565.
15. Hendricks KJ, Adekoya N. Non-fatal animal related injuries to youth occurring on farms in the United States, 1998. Inj Prev 2001;7:307–311.
16. Kipperman BS. The role of the veterinary profession in promoting animal welfare. J Am Vet Med Assoc 2015;246:502–504.
17. Landercasper J, Cogbill T, Strutt P, et al. Trauma and the veterinarian. J Trauma 1988;28:1255–1259.
18. Langley, RL, Hunter JL. Occupational fatalities due to animal-related events. Wilderness Environ Med 2001;12:168–174.
19. Langley RL, Morrow WE. Livestock handling-minimizing worker injuries. J Agromed 2010;15:226–235.
20. Lucas M, Day L, Shirangi A, et al. Significant injuries in Australian veterinarians and use of safety precautions. Occup Med 2009;59:327–333.
21. MacLeay JM. Large-animal handling at the Colorado State University College of Veterinary Medicine. J Vet Med Ed 2007;34:550–553.
22. McGreevy P. Firm but gentle: Learning to handle with care. J Vet Med Ed 2007;34:539–541.
23. McGreevy P, Hawke C, Celi P, et al. Learning and teaching animal handling at the University of Sydney's faculty of veterinary science. J Vet Med Ed 2007;34:586–597.
24. McMillian M, Dunn JR, Keen JE, et al. Risk behaviors for disease transmission among petting zoo attendees. J Am Vet Med Assoc 2007;231:1036–1038.
25. National Association of State Public Health Veterinarians Animal Contact Compendium Committee. Compendium of Measures to Prevent Disease Associated with animals in public settings. J Am Vet Med Assoc 2013;243:1270–1288.
26. National Association of State Public Health Veterinarians. Compendium of veterinary standard precautions for zoonotic disease prevention in veterinary personnel. J Am Vet Med Assoc 2010;237:1403–1422.
27. Patronek GJ, Lacroix CA. Developing an ethic for the handling, restraint, and discipline of companion animals in veterinary practice. J Am Vet Med Assoc 2001;218:514–517.
28. Poole AG, Shane SM, Kearney MT, et al. Survey of occupational hazards in large animal practices. J Am Vet Med Assoc 1999;215:1433–1435.
29. Poole AG, Shane SM, Kearney MT, et al. Survey of occupational hazards in companion animal practices. J Am Vet Med Assoc 1998;212:1386–1388.
30. Stafford KJ, Erceg VH. Teaching animal handling to veterinary students at Massey University, New Zealand. J Vet Med Ed 2007;34:583–585.
31. Van Soest EM, Fritschi L. Occupational health risks in veterinary nursing: An exploratory study. Aust Vet J 2004;82:346–350.
32. White P, Chapman S. Two students' reflections on their training in animal handling at the University of Sydney. J Vet Med Ed 2007;34:598–599.
33. Willems RA. Animals in veterinary medical teaching: Compliance and regulatory issues, the US perspective. J Vet Med Ed 2007;34:615–619.
34. Whittem T, Woodward AP, Hoppach M. A survey of injuries that occurred in Veterinary Teaching Hospitals during 2017. J Vet Med Educ 2021;48:401–416.

2

LARGE ANIMAL BEHAVIOR

DOI: 10.1201/9781003110910-2

Animals are not simply hairier versions of humans. Reacting to animals as if they are humans is called *anthropomorphism*, and anthropomorphism is not effective in establishing a safe and effective relationship with animals. Better animal handling involves the handler assuming a leadership role, having empathy for animals, and having knowledge of the normal behavior and needs of the species involved.

BEHAVIOR AND HANDLING

An important foundation for proper animal handling is learning the normal behavior of the species.

NATURAL INSTINCTS
Knowing the natural instincts of a species is essential to being able to handle, move, and contain them humanely with minimal stress and risk of injury to either the handler or the animals.

BODY LANGUAGE
Most communications between animal species are silent, via "body language."

- **Initial Observation:** Behavior and attitude of animals should be assessed by observing them at a distance before an approach for handling. Animals will be attentive to the handler's appearance and body language upon first sight of the handler and may respond by modifying their own behavior. For example, prey animals will often mask signs of illness or injury, particularly in the presence of strangers.
- **Avoid Appearance of Submissiveness or Being a Predator:** It is essential to not be perceived by animals as either their predator or being of lesser social rank to them.
- **Evaluate for Signs of Aggression:** Most animals will telegraph their intent to display open aggression. The natural tendency is to avoid, if possible, the possibility of injury and death. Therefore, braying or other vocalizations, lunging, pawing, fake charging, and other signals of aggression usually precede an attack on an apparent adversary.

FACILITATING HANDLING
Avoidance of handling resistance in animals requires early socialization with humans and never causing pain or extreme fear (Table 2.1).

Table 2.1	Causes of Irreparable Handling Resistance in Animals
•	Failure to properly socialize animals in their juvenile period of life
•	Infliction of pain at any age
•	Exposure to extremely fearful situations at any age.

PREDATOR OR PREY BEHAVIOR

All domestic animals evolved as either meat eaters (predators) or food for meat eaters (prey). Common large domestic animals, such as horses, cattle, sheep, and goats, are evolutionarily prey. Hogs can be either prey or predator, depending on the circumstances.

PREDATORS

- **Vision:** Predators have eyes that are positioned forward in their skulls, which permits greater overlapping of the field of vision from both eyes and improves depth of vision. Predators stare directly at their prey and are able to track the movement and judge speed of their prey.
- **Pursuit of Prey:** Some predators, for example canids, will quietly pursue prey in groups, encircle them, maintain intense focus, and attack.
- **Stalking of Prey:** Other predators, for example felids, hide motionless until they can ambush their prey.

PREY

- **Vision:** Prey animals have eyes that are located on the sides of their skulls. Prey animals monitor their peripheral environment to detect the presence of predators. They do not stare at predators except to assess their intent and decide on a means of escape.
- **Safety in Numbers:** Most prey animals are gregarious. Living in groups provides more sentinels of danger and sacrificial members for predators.
- **Isolation versus Group Panic:** Group-loving prey animals (cattle, sheep, goats, and horses) are stressed whenever isolated from their own species. Although they should not be separated entirely from herd members, horses, cattle, and hogs should be moved in small groups to avoid mob action by a large group. Sheep can be moved safely in larger groups.
- **Constant Vigilance for Danger:**
  - **Shiny Objects:** Common situations that can elicit fear in prey animals are shiny objects, including sparkling reflections on water or shiny metal.
  - **Squeaky Sounds:** High-pitched sounds are often made by prey captured by a predator, therefore clanging, squeaky, or hissing noises, such as gates, squeeze chutes, dangling chains, exhaust fans, and air hoses are frightening to prey animals.
  - **Rapid, Jerky Movements:** Rapid movements evoke fear, such as blowing plastic bags or fluttering banners or flags. Jerky movements by handlers can scare prey animals, as can fan blades that are turned off and blow with the wind.
  - **Unfamiliarity:** Anything that is unfamiliar in familiar surroundings can be frightening, including clothing, paper bags or cups, different flooring, different panels, puddles of water, or grates in an alleyway.
  - **Impaired Visibility:** Darkness or blinding glare is avoided by prey animals since either can impair their safety from predators.

PERCEPTION OF HANDLERS AS PREDATORS

A handler's body language may unintentionally mimic predator behavior.

- **Vision:** Humans have predator eyes, directed forward. Because of this, staring at prey animals is perceived as a threat. Moving directly toward them is the pushing approach of a pack predator designed to encourage them to run before a kill.
- **Perception as Prey:** A human standing motionless is like that of a stalking predator, especially if the prey animals are being stared at. The least threatening actions are to have relaxed movements while approaching at an angle without looking directly at the animal. This is the demeanor of another grazing prey animal.

ANIMAL HIERARCHY: SOCIAL DOMINANCE

Each animal is an individual, the total of a unique combination of genes and past experiences. General assumptions about behavior might be made based on species, age, gender, and breed, but an individual animal may act and react in a unique fashion.

SOCIAL RANK

- **Assessing Social Rank:** Nearly all domestic animals prefer to live in groups. Within animal groups there is a hierarchy, a social ladder. Knowing the social rank of an individual animal mingling in a group can be helpful in determining the best means of handling or restraint for that animal.
- **Change in Social Rank:** The previous status of a group member, or that of an animal handler, can be altered within a group of animals if the demeanor of the group member or handler is different than usual. Acting ill, injured, or less confident as with advanced age can reduce the status of the individual within a group.

LEADERSHIP

- **Establishing Leadership:** See Table 2.2.

Table 2.2	Establishing Leadership with Large Animals
•	**Control Resources**—Access to food and water
•	**Limit Freedom of Movement**—Provide appropriate confinement
•	**Provide Clear, Consistent Communications**—Requests of change in movement or behavior must be clear, consistent, metered, and within seconds of intended change.

- **Demonstration of Leadership:** Dominant status is conveyed primarily by demeanor, particularly calmness and confidence. Force that inflicts pain is reserved for self-defense or defense of the species, such as conflicts during mating seasons. An effective animal handler must be dominant, by their demeanor, not by applied force or micromanagement, to animals being handled for the safety of both the handler and the animal.
- **Animal Leaders:** Dominance within a group is generally related to height, weight, gender, age, or in the case of ruminants, the size of their horns. The oldest ewe is the most dominant sheep and the oldest doe goat is the herd leader.
  - **Juvenile Play:** Social rank within a group is first established by juvenile play, such as head butting among young goats and bulls and boxing among young stallions.
  - **Deference:** Dominant animals are identifiable by the deference given them by others, not by displays of aggression and force. Higher social rank is usually established by demeanor with direct stares, ritualized aggressive postures, vocalizing, and fake attacks without attempts to cause serious injury.
  - **Elevated Position:** Dominant animals are more calm and confident than others and will seek a position physically above others. For example, dominant horses prefer to be on rises in the land. Dominant individuals within a group of prey animals will seek the center of the group.
- **Maintaining Leadership:** Leaders must remain calm, confident, and appear physically capable to lead. Handlers who attempt to manage animal groups while ill, injured, or acting uncharacteristically timid may be challenged by a group, particularly if the animal group is swine or poultry.

SOCIALIZATION WITH HUMANS

SOCIALIZING LARGE ANIMALS

- **Definition of Socialization:** Socialization of animals is the process of training animals so that they can be kept in close relationship to humans.

- **Critical Periods:** Critical periods for socializing animals for less fear toward humans is lengthened by the degree of species domestication and is later and longer in predators than prey animals. Socialization begins at birth for domesticated prey animals.

RISKS OF EARLY HANDLING

- **Imprinting:** Handling prey animals, generally horses, gently beginning at birth is believed, by some animal handlers, to have a profound beneficial effect in handling the animals with less stress later in life. The process is often referred to as imprinting, although true imprinting is bonding with a mother and acceptance of the proximity of members of the same species.
- **Risks of Socialization:** Exaggerated efforts by humans to "imprint" large prey animals such as horses, cattle, and llamas may cause the animals to lose their respect for humans, and thereby cause them to be more dangerous as they mature.
- **Imitation of the Mother:** More important than imprinting of newborns is the routine handling and grooming of the mothers of young animals, particularly in the first five days of the young animal's life after its eyes have opened, and that the mother responds to humans in a relaxed manner. The young foal, calf, pig, or animal will be profoundly affected for life by how the mother responds to being handled by humans and will develop imitative behavior.

FLIGHT ZONE AND POINT OF BALANCE

Members of all species have invisible borders, *flight zones*, around them in the presence of possible danger.

SIZE OF FLIGHT ZONES

The diameter of an animal's flight zone for humans varies by the animal species involved, its breed, the amount of prior exposure to humans, the quality of prior contact with humans, and the age of the animal when exposed to humans. Flight zones are larger for more dominant individuals. The zone will shrink if the animal is very thirsty and must go into closer proximity to a human than usual to get to water.

MAJOR REACTIONS TO INVASION OF FLIGHT ZONES

- **Flight (Escape):** The least stressful means of moving cattle forward is to calmly and quietly approach their flight zone behind their *point of balance*, also called the drive line, which is an imaginary line just behind the shoulder. The movement produced is like moving a positive pole of a magnet toward the positive pole of another. The approaching magnet at some point repels the other.
- **Fight:** Invading a flight zone does not always result in flight of the animal. If a prey animal cannot find a means of escape, they are likely to fight. This includes an estimation on the ability to outrun a perceived danger. For example, donkeys are more likely to fight than horses because donkeys know they cannot outrun many potential dangers as well as horses can.

MINOR REACTIONS TO INVASION OF FLIGHT ZONES

After a potential threat leaves a horse's flight zone, the horse may exhibit an "adrenaline shake off" from a relief of nervousness or fear.

MANAGEMENT OF FLIGHT ZONES

- **Increase in a Flight Zone:** Fight or flight arousal of prey animals is increased by hunger, sexual arousal, loud noises (barking, stock whips), sight of dogs, having been beaten or shocked by electric prods, and unfamiliar objects or people.
- **Decrease in a Flight Zone:** Familiarity with animals to be handled should be fostered in advance of need whenever possible. Handlers should walk among young livestock to habituate them to seeing and being near people. In addition to humans, desensitization of cattle, sheep, or goats should include desensitization to horses and dogs, if either will be used in herding.

SENSES AND BEHAVIOR

Animal senses activate and modify animal behavior.

OLFACTORY (SMELL)

The sense of smell is more acute in all domestic animals than in humans. Animals monitor the odor of urine, feces, sweat, breath, and special skin organs to identify others, assess their status in a reproductive cycle, and determine their social rank.

- **Species Use of Smell:**
    - **Horses:** Horse herd members defecate where they smell their dominant herd members defecate. These toilet areas are sacrificed from grazing, except when in desperation for food. They also use fecal smell to find their way home or to join other horses.
    - **Cattle:** Cattle have an excellent sense of smell they use to trace the trail of their calves and to differentiate plants to eat. They can tell which is the most dominant animal and members of the herd by their odors.
- **Vomeronasal Organ:**
    - **Location and Structure:** The vomeronasal, also called Jacobson's, organ is located in the roof of the mouth (Figure 2.1). It consists of two sacs that are connected to the nasal cavity by fine ducts. When domestic mammals smell sexual odors, many will lift their upper lip and open their mouth, a procedure called the *flehmen response* (Figure 2.2).

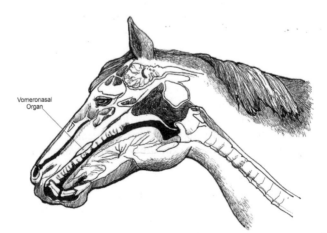

Figure 2.1 Vomeronasal organ.

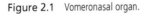

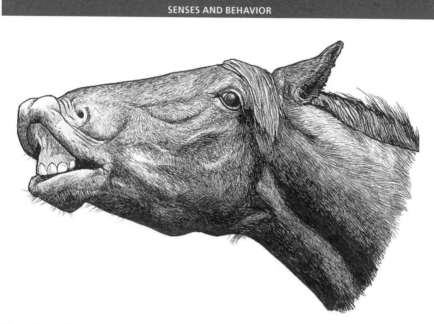

Figure 2.2   Flehmen response.

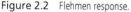

- **Purpose:** The purpose of the flehmen response is to increase the opening of the ducts that carry the smell to the nasal cavity and the olfactory membrane. This enhances the detection of the odor.
- **Species Behaviors:** Male horses do a flehmen response when smelling urine from mares in estrus. Cattle will collect odors in moisture droplets on their muzzle which are licked off with the tongue and detected by the vomeronasal organ.
- **Smell and Handling:**
  - **Smelling Fear:** Animals are sometimes said to be able to smell fear in handlers who are unconfident. In the case of humans, animals "smelling" fear is probably detection of purposeless or unconfident, hesitant body language.
  - **Smelling Submissiveness:** Within the same species and same social group, animals can identify more submissive animals by smell. Because of this, handlers should always handle the most dominant animal in a group first, such as the largest boar in a herd of swine. Otherwise, the smell of subordinate members on the handler may make the dominant member harder to handle.
  - **Odors Repugnant to Animals:** Cologne or other pungent cosmetic odors can also cause animals to resist handling and restraint.
- **Aromatherapy for Handling Animals:** In nature, odors have effects on animal behavior. Their ability to alter behavior to facilitate handling is less clear.
  - **Pheromones:** Pheromones are chemicals used for communication by smell.
    - **In Nature:** Natural pheromones are well-established important communicators of individual identity and reproductive status in many, if not all, vertebrate species.
    - **Synthetics:** Synthetic pheromones and essential oils have been proposed to be effective means of calming horses.
    - **Efficacy:** Aromatherapy is a form of alternative therapy similar to nutraceuticals. Neither are required to prove efficacy to be marketed. Claims of efficacy are usually based on anecdotal statements, studies funded and/or conducted by groups with significant conflicts of interest, or small studies

without sufficient controls and independent evaluations that are required of pharmaceuticals.

- ○ **Pheromotherapy:** The term pheromotherapy has been used to separate the proposed actions of pheromones from other forms of aromatherapy. However, the difference is a matter of semantics rather than action.
- ○ **Short Duration Distraction:** Aromatherapy may be more of a means of non-threatening distraction than a mind-altering drug. If they have any effect, a short duration of effects (less than 30 minutes) should be expected.
- ● **Aromatherapy Agents:** Equine Appeasing Pheromone (EAP) is a pheromone produced by the skin of the mammary gland of mares during the nursing period. A synthetic EAP has been marketed in gel form as an anti-anxiety aromatherapy for horses. However, independent controlled studies have not demonstrated anti-anxiety efficacy for synthetic EAP.

HEARING

Sounds are an important communication method and stimuli that warn animals of potential danger. Animals are able to differentiate each member of their group's voices as well as each of their handlers' voices. They are able to recognize and associate sounds that occur with feeding, distress, and breeding, among others.

- ● **Auditory Communications:** All domestic animals use sound as one means of communication, although not much is known about vocal communications among animals. Most is known about horses.
  - ● **Horses:**
    - ○ **Neigh:** Horses neigh to acknowledge the location of other horses.
    - ○ **Whinny:** Whinnies are louder and more questioning of location.
    - ○ **Nicker:** A nicker is a welcoming sound. At feeding time a nicker means hurry up and do not forget about me.
    - ○ **Snort:** A snort is an alert to all around of a possible danger.
    - ○ **Blow:** A blow is a strong exhale signaling a building of excitement.
    - ○ **Squeal:** Squeals are intended to startle. Mares often squeal to tell another horse to back off.
    - ○ **Grunt:** Grunts are an exclamation of extra effort.
    - ○ **Scream:** Screams mean extreme pain, as in being trapped in a barn fire.
    - ○ **Roar:** A roar is a warning sign of an agitated stallion.
  - ● **Cattle:**
    - ○ **Moo:** Cattle moo to convey their location.
    - ○ **Grunts:** Grunts are used by new mothers as part of the bonding stage in the first days after giving birth.
    - ○ **Bellow:** They use a louder call, a bellow, to locate their calf when separated, warn of possible danger, or express other reasons for distress.
    - ○ **Snort:** Snorting is a sign of agitation and may signal an attack from an angry nursing mother or from an irritated bull.
  - ● **Camelids:**
    - ○ **Hum:** Dams hum to their cria (babies).
    - ○ **Click:** A clicking sound is made to warn of potential danger.
    - ○ **Grumble:** A grumbling sound is made if irritated and before they spit.
    - ○ **Scream:** They will scream if in extreme danger or pain.
  - ● **Hogs:**
    - ○ **Grunt:** Hogs grunt frequently. When excited, the grunts are short in duration. Long grunts are used when content or calling to establish location of other hogs.

- ○ **Squeal:** Pigs squeal when disturbed.
- ○ **Scream:** When hurt or frightened.
- ○ **Bark:** Dominant hogs will bark at a subordinate to make them move, establishing or re-establishing their superior social rank.
- **Chickens:**
  - ○ **Cluck:** Both hens and roosters will cluck if grouping chicks or announcing the presence of food or something else of curiosity.
  - ○ **Cackle:** Hens will cackle after laying an egg and may be joined by other nearby hens.
  - ○ **Growl:** A growl is a warning from hens of an invasion of personal space, especially if protecting eggs or chicks. It may be followed with aggressive pecking.
  - ○ **Squawk:** Both hens and roosters will squawk if frightened. Other nearby chickens may also squawk and run toward or away from the threat.
  - ○ **Crow:** Adult roosters crow to announce their territory and an intent to defend it.
- **Turkeys:**
  - ○ **Bark:** Turkey hens bark when in an unfamiliar area to keep the flock together.
  - ○ **Wheat:** A wheat-sounding alert is made if a threat may be near.
  - ○ **Gobble:** Male (tom) turkeys make the gurgling gobble sound to make their presence known to the hens.
  - ○ **Purr:** A tom will make a purring sound if intending to attack.
- **Three Aspects of Hearing:** See Table 2.3.

Table 2.3	The Three Aspects of Hearing
•	**Intensity**—Amplitude, measured on a logarithmic scale in decibels (dB)
•	**Frequency**—Number of vibrations per second, measured in Hertz (Hz) units
•	**Directional Ability**—Discerning the origin of a sound.

- **Intensity:**
  - ○ **Soft Sounds:** Low-toned soft sounds are soothing to animals. Soothing background music can calm animals and is often used in milking parlors and horse stables. On the other hand, raucous music is not beneficial to animal handling.
  - ○ **Loud Sounds:** Yelling with a high-pitched voice causes prey animals (horses, cattle) to panic and attempt to flee. To reduce fear in livestock, it helps to attach rubber bumpers to metal gates and lubricate hinges, fans, and other moving equipment to control high-pitched noises during handling.
  - ○ **Appropriate Means to Induce Movement:** Yelling and waving arms should not be used to move animals, especially if they are in confinement. Cattle can be moved more efficiently and quietly by avoiding yelling and instead using canes, whips, or paddles as visual extensions of the handler's body without contacting the animal's body.
- **Frequency:** The auditory range of humans is approximately 20 to 20,000 Hz. Horses and livestock have upper ranges of 35,000 to 40,000 Hz.
- **Direction:**
  - ○ **Point of Attention:** The ability to hear can be enhanced by moving external ear position in the direction of the sound source. Horses and cats turn their external ears in the direction of their current point of attention. Horses' ears moved toward a handler indicate that the handler has their attention.

○ **Indication of Behavior:** Ear position is an indication of expected behavior. Laid back ears can be an indication of aggressiveness in horses and llamas. However, horses will lay their ears back when highly focused on any task, including working with great intensity, such as running hard or being intensely serious about wanting to eat grain.

VISION

Vision is the primary sense used for detecting danger for many species. It is adapted for the needs of a species, particularly the needs of defense and communications. Impaired vision can affect an animal's tractability, such as diurnal birds being more easily handled in subdued lighting and blindfolds improving the ability to handle horses, raptors, and ratites (Table 2.4).

Table 2.4   Vision Components
• Field of view
• Depth perception (judgment of distances)
• Acuity (focus)
• Perception of motion
• Color differentiation and night vision.

- **Field of View:**
  - **Grazing Animals:** The eyes of grazing/prey animals (horses, cattle, sheep, goats, rabbits) are located on the sides of their heads and protrude slightly in comparison to predator eyes. The side location and protrusion of their eyes allow grazing prey animals even greater horizontal peripheral vision. The horizontal vision of grazing animals is approximately 200 degrees, or more, with their heads raised, and up to about 340 degrees, with their head lowered in grazing position (Figure 2.3).
  - **Swine:** The distance and peripheral vision of swine, a prey and predator, is poor.

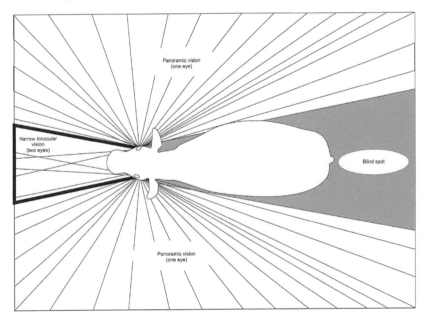

Figure 2.3   Range of vision in a cow.

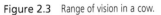

- **Pupil Shape and Light Accommodation:**
  - **Pupil Shape:** The pupil of prey animals adapted to living on open grassland is often horizontally oval, which further enhances peripheral vision (Figure 2.4).
    - ○ **Vertical Vision:** However, the vertical vision (being able to see above or below) is less in grazing prey animals than in humans or predators. Prey animals' range of vertical vision is only about 60 degrees. To properly place their feet on unfamiliar ground or to step into unfamiliar water, they have to lower their head.
    - ○ **Horizontal Vision:** Horizontal pupils enable prey animals to see vertical lines better than horizontal lines. Containment fencing with more vertical lines is a more effective psychological barrier for grazing animals than the more common fences that have long sections of horizontal planks or rails.
  - **Speed of Accommodation to Light:** Dilation and constriction of the pupil are the primary means of accommodating to changes in lighting. Livestock, diurnal species, have pupils that accommodate slowly compared to humans.

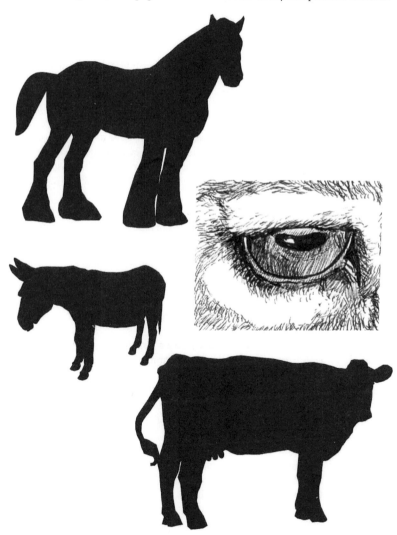

Figure 2.4   Horizontal pupils in prey, grazing animals.

- **Depth Perception:** Depth perception (stereopsis, i.e., judgment of distances) requires overlapping fields of vision from each eye. Humans and predator animals have binocular vision. They always focus on objects with both eyes.
  - **Grazing Livestock:** Prey animals have monocular vision and can focus on objects on both sides of their body at the same time but with little depth perception to monitor for predators while grazing. When looking forward, prey animals can view the same object with both eyes using binocular vision which is needed for depth perception. Horses have an overlap of 65 degrees but 350 degrees of panoramic vision.
  - **Distance Vision:** Horses and most other grazing prey animals have good distance vision, especially for moving objects, but their ability for depth vision and the ability to focus on near objects is slow and poor, requiring them to face the object of interest.
  - **Near Vision:**
    o **Holes and Shadows:** In prey animals, shadows appear as holes, and water depth cannot be determined. Because of this, it is important to keep surfaces for them to walk on dry and lit by diffuse, shadow-eliminating lighting.
    o **Inclines and Declines:** Loading ramps that slant upward are easier for grazing prey animals to negotiate than steps.
    o **Color, Shading, and Texture:** Consistent color, shading, and texture to prey animals' floors are important to keep them from balking. A change in the color, shading, or texture of the surface of flooring will cause the animals to stop to reassess if there might be a change in the depth.
    o **Location Blind Spot:** Grazing animals have a cone-shaped blind spot 4 feet directly in front of their face. They also cannot see directly below their jaw. Objects that suddenly appear from a blind spot may startle them, particularly horses.
- **Acuity and Perception of Motion:**
  - **Visual Acuity:** Visual acuity (focus) is the ability to see details. Domestic mammals do not have the visual acuity of humans. Normal humans have 20/20 acuity while horses have 20/33, which means normal humans can see clearly at 33 feet with the clarity that horses see at 20 feet.
  - **Motion Detection:**
    o **Predators:** In most predators the area of greatest acuity is a circular area in the retina, called the fovea or *area centralis*. To visually evaluate the greatest detail, predators have to hold their head still and concentrate the image on the fovea.
    o **Prey:** Grazing prey animals have a *visual streak*, an elongated band that runs across the retina. This permits grazing animals to better detect motion in their peripheral vision.
- **Color Differentiation and Night Vision:** Most animals see better in low light than do humans but perceive fewer colors.
  - **Retinal Light Receptors:** The retina of the eye contains two types of light receptors: rods and cones.
    o **Rods:** All mammals have more rods than cones and animals have more than humans. For example, humans have nine rods/cone while horses have 20 rods/cone.
    o **Cones:** Cones perceive objects best in bright light and can differentiate colors. The *area centralis* or visual streak contains the highest concentration of cones and the lowest concentration of rods.

- **Color Vision:**
  - ○ **Humans:** Humans have three types of cones which permit trichromatic color vision (tones of red, green, and yellow).
  - ○ **Domestic Animals:** Most domestic animals that are active during daylight have two types of retinal cones and *dichromatic color vision* (yellow and blue). They cannot distinguish colors in the range of 510 to 590 nm, the red wave length.
  - ○ **Dichromatic Color Vision:** Dichromatic color vision in animals is similar to humans with red-green color blindness. Animals with dichromatic vision appear to see blue and yellow best and have trouble perceiving red and green. Dichromatic vision may aid in seeing sudden movements and objects in low light.
- **Night Vision:**
  - **Retinal Rod Cells:** Retinal rod cells are responsible for magnifying light impulses. Rods are able to detect low intensity light and motion and differentiate shades of gray, but they provide poor resolution. Most domestic animals, especially nocturnal foragers (horses), have many more rods than do humans.
  - **Tapetum Lucidum:** Species that are scoptic (have vision in dim light) or nocturnal also have a *tapetum lucidum* (reflective structure in the retina that increases the gathering of light). This results in superior night vision and more intense differences in grays, plus better detection of motion. Horses and most other grazing animals are believed to see approximately up to 4 times better at night, after accommodation to lighting, than can humans.
  - **Swine:** Swine have forward-placed eyes, round pupils, no tapetum, and are dichromats. Hogs are nearsighted and cannot see well in dim light. Their depth perception is good for close objects which aids their quest for food on forest floors.

TACTILE (TOUCH)

- **Communication:**
  - **Among Animals:** Animals communicate with each other with a range of touches. Soothing or grooming touches reinforce the bonding within a group. Quick metered blows or bites are to reinforce early visual or vocal warnings of needed behavior change of another member of the group.
  - **With Handlers:** Excessively light touching by handlers may be perceived as fear by horses and cattle. Moderately firm stroking conveys a better impression of confident leadership of a good handler. Horses should be gradually desensitized to pats and gentle slaps for the safety of handlers who may slap horseflies on the horse to protect themselves or the horse, or who might unintentionally slap a horse with tack.
- **Spatial Orientation—Vibrissae:**
  - **Definition:** Whiskers (vibrissae) are large, long, well-innervated hairs surrounded by a vascular sinus.
  - **Location:** Most species have vibrissae on the upper (maxillary) lips. Vibrissae on the muzzle of horses is trimmed for some show events. This can alter normal spatial sensations causing some horses to temporarily quit eating or drinking.
  - **Function:** The function of vibrissae is to feel spatial limits and air movements.

RESISTANCE BEHAVIORS

Resistance to handling may be manifested as avoidance or aggression. Aggressive behavior can be caused by irritability or pain (Table 2.5).

Table 2.5 Causes of Aggression	
•	Maternal
•	Pain
•	Predatory
•	Territorial (Possession)
•	Fear-induced
•	Intermate
•	Dominance.

MATERNAL AGGRESSION

Animal mothers will protect their young when the mother may not be willing to protect herself. This is most acute after birth to the time of peak milk production. A cry from a young animal of any species may precipitate an attack on the handler from the animal's parents or other adults of the group.

- **Swine:** Before handling nursing pigs, sows should be separated from the pigs at a distance that all sows cannot hear the pigs squeal.
- **Horses:** Unlike with swine, foals should be kept within sight of mares or both will become frantic.

PAIN-RELATED AGGRESSION

Feeling pain or just anticipating pain can cause aggression.

- **Perception of Pain:** Pain-related aggression is a natural response to noxious stimuli. Pain from saddle sores or arthritis are common causes for formerly mild-mannered horses to act resentful of handling or being ridden.
- **Anticipation of Pain:** Anticipation of possible pain can induce fear aggression. Frequent gentle handling of all parts of an animal's body, with no other purpose than training, can desensitize animals to anticipated pain aggression.

TERRITORIAL AND POSSESSION AGGRESSION

- **Territorial Aggression:** Mature bulls can become aggressive in protecting what they perceive as their territory such as a pen or pasture.
- **Food Aggression:** Horses assert dominance within their herd over individual feeding territory. Hay piles have to be separated into piles equal or exceeding the number of horses to prevent or minimize possession aggression. Hogs become more aggressive at feeding time, especially when feeding times are unpredictable.

FEAR-INDUCED AGGRESSION

- **Incidence:** Fear can induce aggression in all animals. Handlers should always avoid causing intentional fear.
- **Intentional Fear:** The fighting bulls of Spain have been associated with bravery, but they fight humans not from predatory aggression but from fear of the unknown and pain.

They are induced to fight by never being allowed to see a human on the ground until they are in the bullring, by being separated from other cattle, and with lances and barbed sticks (banderillas) that are thrust into the neck muscles by picadores and the matador, respectively.

- **Response to Fear Aggression:** When a handler who has unintentionally created fear in an animal withdraws, the aggression is rewarded and the animal will intensify its aggression the next time it feels threatened.

INTERMATE AGGRESSION

Intermate aggression can endanger handlers. Bulls, boars, rams, bucks, and stallions are particularly dangerous during mating season. Female animals in estrus will intensify male agitation and aggression.

DOMINANCE AGGRESSION

The social status among large animals is affected by age, weight, sex, and breed. With horned species, the presence of horns increases social dominance. Adult, sexually intact males tend to be more dominant than females (Table 2.6).

Table 2.6 Major Factors in Exhibiting Dominance Aggression
• Selective breeding for dominance tendency
• Larger than typical body size
• Influence of male sex hormones.

- **Body Size:**
  - **Cattle:** Larger size means more food has been needed and successfully attained in a competitive environment. Larger individuals are more dominant than small individuals of the same breed, and larger breeds are more dominant to smaller breeds. Larger breeds of dairy cattle are dominant to smaller breeds, but breed dominance in beef cattle is not as closely linked to body size.
  - **Swine:** The size of a hog is directly related to its degree of exerting dominance within a group.
- **Male Sex Hormones:** Male sex hormones are also major influences on displays of dominance.
  - **Effects of Castration:** Castration, prior to puberty, does not eliminate the possibility of dominance aggression, but it significantly reduces it. Postpubertal castration effects are less impressive since adult male behavior may become ingrained on the nervous system before the removal of male hormone stimuli.
  - **Bulls:** Bulls display dominance aggression by pawing the ground, shaking their head, and displaying the silhouette of their side. A bull that is ready to attack will stand with his side displayed to demonstrate how big he is to his opponent. A bull that charges a person in an open pasture should be culled for slaughter and not sold at auction putting others at risk of danger.
  - **Male Small Ruminants:** Unprovoked aggression against a human by a ram, buck goat, or stud camelid should be reason to cull them.
  - **Stallions:** Most aggression from stallions is the result of improper handling.
    - **Need for a Stallion:** Stallions should always be castrated if there is not an established breeding value and plan for breeding.
    - **Correct Bad Manners without Hesitation:** An intentional breach of a handler's personal space by a stallion necessitates a reassessment of handling techniques, need for retraining, or elimination from a herd.

- **Isolated Male Aggression:** Many owners will not risk a young stallion or bull possibly getting hurt during socialization with older, larger animals and will raise them in isolation from their own species.
  - ○ **Orphans:** Orphaned male grazing animals should be castrated early or placed in a social group with their own species by 6 weeks of age.
  - ○ **Manners Taught by Peers:** Stallions or bulls are more easily handled if they are raised with other horses or cattle, including older males of their species. Older or larger males teach the challengers that they cannot easily bully others. If raising young males together, sufficient room must be provided to allow subdominant males to escape a losing fight.
  - ○ **Minimize Isolation of Males:** When stallions must be kept in stalls, the stall should be as large as possible and as visually open as possible with good ventilation. At a minimum, they should be turned out daily in stallion-appropriate (at least 7 ft tall) pens where they can see other horses and be provided with forms of environmental enrichment. Similar exposure of males to others of the same species is helpful in handling bulls, boars, and other prey animals.
- **Genetic Aggression:**
  - **Natural Genetic Selection:** Well-adjusted dominant animals only become aggressive if they have to protect themselves or their group. Within a species, animals do not risk serious injury or death to establish dominance, except for mature males during breeding seasons.
  - **Selective Breeding:** Some breeds are more aggressive than others. For example, Angus cattle and Brahmans are usually dominant to Herefords and Shorthorns. Ayrshires are dominant to Holsteins, which are dominant to Jerseys.
- **Handler Response to Animal Dominance:** Handler response to animal dominance actions will affect subsequent interaction with the animal.
  - **Submission Is Dangerous:** Attempting to run away from an aggressive large animal is usually dangerous for the handler. Running away will also intensify the animal's future aggression.
  - **General Response to Dominance Aggression:** Handlers should protect themselves first from possible injury from an animal with dominance aggression. Following that, indications to the animal that it can control the handler's movements should be avoided. For example, a horse that invades the handler's personal space in an attempt to move the handler should be backed away and then the handler should make the horse briskly move its hindquarters to one side and then the other to reinforce the handler's leadership over the horse's movements.

SPECIES' DIFFERENCES IN AGGRESSION AND AVOIDANCE

HORSES

Horses kept in stalls and those maintained without direct interaction with other horses are most likely to be aggressive.

- **Stallions:** Stallions and horses that are handled in small confinements, or with training techniques that restrict natural movement, are more likely to be aggressive.

- **Mares:** Mares with foals can be very protective even if they are docile in other situations. Snappy swishing of the tail to each side can be a sign of frustration and irritation.

CATTLE
- **Dairy Breeds:**
  - **Bulls:** Dairy bulls are the most dangerous of all domestic animals. They are unpredictable and extremely strong. They will inflict injury by crushing, goring, pinning on ground, and smashing the victim. Dairy bulls are typically hand (bottle)-raised which leads them to losing their flight zone and natural respect for humans.
  - **Cows:** Dairy cows are usually handled frequently and become docile, if handled well.
- **Beef Breeds:**
  - **Bulls:** Beef bulls, although also dangerous, are more predictable and respectful of human space. Being raised with other bulls and cows, beef bulls concentrate more on establishing their dominance on cattle, not people.
  - **Cows:** Beef cows vary depending on frequency and quality of handling. Nursing cows are more likely to be aggressive whether they are beef breeds or dairy breeds.

SMALL RUMINANTS
- **Sheep:** Sheep defend themselves by tightly flocking together and moving as a unit. Rams may attempt to butt handlers and can be dangerous, particularly during breeding season.
- **Goats:** Dominance in goats depends on their age, gender, body size, and whether they have horns, and if they do, the size of their horns directly increases the goat's social status.

SWINE
- **Boars:** If not socialized properly or deprived of social interactions with other hogs, boars can be very aggressive.
- **Sows:** Nursing sows are always aggressive if they hear any piglets or pigs squeal.
- **Pigs:** Young pigs should be penned in small groups since they huddle, climb, and shove each other. Introducing one new pig or hog into an established group will often initiate life-threatening aggression by the dominant members of the group.

POULTRY
Chicken pullets and turkey poults, in extreme confinement, have their beaks trimmed because of dominance and territorial aggression resulting in feather picking and cannibalism. Turkeys, and some chicken hens, can become aggressive toward handlers who are timid in their body language when handling a flock.

TRAINING METHODS FOR HANDLING LARGE ANIMALS

Training animals to be handled should be the major part of preparing young animals to become socialized with humans. The most effective means of training depends on species and what is to be learned. Success at training is dependent on animal genetics, observational learning from its mother, and the quality of handling it receives prior to puberty (Table 2.7).

Table 2.7	The Foundation for Success at Handling and Training Animals
•	Selection of a young animal that is an offspring of parents that have been willingly receptive to their own training
•	A mother that has been properly socialized to humans and is quietly handled in the offspring's presence (observational training of offspring)
•	Gentle, repeated but infrequent handling of the young animal during its critical socialization period.

REINFORCEMENTS

Either *positive reinforcement* (adding a reward such as food treats) or *negative reinforcement* (removal of a noxious stimulus) are used to instill trained behaviors.

- **Timing Is Critical:** The timing of either reinforcement is critical (i.e., within 3 seconds of the behavior to be reinforced with a treat or discouraged with a reprimand). Late negative reinforcement becomes simply punishment, which can lead to the animal becoming aggressively defensive or developing a helplessness attitude that inhibits further learning.
- **Positive Reinforcement:**
  - **Food Rewards:** Large prey animals (horses, cattle) can be trained to do "tricks" with positive reinforcement (food treats).
  - **Hazardous Disadvantage:** Food rewards can teach large animals to be a nuisance and dangerous since it can eliminate the animal's respect for human personal space that is needed for safer handling of large species.
  - **Impracticality for Training to Work:** Food rewards are impractical for training horses for work or performance since carrying and providing treats is not possible when the work or performance is in progress. Herd leaders of prey animals do not provide treats for acceptable behavior. They lead to food sources, provide protection from dangers, and expect respect from less dominant members of the herd.
- **Negative Reinforcement:**
  - **Rest as a Reward:** Herd animals are also rewarded by being left alone by the more dominant member of the herd. Work and performance horses are trained by providing a stimulus to elicit an action. The reward is an opportunity to rest.
  - **Pressure and Release:** Behaviorists' terminology of "negative reinforcement" carries an erroneous connotation that punishment is involved. Pressure and release is a more descriptive phrase than negative reinforcement for training of large animals.

SHAPING AND CHAINING

Advanced training of maturing or mature domestic animals involves *shaping*, breaking a task to be learned into small pieces, which are gradually refined. The refined small pieces of a trained activity are then performed in sequence, a process referred to as *chaining*.

COUNTERCONDITIONING

Counterconditioning is rewarding no response. It is useful in training animals to accept something that might cause a fearful reaction. For example, allowing a horse to rest if it does not shy from a balloon that it had been fearful of is counterconditioning.

HABITUATION AND DESENSITIZATION

Habituation and *desensitization* are similar training methods. Habituation is providing a steady stimulus that causes an undesired response until no response occurs. Desensitization is using a repeated stimulus with increasing intensity until no response occurs. Habituation and desensitization are often used to eliminate a flight reaction to a previously fearful stimulus in prey animals, particularly horses.

AVERSIVE TRAINING METHODS

Aversive training methods should be avoided, but sometimes what is aversive is conditional.

- **Abusive Use of Training Aids:** Spurs are used to train horses for lateral movement. Spurs can be aversive, but they are not if used with the correct timing and with the minimum effort to elicit an intended response. Excessive handling can be harmful by exhausting young animals physically and mentally and may break down respect for the handler and the handler's personal space.
- **Exhaustive Training Methods:** A training technique called *flooding* is used to habituate or desensitize an animal by rapidly presenting several stimuli until mental exhaustion and no response occurs. Flooding is used in colt-starting contests to demonstrate rapid results for entertainment purposes, but flooding is a poor training technique with short-lived results if not followed by longer-term training of lower intensity.

HEALTH AND BEHAVIOR

Illness or injury can markedly alter the animal's tolerance to handling.

ASSESSMENT OF HEALTH

Handlers should always make an assessment of an animal's health before attempting to handle it (Table 2.8).

Table 2.8 Practical Assessments of Animal Health
• Overall appearance (body condition, hair coat condition)
• Locom'otion
• Interactivity with other animals
• Consciousness of the environment
• Evidence of food and water consumption
• Presence of fecal matter and appropriateness of the character of feces relative to the animal's own species
• Appearance and quantity of voided urine.

PREY ANIMAL HEALTH BEHAVIORS

Prey animals tend to attempt to hide their illnesses by fake eating and minimizing lameness. They will become more social so that they do not stick out from the herd. True behavior of sick or injured animals, particularly prey animals, often requires containment in familiar surroundings and monitoring behavior unobserved with hidden video cameras.

STEREOTYPIC BEHAVIOR AND ENVIRONMENTAL ENRICHMENT

IMPERFECT METHODS TO QUANTIFY STRESS

- **No Exact Measurements of Psychological Stress:** The determination of psychological stress in animals is qualitative. This tempts some people to anthropomorphize that certain situations are mentally stressful to animals, which may or may not be the case. Surveys of owners' opinions are bias prone.

- **Cortisol Measurements as Indication of Stress:** Efforts at quantitative measures have traditionally relied on the measure of cortisol levels and heart rates, both measures of parameters that change within minutes and are affected by multiple stimuli. Meta-analysis of salivary cortisol studies in animals has indicated that cortisol as a single parameter and without context of duration of possible stress, gender, and other effectors of cortisol concentrations is unreliable as an indicator of stress or welfare.

PRAGMATIC MEANS TO MEASURE STRESS

- **Visible Changes to Normal Behavior:** Visible reactions of animals to situations that induce apprehension, fear, trust, respect, and pain are very similar to observable human reactions. Experienced animal handlers can recognize these primitive basic feelings in animals as well as any human can recognize the visible signs of fear, pain, and other basic reactions in another human.
- **Recognition of Stereotypic Behaviors:**
  - **Ethograms:** An ethogram is a catalog of behaviors exhibited by an animal. Changes in grooming, foraging, resting and sleeping, attempts to thermoregulate in an environment, or playing can be used to semi-quantitatively assess welfare in animals.
  - **Dysfunctional Behaviors:** Failure to appropriately thrive and repetitive alterations in normal behavior are reliable indicators of stress in animals. *Stereotypic behavior* is dysfunctional behavior, usually induced by stress and influenced by genetics.
  - **Manifestations:** Stereotypic behaviors are characterized by repetitive actions having no obvious purpose. Common types are usually forms of pacing or oral behaviors (Table 2.9).

Table 2.9 Example Stereotypic Behaviors
• Cribbing and weaving in horses
• Tongue rolling in cattle
• Bar biting in sows as well as belly nosing and tail and ear biting in pigs
• Wool eating in sheep.

  - **Causes of Stress:** The stresses are often excessive confinement; barren, boring environments; or isolation from their own species.
    - **Common Stereotypic Behaviors:** Stereotypic behaviors are most common in stabled horses without turnouts, crate-confined hogs and pen-confined hogs without environmental enrichments, and chickens confined to battery cages. These behaviors are not seen in wild animals or those with relative freedom and adequate stimuli for mental exercises.
    - **Degree of Stresses:** The percentage of confined animals that show stereotypic behaviors can be an indication of the degree of stress from excessive confinement.
  - **Prognosis:** Observed stereotypic behaviors may relate to current environment or past environment. Once the behavior has been established, it may be permanent due to alterations in primitive brain locations.

NUTRACEUTICALS FOR THE CONTROL OF ANXIETY

EFFICACY AND SAFETY OF NUTRACEUTICALS

Nutraceuticals are over-the-counter food substances administered orally with the intention to improve health or provide medicinal benefits. They are not considered pharmaceuticals and therefore are not regulated the same as drugs.

- **Efficacy:** Scientific studies of efficacy in correcting health problems or altering behavior are not required of nutraceuticals and seldom established by independent investigators.
- **Safety:** Nutraceuticals are regulated by the U.S. Food and Drug Administration's reaction to public complaints involving egregious medical claims, misleading marketing, and contamination with hazardous materials.

ANTI-ANXIETY NUTRACEUTICALS

- **Common Use:** Nutraceuticals for altering behavior in large animals are primarily marketed as sedatives for horses. True sedatives can make horses dangerous to their riders. Only stabled horses should be sedated for non-medical reasons.
- **Control of Anxiety in Horses:** See Table 2.10.

Table 2.10 Control of Excessive Anxiety in Horses without Drugs
• Selectively breed horses without excessive anxiety tendencies
• Provide proper training
• Handle frequently and calmly expose to new objects, situations, and environments
• Allow optimal time in pasture with other horses
• Give constant access to low calorie forage (pasture grass or grass hay).

- **Nutraceuticals Marketed for Anti-Anxiety**
  - **L-Tryptophan and 5-HTP**
    - **L-tryptophan:** Tryptophan is a large amino acid that is a precursor to serotonin. Tryptophan dietary supplements are administered with the expectation that serotonin levels in the brain will increase, improving mood and behavior.
    - **5-HTP:** 5-hydroxytryptophan (5-HTP) is generally recommended over L-tryptophan because it crosses the blood-brain barrier better and is more effectively converted to serotonin. However, the clinical benefits in humans are insignificant and behavior improvement in treated horses has not been scientifically validated.
  - **Melatonin:** Melatonin is a hormone produced by the pineal gland in the brain and also by plants. Oral melatonin administration is proposed to treat insomnia in people and modulate fear in horses, but proof of efficacy is currently insufficient.
  - **Alpha-Casozepine:** Alpha-casozepine is a trypsin hydrolysate of the mammalian milk protein, casein. It is marketed as an anti-anxiety supplement for horses, but evidence of clinical efficacy from independent, controlled studies is lacking.
  - **Magnesium:**
    - **Method of Action:** Magnesium can block N-methyl-D-aspartate (NMDA) receptor, an ion channel found in neurons as well as calcium receptors. This effect helps regulate neural and neuromuscular activity.

- ○ **Uses:** Magnesium, particularly magnesium bromide, has been used in humans as a mild oral sedative. It was used as an intravenous anesthetic in horses but has since been replaced by much better anesthetics.
- ○ **Efficacy:** Deficiency of magnesium can cause tremors and anxiety which is ameliorated by magnesium supplementation. More studies by independent investigations are needed on the efficacy of magnesium supplements as a treatment for anxiety in horses that are not deficient in dietary magnesium.
- **L-Theanine:**
  - ○ **Source:** Theanine is an amino acid found in tea leaves.
  - ○ **Efficacy:** Reduction of anxiety in horses has been attributed to the oral administration of theanine, but more studies are needed to confirm these claims. Health claims in humans were not substantiated by the European Food Safety Authority. The European Union now prohibits L-theanine health claims for humans.
- **Valerian:** Valerian or valerian root extract is also an herb promoted for the control of anxiety in humans based on anecdotal evidence. Scientific evidence is inconclusive. Its efficacy in horses is unknown.
- *Magnolia officinalis*: *Magnolia officinalis* is a flowering tree that grows in the mountains of China. It contains honokiol, which has been claimed to have anti-inflammatory and antioxidant effects. There are no independent scientific studies that have demonstrated the anti-anxiety efficacy of *Magnolia officinalis* in horses.
- **Ashwagandha:** Ashwagandha (*Withania somnifera*) is an evergreen shrub that grows in India. Its name translates as "horse smell." There is no scientific proof that ashwagandha has any anti-anxiety effects in horses nor any proof of its safety.
- **Cannabidiol:** Cannabidiol (CBD) is one of more than 100 cannabinoids in the *Cannabis sativa* (marijuana) plant. If purified, it does not have the psychoactivity of tetrahydrocannabinol (THC).
  - ○ **Proposed Benefits and Known Risks:** CBD is marketed as a calming and pain-relieving agent but independent controlled efficacy studies are lacking. However, depression, liver damage, diarrhea, and altered metabolism of some concurrently administered medications are established potential adverse effects.
  - ○ **Confusing Regulations:** Because the regulation of cannabis products in the U.S. is a fluid, conflicting, and confusing mess, false claims of medicinal effects and mislabeled products containing little to no CBH are common.
  - ○ **Federal Versus State Regulations:** Cannabidiol extracted from marijuana is classified federally as a Schedule I Controlled Substance. However, some states have passed laws to allow CBD sales, while federal enforcement of sale as a federally controlled drug superseding state law is inexplicably ignored.
  - ○ **Recommendations Allowed:** Veterinarians may recommend CBD veterinary products under the Animal Medicinal Drug Use Clarification Act.

ANIMAL BEHAVIOR SPECIALISTS

Knowing basic animal behavior is essential for anyone to become a good animal handler. Animal behaviorists and animal handlers are not synonymous, however. Some excellent animal handlers may only be able to describe normal animal behavior in colloquial language while some excellent animal behaviorists may be less than average animal handlers.

ANIMAL BEHAVIORIST TRAINING

There are no state or federal regulations for people to claim to be an animal behaviorist or trainer. Certification of training can be reputable, or not.

CERTIFICATION AS AN ANIMAL BEHAVIORIST

- **Veterinarians:** A certified animal behaviorist veterinarian is trained in the investigation of how and why animals behave as they do. A certified animal behaviorist who is a veterinarian is the best source of information on how to diagnose abnormal behavior and what corrective measures to prescribe. The American College of Veterinary Behaviorists (ACVB) establishes the requirements for formal education and evidence of acquired knowledge and skills for becoming a certified animal behaviorist.
- **Veterinary Technicians:** Certified or Registered Veterinary Technicians can go through specialty training to become a Veterinary Technician Specialist in Animal Behavior. The Academy of Veterinary Behavior Technicians (AVBT) certifies veterinary technician specialists in animal behavior.
- **Reputable Animal Behaviorist Organizations:** For more information on becoming a behaviorist or on behavior problems in animals, contact the ACVB at www.dacvb.org or AVBT at www.avbt.net.

BIBLIOGRAPHY

1. Berger JM, Spier SJ, Davies R, et al. Behavioral and physiological responses of weaned foals treated with equine appeasing pheromone: A double-blind, placebo-controlled, randomized trial. J Vet Behav 2013;8:265–277.
2. De Paula RA, Aleixo ASC, da Silva LP, et al. A text of the effects of the equine maternal pheromone on the clinical and ethological parameters of equine undergoing hoof trimming. J Vet Behav 2019;31:28–35.
3. Falewee C, Gaultier E, Lafont C, et al. Effect of a synthetic equine maternal pheromone during a controlled fear-eliciting situation. App An Behav Sci 2006;101:144–153.
4. Hart KA. The use of cortisol for the objective assessment of stress in animals: Pros and cons. Vet J 2012;192:137–139.
5. Houpt KA. Domestic Animal Behavior for Veterinarians and Animal Scientists. 5th edition. Blackwell Publishing, Ames, IA, 2010.
6. McDonnell SM, Miller J, Vaala W. Calming benefit of short-term alpha-casozepine supplementation during acclimation to domestic environment and basic ground training of adult semi-feral ponies. J Eq Vet Sci 2012;33:101–106.

3

ROPES, KNOTS, AND HITCHES

DOI: 10.1201/9781003110910-3

Ropes are essential tools for working safely with livestock and horses. They can save a handler's life or endanger it, depending on the judgment and skill exercised in using them.

TERMINOLOGY AND ROPE CONSTRUCTION

DEFINITION OF TERMS

- **Ropes:** Ropes are more than 5/12 inches in diameter. Smaller fiber diameters are referred to as cord twine, string, or thread. Ropes are made of natural fiber or synthetic fibers.
- **Lariat:** A rope that is used to handle or restrain livestock and horses is called a *lariat* from the Spanish word for the rope, *la reata*. A lariat may have a running noose for catching animals or no noose for tying (tethering, picketing) animals. The word *lasso* comes from the Spanish word *lazo* meaning noose or snare.

NATURAL FIBER ROPE

- **Fibers:**
  - **Manila and Hemp:** Among natural fibers, manila and hemp are the strongest plant fibers for ropes. Hemp is smoother than manila and is the oldest rope fiber, but its use declined approximately 200 years ago due to preference for the stronger manila rope.
  - **Cotton and Flax:** Cotton and flax are both softer and more manageable than manila and hemp, but cotton and flax will stretch and rot. Cotton continues to be widely used for lead ropes and is the preferred type of rope for restraining animal legs.
  - **Jute and Sisal:** Jute and sisal are less expensive, weaker plant fibers. Jute and sisal are natural fibers more often used for making twine.
  - **Leather:** Leather was used by Spanish and Mexican vaqueros to plait four to 12 strands of leather into 3/8-inch diameter rope called a reata (riata is an Americanized spelling of reata) of 50 to 65 feet in length. However, they require frequent treatment with tallow to prevent sunlight or water damage. Leather reatas are also about 10 times more expensive than other ropes.
  - **Maguey:** Maguey ropes (from fibers of the maguey plant) are handmade 4-stranded ropes, 3/8 inches in diameter from the maguey plant in Mexico. These have a smooth surface and are relatively firm, which aid in forming loops. Reatas and maguey ropes should be dallied (wrapped around an object) rather than tied due to the risk of breaking if jerked on with large animal force.
- **Advantages and Disadvantages of Natural Fibers:**
  - **Advantages:** The advantages of natural fiber ropes are a hairy-like rough surface that provides better traction and an easier grip.
  - **Disadvantages:** The disadvantages of natural fiber ropes are that they absorb water and swell, making knots difficult to untie. They can support mildew and rot, and they become brittle from strong sunlight or salt.
- **Construction:**
  - **Twisted (Laid) Formation:** Natural fiber rope is always twisted (also called laid) to increase strength from alternate twisting ("laying up") of components. Synthetic fiber rope is occasionally twisted.
    - **Fibers:** Fibers are twisted commonly to the right to form yarn.

- ○ **Yarn:** Three yarns are twisted to the left to form strands.
- ○ **Strands:** Three strands are twisted to the right to form the rope.
- **Advantages of Twisting:**
  - ○ **Easy to Grip:** Twisting creates a knobby exterior that is easier to grip and less likely to let a knot or hitch slip.
  - ○ **Splicing:** A *splice* is interweaving sections of untwisted rope. Twisted rope can be untwisted in sections to form a loop on an end of a rope with an eye splice or to join two ropes together by a short splice of the end of each rope.
- **Disadvantage of Twisting:** The disadvantage of twisted rope is that there is no protective outside layer. Every fiber twists to the outside multiple times being exposed to abrasion, moisture, and sunlight.

SYNTHETIC FIBER ROPE

- **Fibers:** Synthetic ropes vary in material and in strength (Table 3.1).

Table 3.1	Synthetic Fiber Types in Decreasing Order of Strength
•	**Nylon (Polyamide)**—Strongest and very elastic, but absorbs water
•	**Polyester**—Less elastic, more UV resistant, resistant to water
•	**Polypropylene**—Weaker, susceptible to UV damage, and can melt with heat from friction.

- **Advantages and Disadvantages of Synthetic Fibers:**
  - **Advantages:**
    - ○ **Strength:** Because synthetic rope is generally made of continuous fibers that run the length of a rope, synthetic ropes are stronger than natural fiber ropes. Natural fiber ropes are composed of short fibers that do not extend the length of the rope.
    - ○ **Durability:** Most ranch ropes are a nylon-polyester combination for strength with moderate elasticity in a twisted pattern. Synthetic ropes are lighter, stronger, and less expensive than natural fiber ropes. In addition, they do not rot or become brittle.
  - **Disadvantages:** The disadvantages of synthetic fiber ropes are that heat, even friction, can cause them to melt and that their smoothness, if not twisted, can cause hand grips and knots to slip.
  - **Construction:**
    - ○ **Variety:** Synthetic fiber ropes are constructed in a variety of patterns. They may be twisted, as with natural fiber ropes, *plaited* in four- to eight-stranded solid plaits, or *braided* in 16 or more strands (the *mantle*) around a core of long twisted center fibers, called the *kern* (Figures 3.1–3.2).
    - ○ **Mantle Protection:** The mantle of braided rope protects the inner fibers while all fibers of twisted or plaited rope are exposed to the elements.
    - ○ **Smooth Exteriors:** Due to their smooth exteriors, plaited and braided ropes do not hold knots and hitches as well as twisted rope.
    - ○ **Shoof Vet-Rope:** The Shoof Vet-Rope is a marine-grade polyester, oval-shaped rope that is woven with a hollow center, which causes it to flatten with tension. The Shoof rope is used for leg restraint of large animals and permits greater comfort to the animal and the handler. However, its construction also allows it to stretch more than conventional twisted rope, which can be disadvantageous in some restraints.

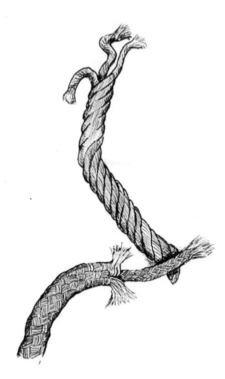

Figure 3.1 Twisted rope (top) and braided rope (bottom) which shows mantle and kern.

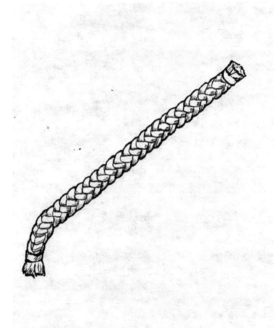

Figure 3.2 Plaited rope.

ROPE PARTS

- **Terminology:** Ropes have a *working end*, *standing part*, and *standing end*. A 180-degree bend in a rope is called a *bight*. A circular bend is a *loop* (Figure 3.3).
- **Hondas:** A sliding loop (noose) can be made with a knot, called a *honda*, that forms a small, fixed loop or channel for the rope's standing end to slide through.
  - **Rope Hondas:** Rope hondas may have a small leather wrap called a "burner" around the honda loop to reduce friction as the slip loop slides through. Other rope hondas may have a metal lining inside the tied loop to permit better sliding similar to a complete metal honda.
  - **Metal Hondas:** Hondas may also be metal (aluminum or stainless steel) or plastic.
    - ○ **Horse Training:** Metal hondas allow the rope to slip back and forth more easily to provide immediate pressure release when a horse stops resisting restraint. If to be used around the neck of a horse, a double-overhand knot can be tied in the rope (2 ft from the honda for 2-year-olds and 18 inches for weanlings and yearlings) to prevent the loop from completely closing and squeezing the neck of young horses. Metal hondas are also more reliable in wet conditions than rope hondas.
    - ○ **Quick Release Hondas:** A quick release honda is a metal honda that can be opened to release a caught animal without the need to loosen the slip loop (Figure 3.4). Quick release hondas have a finger latch to quickly open the metal honda. The finger latch has a hole in it so that a leather string can be grabbed to open the latch rather than putting a finger in the honda and endangering that finger if the animal moves while the finger is entrapped (Figure 3.5).

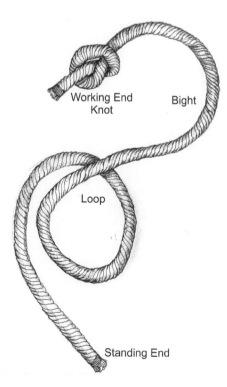

Working End
Knot

Bight

Loop

Standing End

Figure 3.3 Parts of a rope.

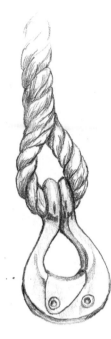

Figure 3.4   Quick release honda.

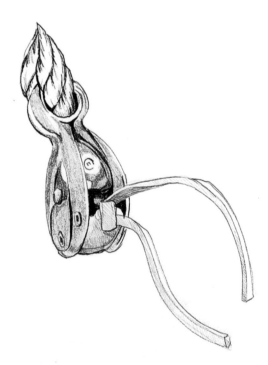

Figure 3.5   Leather tether for opening a metal honda's latch.

EQUIPMENT MAINTENANCE

STABILIZING THE ENDS OF ROPES

The ends of ropes will fray or unravel if not fixated.

- **Stopper Knots:** A *stopper knot*, such as an overhand, figure 8, or blood knot (a multiple wrapped overhand knot) can prevent unraveling and create a 'knob' at the end of a rope. A stopper knot can be valuable to reduce the chance of the rope being pulled and running through a handler's grip. However, an end knot can be an impediment to tying other knots or hitches.
- **Crown Knot:** Unraveling the end of a twisted rope a short distance allows the strands to be interwoven back (back spliced) on the rope end to form a *crown knot*. A crown knot doubles the diameter of the rope but does not create an obstructive knob to the same degree as an overhand or figure 8 knot.
- **Whipped, Back Spliced, and Melted Ends:** To create smooth ends on a twisted rope, rope ends may be whipped, back spliced, or melted (if synthetic).
    - **End Preparation:** Wrapping a section of rope with electricians' or duct tape, then cutting through the tape and rope together with a sharp knife, prevents the ends from unraveling until a more permanent means of fixating the ends is applied.
    - **Whipping:** The ends of twisted ropes can be wrapped (*whipped*) with string hiding the ends of the string underneath the wrapping (Figure 3.6). Natural fiber string should be used to whip natural fiber ropes and synthetic string used to whip synthetic ropes.

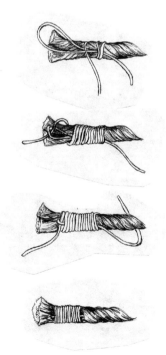

Figure 3.6   Whipping a twisted rope end.

- **Back Splicing:** Twisted ropes can be back spliced at their ends to prevent unraveling.
- **Melting (Burning):** Nylon and polypropylene twisted, plaited, or braided ropes can be burned on the end to melt the fibers together by open flame or hot irons or hot plates. If not melted evenly and carefully, rough or sharp strands may develop and be dangerous to the handler's hands.
- **Ferruled:** Some twisted ropes are prevented from unraveling by bending a band or ring of metal, a *ferrule*, around the end. Ferruled ropes should not be used for animal restraint due to risks to the animal or handler from the metal developing sharp edges.
- **Dipped:** Dipping rope ends into lacquers and similar liquids that dry into a hard encasement can also produce a rough, sharp surface that can be hazardous. Dipped end ropes should also not be used for animal restraint.

STORING ROPES

Ropes cannot be sanitized, but they should be rinsed thoroughly after use, dried with a towel, and stretched out to dry before being hanked or coiled.

- **Hanking:** Ropes not in use should be stored properly. Softer, twisted ropes are coiled, and the coil is collapsed, wrapped, and tied. This is called *hanking* a rope (Figure 3.7). Hanked ropes prevent tangling when releasing the coil.
- **Hanging:** When hung up for storage, ropes and leather restraints should never be hung over a thin peg or nail which causes a sharp bend and weakens the fibers. When hanging hanked ropes, the rope should be hung over a tack knob, a 2- to 4-inch diameter hanger.
- **Rope Cans:** Synthetic material lariats are stiff and need to maintain their curve. These are coiled and stored as circular coils, not hanked. Ropes with strands twisted to the right need to be coiled in a clockwise direction.

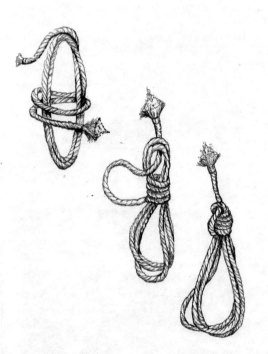

Figure 3.7 Hanking a rope for storage.

LEATHER QUALITY AND CARE

Leather is tanned animal skin. Most leather in the U.S. comes from cattle hide. Thick, strong leather for safe tack comes from select steers, not heifers, and is vegetable tanned.

- **Tanning:** Tanning makes leather more durable, pliable, and resistant to wear and rot. The most common methods of tanning are vegetable tanning and chrome tanning.
  - **Vegetable Tanning:** Vegetable tanning produces leather that is non-corrosive to metal, non-irritating to the skin, can be carved or molded, and is strong, if thick. Vegetable tanning is used for saddle and other tack construction. The Hermann Oak Leather Company, founded in 1881, in St. Louis, Missouri is the leading vegetable tanned leather manufacturer in the U.S. and tans only high-quality steer hides.
  - **Chrome Tanning:** Chrome tanning is less time-consuming and less expensive than vegetable tanning and more commonly used. It produces leather that is soft, pliable, and strong when thin. It is often used for making leather clothes.
- **Leather Maintenance:** Well-tanned quality leather can last generations if treated properly. It should not be constantly stretched, repeatedly soaked with water, or allowed to dry out.
  - **Shaping:** Leather can be shaped by wetting it to create the desired shape, but must be dried slowly with gentle ventilation. It should not be heated during the drying process.
  - **Moisturizing:** Leather should be moisturized 1 to 4 times per year with warm oil, usually a variable combination of lanolin or neatsfoot oil, mink oil, cedar oil, beeswax, and a petroleum-based solvent, and then beeswax is added to the surface. This lubricates the internal fibers and inhibits drying leading to cracking. The frequency should be more often if exposed to moisture, drying, or dust.
  - **Surface Cleaning:** Leather should be cleaned with a damp cloth as often as needed based on its use. Abrasion can wear the external surface of leather, and small particles of grit ground into the leather can abrade internal fibers.
  - **Storage:**
    - **Avoid Mold:** Leather should never be stored in a plastic bag where it would likely mold. Exposure to extreme heat and very low or high humidity should be avoided. Exposure to air and gentle ventilation reduces the risk of mildew.
    - **Avoid Excessive Exposure to Sunlight:** Leather should not needlessly be exposed to sunlight. It should be stored in shade or indoors when not in use.

CLEANING ROPES

- **Need for Cleanliness:** Animal handling ropes cannot be sanitized, but with basic cleanliness, the same rope may be used on multiple healthy-appearing animals with little risk of transmitting disease. Keeping ropes clean cannot only reduce the risk of transmitting disease but can also remove sand and other abrasives or chemicals that can break down the fibers of rope.
- **Methods:**
  - **Natural Fiber Ropes:** Urine, manure, and saliva should be rinsed from natural fiber ropes with only water. The uncoiled damp rope should be laid over hay bales or tied between two objects to dry on all sides of the rope before recoiling or hanking.
  - **Synthetic Fiber Ropes:** Synthetic fiber ropes can be washed with water and a mild soap, and then thoroughly rinsed. Synthetic fiber ropes should be air dried uncoiled as with natural fiber ropes before they are coiled for storage.

EQUIPMENT SAFETY

MANAGE ROPES ON ANIMALS

Any time ropes are used to handle or restrain large animals, the handler should never allow a rope attached to the animal to become wound around a hand, arm, or leg. When tying an animal by a halter, if the tail of the lead rope is long enough to be a hazard, a *daisy chain* (chain sinnet, monkey braid) can be tied to shorten the length of the lead rope. Daisy chains are formed with a series of loops and bights.

MONITOR EQUIPMENT WEAK POINTS

- **Check for Weak Spots:** Before each use, all handling equipment should be reinspected for weaknesses that might cause breakage.
- **Metal Quality Is Important:** Lead snaps are often die-cast, created in molds that can permit air to be entrapped in the metal, which is often zinc, and make it weak. Steel or iron snaps, those that are attracted to a magnet, are more reliable.

ALWAYS CARRY A SHARP KNIFE

- **Need:** A sharp knife should always be carried by animal handlers who use ropes to free entangled animals, an assistant, or the handler. In addition, quick release hitches can be pulled tight enough by a horse that the hitch cannot be untied and must be cut.
- **Easily Retrieved and Deployed with One Hand:** The knife should be retrievable by one hand and either a fixed blade in a scabbard or an assisted opening folding knife with a cord that extends from the handler's pocket for quick retrieval, in case one of the handler's arms is entrapped or incapacitated. The blade should have a partially serrated edge for cutting thick ropes.

USEFUL KNOTS, BENDS, AND HITCHES FOR ANIMAL HANDLERS

DEFINITION OF TERMS

See Table 3.2.

Table 3.2 Terms Used in Rope Tying	
•	**Knot**—Intertwining a rope to itself
•	**Bend**—Intertwining a rope to another rope or two ends of the same rope
•	**Hitch**—Intertwining a rope to another object, such as a hitching ring
•	**Splice**—Unwinding the strands of a twisted rope so that they can be interwoven with the strands of another rope or to create crown knots, halters, and other rope handling tools.

CHALLENGES IN TYING KNOTS, BENDS, AND HITCHES

- **Learning and Maintaining:** Tying knots, bends, and hitches is more difficult than they appear. Practice is required to acquire and to maintain the skills. If not used frequently, monthly practice of tying knots and hitches should be planned.
- **Importance of Proper Pull Down:** Forming the knot, bend, or hitch is just the first part. For many knots, bends, and hitches, how they are pulled tight is just as important. A flip or twist in the pull down or a lack of proper pull down (tightening) can ruin a knot's or hitch's effectiveness.
- **Selection of the Appropriate Knot, Bend, or Hitch:** Each knot, bend, or hitch has a different purpose. The selection of which knot to use is based on its ability to remain secure, the ease of tying and untying, and its size.

OVERHAND KNOT (THUMB KNOT) AND OTHER STOPPER KNOTS

- **Overhand Knot:**
  - **Purpose:** The *overhand knot* is the simplest knot. It is used as a stopper knot to keep the end of a rope from fraying or to put knobs in the length of a rope to add traction points and prevent the end of ropes from pulling through a handler's grip.
  - **Method:** The overhand knot is made by making a circle with a rope and bringing one end over the top of the loop and through the loop (Figure 3.8).
- **Blood Knot:** Bulkier stopper knots may be created by going through the loop 2 or 3 times. The triple overhand knot was called the blood knot because it was used on the ends of the British cat o'nine tails, a whip used to flog sailors for punishment.
- **Figure 8 Knot:** The figure 8 knot is another stopper knot (Figure 3.9). It is formed by creating a bight at the end of a rope, twisting the bight 180 degrees, and then inserting the working end of the rope through the formed loop.

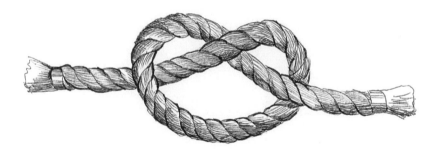

Figure 3.8   Overhand knot.

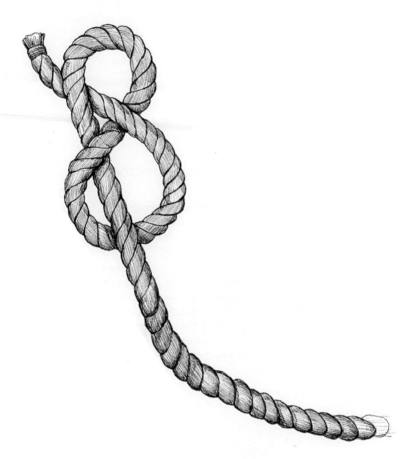

Figure 3.9   Figure 8 stopper knot.

SQUARE KNOT

- **Square Knot:**
    - **Purpose:** The square knot is popular for tying two ropes of an equal diameter together. It will not slip or jam, but it should not be used in potentially dangerous situations because it creates sharp bends that weaken ropes. It may have caused more deaths and injuries than other knots because of its popularity and misuse.
    - **Method:** The square knot is an overhand knot tied on an overhand knot (Figure 3.10). It is tied right over left, then left over right. When tied properly the shorter free ends will be in line with the tied or taut lines.

- **Variations on the Square Knot:**
  - **Surgeon's Knot:** A double overhand knot (the working end goes around the rope twice) is the first half of a surgeon's knot (Figure 3.11). A surgeon's knot inhibits slippage while the second overhand is tied, completing the surgeon's knot.
  - **Reefer Knot:** A *reefer knot* (reef is a name for a type of sail) is a square knot with a bight in one of the short ends. This acts as a slip knot to quickly untie the square knot. Shoelaces are typically tied with double reefer knots.
  - **Granny Knot:** The *granny knot* (right over right or left over left) is similar to a square knot but will slip under tension or will jam (Figure 3.12). Pulling on the longer ends of a granny knot will make the short free ends go out of line with the long ends to form an "X" or cross. Granny knots are improperly tied square knots and have no useful purpose.

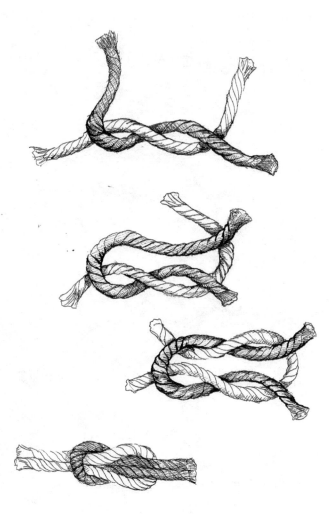

Figure 3.10   Square knot.

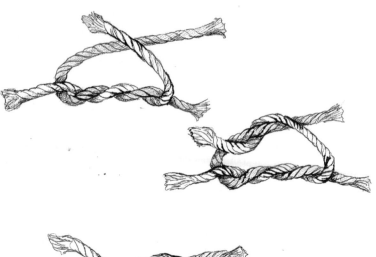

Figure 3.11   Double overhand in a surgeon's knot.

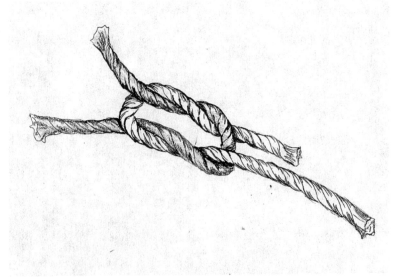

Figure 3.12   Granny knot.

QUICK RELEASE HITCHES (LEAD ROPE TIES)

- **Standard Quick Release Hitch:**
  - **Purpose:** The most common quick release hitch, also called the *halter hitch*, is the standard lead rope tie. It is the most commonly used hitch for lead ropes in handling horses. This hitch allows the working end to be pulled to the side, which is the easiest direction to release a quick release hitch.
  - **Method:**
    - ○ **Tie to a Stout Object:** This tie is performed after the end of the lead rope goes through a tie ring or around a stout horizontal post.
    - ○ **Making the Hitch:** With the standing end that goes through the tie ring, a loop is made on the left side of the lead rope going to the horse's halter. The standing end of the lead is taken under the lead to the horse and bent into a bight. The bight goes over the lead to the horse and through the loop (Figure 3.13).
    - ○ **Pull Down Properly:** The hitch is tightened around the lead and then slid up to the tie ring.
  - **Preventing Horse Escapes:** When horses that may untie hitches are tied, the working end of the lead rope should be dropped through the bight of the hitch to prevent pulling on the end from untying the hitch. Alternatively, a bowline should be used to tie horses that untie quick release hitches.
- **Manger Hitch:** A variation of the quick release hitch is a shoelace-like tie (a double reefer knot), called the manger hitch. This variation requires pulling the working end toward the tie ring and is much more difficult to release the hitch in a hurry than the standard hitch for lead ropes. It is not recommended as a substitute for the true quick release lead rope hitch.
- **Highwayman's Hitch:** The highwayman's hitch, also called the "draw hitch," is a quick release using a bight around the object (Figure 3.14). The highwayman's (an old term for bandit) hitch was reputedly used in the past by bank robbers to tie their horses for a quick getaway.
  - **Method:** The highwayman's hitch is performed by putting a bight through the tie ring. The end of the lead is wrapped around the lead line and lead line bight and then a second bight is put into the first and the hitch is pulled down tight to the tie ring.
  - **Advantage and Disadvantage:**
    - ○ **Advantage:** The advantage of this hitch is that it permits a quick tie of a very long rope and a quick release. Unlike the standard quick release hitch which requires the length of the lead to run through a tie ring and then regrasping the lead, a highwayman's hitch is released with a pull with one hand and the grip can be retained on the rope after its release from the hitch ring.
    - ○ **Disadvantage:** The disadvantage is that horses that can untie themselves from a highwayman's hitch will become completely loose compared to untying the standard quick release tie that leaves the lead rope draped through the tie ring. Most seasoned horses, even if untied, will stand in place if the lead line is still running through the tie ring.

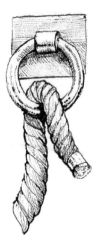

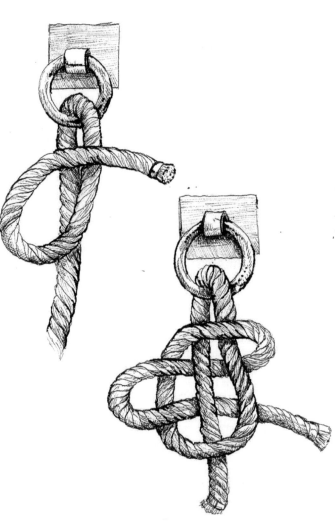

Figure 3.13   Quick release lead rope hitch.

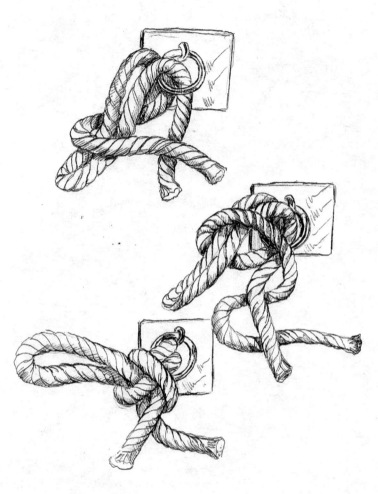

Figure 3.14 Highwayman's hitch.

HONDA KNOT

- **Purpose:** A honda is a small, fixed loop, a channel for the other end of the rope at the end of lariats for livestock and horses (Figure 3.15).
- **Method:** A honda knot is recreated by making an overhand knot in the end of the rope as a stopper knot and then making another overhand knot a few inches up the rope. Before tightening the second overhand knot, the stopper overhand knot in the end is put inside the loop of the overhand knot and trapped by pulling the second knot tight.

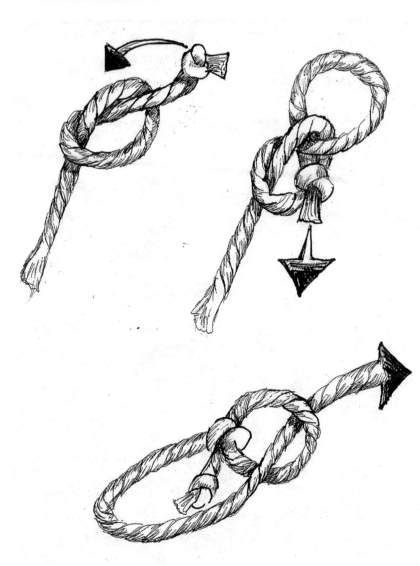

Figure 3.15   Honda knot.

SHEET BEND (WEAVER'S KNOT; TAIL TIE)

- **Purpose**
  - **Tying Rope Ends Together:** A sheet bend is used to tie two ropes together (Figure 3.16). This simple bend is secure, even if the ropes are of different sizes.
  - **Tail Tie:** It is also used to tie cords to cattle or horse tails to restrain the tail.
  - **Lead Tie to Halter:** A double sheet bend can be used to tie a lead rope to a horse halter. It is lighter, softer, and stronger than a typical metal fastener for a lead rope.
- **Method:** The sheet bend is created with a bight in one end of a rope while the other rope end goes through the bight, is wrapped completely around the bight, and then trapped underneath itself where it first emerged from going through the bight. A double sheet bend is wrapped around the bight twice before going under itself.

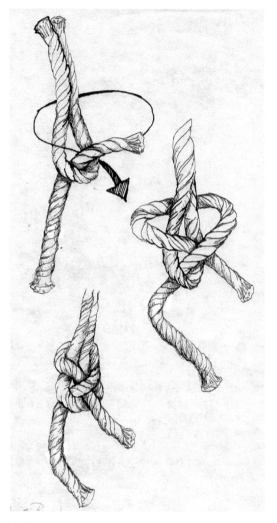

Figure 3.16 Sheet bend knot.

BOWLINE ("KING OF KNOTS")

- **Purpose:** The bowline (pronounced "BO-linn") knot has many uses since it creates a loop that will not slip, bind, and risk choking an animal if around its neck. It is the preferred knot to tie the lead line of a horse that can untie hitches since it cannot be untied by horses and does not bind. It is probably the most versatile knot used in handling large animals (Figure 3.17).
- **Method:** The knot can be tied with one hand, but most people learn to tie the knot by memorizing "the rabbit comes out of the hole, goes around the tree, and back down the hole."
  - **The Rabbit's Hole:** A bight is created first and twisted 270 degrees to create a loop.
  - **The Rabbit Comes out and Goes around the Tree and Back down the Hole:** The end of the rope goes through the loop, circles around the standing part of the rope and goes back through the loop. The loop is then pulled closed finishing the bowline knot. Making two loops for the "rabbit's hole" will create a double bowline that is even stronger than an ordinary bowline.

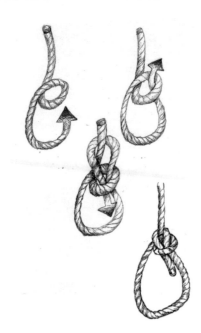

Figure 3.17   Bowline knot.

BOWLINE ON THE BIGHT

- **Purpose:** A bowline on the bight knot is useful for making a rope collar in the middle of a long rope with two trailing lines, as needed for breeding hobbles, or one trailing line for creating a Scotch hobble (Figure 3.18). The knot will not slip and choke the animal. It is easily untied even after tension has been on the knot.
- **Casting Horses:** The bowline on the bight knot has been used for *casting* (laying down) sedated horses for surgical procedures, but less commonly since the advent of newer injectable anesthetics that produce relatively smooth inductions and recoveries.

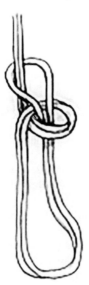

Figure 3.18   Bowline on the bight.

HALF HITCH

- **Purpose:** A half hitch is a quick means of tying to an object, but it is generally unreliable (Figure 3.19). It can be a reliable knot if tied repeatedly over itself as when tying legs on a recumbent animal or on a cattle chute cleat (then called the *cleat hitch*).
- **Protect Fingers:** Wrapping figure 8s with a rope around a cleat on a cattle chute should be done with the heel side of the hand to keep fingers less vulnerable of being trapped in the wraps. The same grip also provides greater strength to pull the rope around the cleat.

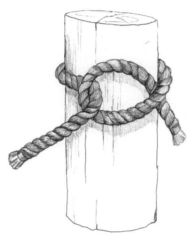

Half hitch

Figure 3.19   Half hitch.

CLOVE HITCH

- **Disadvantage:** The clove hitch works by friction and is generally unreliable for tying animals with a rope (Figure 3.20). If an animal rocks the rope back and forth with head movements, it will loosen a clove hitch.
- **Improved Reliability:** If the lead is first wrapped around another post and then tied to another post with a clove hitch, the hitch is reliable. This confines rocking effects to the wrap and prevents a rocking effect on the hitch which could loosen it.

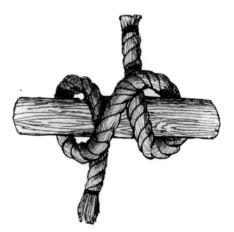

Figure 3.20   Clove hitch.

PICKET LINE HITCH

- **Purpose:** Sometimes the most convenient place to tie horses is to a rope tied horizontally between two secure objects such as trees. This is called a picket line. Picket lines may be chest height, but overhead picket lines will reduce the risk of pulling the line down or becoming entangled.
- **Method:** A picket line hitch is similar to the clove hitch but is much more secure because the working end is trapped under itself (Figure 3.21).

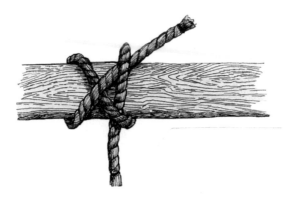

Figure 3.21 Picket line hitch.

ROPE HORSE HALTER TIES

- **Purpose:** Rope halters for horses can apply more pressure to the poll and bridge of the nose than leather or nylon band halters. As a result, a clearer correction for misbehavior can be delivered, and horses will not pull or lean on the halter and lead rope (Figure 3.22). Rope halters also require less room to store and do not trap moisture that can promote bacterial or fungal infections compared to leather halters.
- **Method:** The knot used to tie a horse's rope halter is a sheet bend (Figure 3.23). A double sheet bend can be used to attach the lead line to the halter rather than a metal clip.

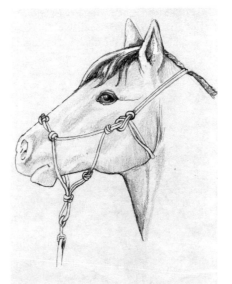

Figure 3.22 Rope halter.

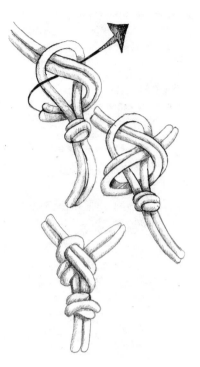

Figure 3.23   Rope halter tie.

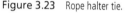

USING A LARIAT

VALUE DEPENDS ON EXPERIENCE

- **Skill Requires Much Practice:** Throwing a lariat loop is sometimes necessary for capturing livestock and horses. Some handlers consider lariats as the least stressful option for untrained animals and others consider lariats as the last resort for capturing an animal.
  - **Value:** Opinions on the value of using a lariat are affected by the handler's skill in using one. The proficient use of lariats must be routinely practiced. Ability of the handler is the dominant factor in how soon, how often, or if throwing a lariat is used in capturing animals.
  - **Initial Practice on Inanimate Objects:** The skill must be acquired by much practice on inanimate objects before ever attempted on animals.
- **Pros and Cons:**
  - **Cons:** Poor use of a lariat can instill fear in animals of human approach. Injuries to an eye can result, especially with metal quick release hondas, or a leg may be accidentally caught increasing the risk of a broken leg or neck. On the other hand, throwing a lariat loop can be the only practical available means of capturing range cattle or untamed horses.
  - **Pros:** The correct rope in the hands of an experienced roper can be less stressful on managing calves than alleys, chutes, and head catches. Rodeo calf and steer roping events that are exciting and flashy are sometimes inhumane are for entertainment only. Good cattle and horse handling with ropes is slow, quiet, and can be boring to watch.

- **Horseback Roping Styles in the United States:**
  - **Texas-style:** Small loops are thrown with speed in Texas due to the brushy environment in south Texas and the need to catch cattle quickly.
    - **Shorter Ropes:** Common lariats used in Texas-style roping are stiff ropes 5/16 or 3/8 inches in diameter and 28, 30, or 35 feet long.
    - **Smaller Diameter Saddle Horns:** Roping from horseback is done with saddle horns with a small diameter designed for tying.
  - **Californio-Style:** Big loops are used in California and Basin and Mountain states where the land is more open and better permits large, slowly tossed loops.
    - **Long Ropes:** Californio-style roping is done with softer ropes at greater distances. Cattle are quietly roped from outside their flight zones. Leather reatas or Mexican maguey ropes 50 to 60 feet long are used for Californio-style roping.
    - **Large Diameter Saddle Horns:** Saddles are used with large diameter saddle horns (*gourd horn*) that are more effective for *dallying* (wrapping the rope without tying). Dallying the rope is easier on the cattle being handled than tying.
- **Tossing or Throwing a Lariat on Foot:**
  - **Purpose:** Throwing a rope while the handler is on the ground is used to capture and sort cattle when chutes and other handling facilities are not available. It may also be used as an early tool in horse training.
  - **Dally Post:** Prior to throwing a lariat from the ground, a stout stationary object should be selected as a potential dally post, and gloves should be worn. Smaller animals may be restrained by taking the rope behind the handler's seat (a half dally). This allows the handler to grip with the rope wrapped behind the handler's back and to push backwards with the legs rather than try to pull with the arms and maintain just a hand grip on the rope.

ANATOMY OF A LARIAT LOOP
- **Loops:** Lariat loops (also called nooses) consist primarily of a base, tip, honda, and spoke.
  - **Base:** The *base* is the top part of a loop and the bottom portion is the *tip*.
  - **Tip:** The tip is the bottom portion of a loop.
  - **Spoke:** The *spoke* is the portion of the rope that has passed through the honda and extends to the portion that is held with the base by the throwing hand.
  - **Strands:** The *bottom strand* of the loop is the section of rope from the honda side of the base to the tip. The *top strand* is the section of loop from the tip to where the rope goes through the honda (Figure 3.24).
- **Hondas:**
  - **Construction:** Hondas on lariats should be natural or synthetic fiber, leather, or lightweight metal.
  - **Fiber or Leather Hondas:** Fiber or leather hondas are lightweight, relatively soft hondas used on traditional lariats to catch horses or cattle.
  - **Metal Hondas:**
    - **Lightweight Metal Hondas:** Heavy metal hondas on ropes to be thrown can injure the animal's eyes, ears, or facial bones. Lightweight metal hondas are useful in training horses and other animals to give under pressure. When the animal quits pulling on the rope, there is an immediate release (reward).
    - **Quick Release Metal Hondas:** Quick release hondas unsnap, preventing the need to loosen the rope first. These hondas can be useful in restraining cattle, but they can be dangerous to handler's fingers if the handler uses a finger to unclasp the latch when freeing the animal. Rather than putting a finger in the honda to release the snap, a rawhide string to pull the snap open should be used.

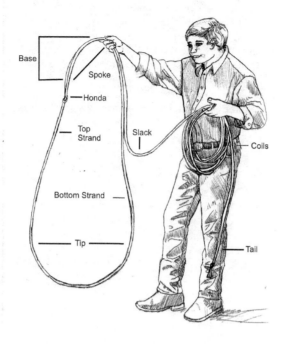

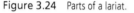

Figure 3.24   Parts of a lariat.

THE THROWN LOOP (TOSSED LOOP)

- **Preparation of Surroundings:** Occasionally there is no other realistic option than roping for capture, particularly with cattle. If cattle are to be caught with a lariat, they should first be herded into the smallest holding area that is strong enough to contain a group of pushing cattle. A dally post should be identified and its strength inspected before attempting to catch and snub a cow or calf.
- **Preparation of the Loop:** In preparation of a catch, the group is approached at an angle quietly on foot with a loop ready and held low, dragged on the ground, and held slightly behind the right leg for a right-handed roper. The spoke should be held to extend about one-fourth down the top strand.
- **The Toss:**
    - **Quiet Cattle:**
        - **Do Not Swing the Rope:** It is preferable to catch cattle with a lariat before they become agitated. Swinging the rope before a toss will frighten cattle. The loop is dragged behind the handler.
        - **A Gentle Flip:** The toss is a silent, smooth upward movement of the arm with a slight flip of the wrist. The loop should make one-half turn by the time it reaches its target with the tip of the loop falling over the target. The honda should fall in front of the target and not hit it.
    - **Agitated Cattle:**
        - **Swing the Rope for Momentum:** If the cattle are not quietly settled and run from the quiet approach of the handler, a thrown loop must have momentum to quickly get to the animal to be caught. One swing of the loop is generally enough.

      ○ **Dally and Snub:** As soon as the animal is caught, the handler has to pull it in a circle close enough to make a dally (loops/wraps) around the dally post. Once caught and snubbed, the animal is driven toward the dally post while the slack is taken up in the rope.

      ○ **Switch to a Halter:** If the reason for catching the animal requires that it be held for more than a minute, a halter should be placed on the animal and tied to the post. The neck loop should then be loosened or removed to prevent the animal from choking.

- **Tossing a Quick Release Honda:** Ropes with quick release metal hondas can be tossed, but they should not be swung and thrown. The weight of the honda unbalances the loop and can cause injury to the animal if thrown with speed.

THE HOOLIHAN LOOP

- **Purpose:**
  - **Catching Horses with a Lariat:**
    - ○ **Horse Agility:** Because of their quick movements and long neck, horses can easily duck and avoid a thrown lariat loop if they see it coming directly toward their head.
    - ○ **Range Horses:** Range horses that are broke to ride are trained to be gathered in rope corrals and stand side by side with their rumps to a *wrangler* (western-style horse handler) while the handler selects and ropes individual horses for work. This is much safer than milling among a herd of 20 or more riding horses, called a *remuda* in the Southwestern U.S. or *cavvy* in the Great Basin states, early in the morning.
    - ○ **The Loop:** The type of loop thrown to select the horses from a remuda is called a *hoolihan*, which is thrown off the index finger after swinging the loop once smoothly and quietly around and above the roper's head. Ideally, the loop is thrown from behind the horse near its blind zone and drops down over its head from behind.
    - ○ **Catching Cattle:** The hoolihan loop can also be used to catch cattle in a pen. The advantage of a smooth, quiet swing to develop momentum and a large loop may be helpful in catching cattle in some situations. However, more room is needed to swing the loop around the thrower's body than is required of many other loops.
- **Method:**
  - **At Ready Position:** A right-handed roper holds the loop over the roper's left shoulder. This allows a large loop to be held close to the body and not be dragged on the ground. The spoke should be held so that it extends about three-fourths down the top strand.
  - **The Throw:** The throw begins with smoothly swinging the loop clockwise around the body. The loop is released when the right hand is over the handler's head and in approximate line with the left ear. The loop should make one-half turn and the tip should drop over the target.
  - **Training Horses to Be Caught:** Only the best, most experienced ropers catch horses from a remuda for the other wranglers. Horses unaccustomed to ropes should only be caught with a rope in a small round pen with solid, high walls by a skilled roper and soft ropes.

LOOP ON A STICK (UURGA)

- **Purpose:** The uurga is a traditional horse capture tool of Mongolian horsemen. Still today, the loop on a stick, an improvised uurga, can sometimes be more effective and simple than throwing a lariat.

- **Method:** A telescoping pole, available at most home care stores, can be easily transported and adjusted to desirable lengths. Attaching the loop with Velcro strips will hold the loop open until quietly placed over its target (Figure 3.25). The pole can then be removed and the animal captured by dallies around a stout post or running the standing end of the lariat through a tie ring.

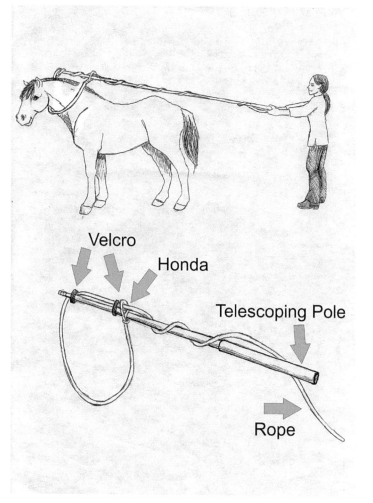

Velcro

Honda

Telescoping Pole

Rope

Figure 3.25   Improvised uurga.

BIBLIOGRAPHY

1. Bigon M, Regazzoni G. The Morrow Guide to Knots. William Morrow and Company, Inc., New York, 1982.
2. Costantino M. The Knot Handbook. Metro Books, New York, 2010.
3. Owen P. The Book of Outdoor Knots. The Lyons Press, Guilford, CT, 1993.
4. Sharp J. Knots, Hitches, and Their Uses. Central Oregonian, Prineville, OR, 1966.

4

HORSES, DONKEYS, AND MULES

DOI: 10.1201/9781003110910-4

After becoming domesticated more than 6,000 years ago, horses provided unsurpassed mobility to humans until the development of steam engine locomotives. Horses enabled the spread of languages and cultures and the advancement of human civilization. The United States has more horses than anywhere else in the world.

Table 4.1   Age and Gender Terminology for Horses
• **Stallion**—Adult, sexually intact male
• **Gelding**—Castrated male
• **Mare**—Adult female
• **Foal**—Nursing baby horse
• **Weanlings**—Horse of either sex between weaning and 1 year of age
• **Yearling**—Horses between 1 and 2 years old
• **Colt**—Young male horse under 4 years of age
• **Filly**—A young female horse under 4 years of age.

NATURAL BEHAVIOR OF HORSES

Horses are highly social prey animals that prefer to live in groups and defend themselves primarily with their ability to detect distant motion of predators and flee rapidly.

INHERENT HERD BEHAVIOR

Horses in the wild prefer to form small *bands* of three to 30 horses, usually a stallion and four to six mares with foals, that share a grazing territory. The sexually mature mares within a band are called the *harem*.

- **Dominant Mares:** Each band of mares and immature horses is led by an older dominant (*boss* or lead) mare.
    - **Herd Guide:** Dominant mares lead the band to water and grazing sites.
    - **Disciplinarian:** The boss mare occasionally reinforces her social position by roaming through the herd checking the deference given her. An insufficient response to move elicits controlled aggression to reassert the recognition of her role in the herd.
- **Dominant Stallions:** The band also has a dominant or *lead stallion*.
    - **Herd Guardian:** The lead stallion guards the periphery of the herd and the slowest of the band against predators when the band is moving.
    - **Controls Genetic Superiority:** Young stallions nearing puberty at about 2 years of age are forced out of the herd. Bachelor stallions follow bands at a distance. During breeding seasons, some bachelors will occasionally challenge the lead stallion for his position as band sire.
- **Herd Dynamics:** After the dominant mare and stallion, the remainder of the herd is in a linear hierarchy.
    - **Social Status Based on Assertiveness:** Physical contact among band members is usually avoided by the use of threatened bites and posturing as if to kick. Ignoring this body language will lead to meaningful bites or kicks.
    - **Violent Reactivity:** Like other animals, the rank of horses in a herd is primarily based on deference, not by actual fighting. Fights that can result in serious injury are most often between adult stallions or between a nursing mare and any perceived threat that might endanger her foal.

- **Herd Socialization:** The opportunity to socialize with other horses, to feel the security of other horses being present, and to graze 12 to 17 hours per day is essential to horse mental health. Each of these opportunities beneficially affects their ability to be handled by humans.
  - **Grazing:** Freedom to graze in groups is a great stress reliever in horses.
  - **Mutual Grooming:** Another stress reliever is mutual grooming, such as standing nose-to-tail with a herd buddy, nibbling each other's withers, and swishing flies away from each other's face.
  - **Surrogates:** Devoid of companionship with other horses, some horses will develop a bond with goats, ponies, or donkeys, among other animals. If goats are used, meat breeds such as the Boer or large dairy breeds (Alpine, Saanen, LaMancha, or Toggenburg) should be selected rather than small or miniature breeds.

GENDER BEHAVIOR

- **Mares:** Boss mares can be particularly difficult to handle if allowed to control the movement of a handler or access to food (i.e., food possession aggression).
- **Stallions:** Stallions may be more receptive to handling than boss mares if they do not feel the need to assert their social status with a human handler because of breeding seasons or if handled roughly.
- **Kick, Bite, or Strike:** Fillies and mares are more likely to kick. Colts and stallions are more likely to bite or strike.

CURIOSITY

Horses have a high degree of curiosity in new objects. In addition to exploring new objects with their lips, horses use their nimble lips to gather grass to bite with their incisors when grazing. This ability allows many horses to learn to open latches on stalls, pick up one grain of corn from a feeder, and untie knots, among other feats of lip dexterity.

DEFENSE

Horses' primary defense is to flee danger. When necessary, they will bite, strike with their forelegs and kick with their hind legs. Bucking is sometimes needed as a defense tactic against predators.

- **Bucking off Predators:** Large predators of horses usually jump on the horse's back and neck to which the horse responds with violent bucking to become free of the attack. If successful in escaping, the horse will be more inclined to buck with greater effort the next time.
- **Bucking off Riders:** Analogous actions occur if young horses started under saddle are allowed to buck, especially if they are successful in ridding themselves of the rider. Ideally, during early training, a saddle horse is tacked up securely so that when bucking with an empty saddle first occurs, they are not successful in ridding themselves of the saddle until the handler removes it when the horse is quiet. This is a major step in lessening the horse's urge to buck with a rider.

SLEEP

- **While Standing:** Horses sleep only a few hours, most of it dozing in a standing position since they are able to fixate their legs in extension with their *stay apparatus*. If startled while dosing, they are likely to kick. The sleep time is usually in multiple short periods of approximately 15 minutes each.
- **REM Sleep:** To achieve REM sleep, they must lie down to sleep for an hour or two every few days, and in a herd, they typically will not lie down unless another trusted horse is near and remains standing as a sentinel to guard against predators.

COMMUNICATIONS

- **Body Language:** The most frequent communication among horses is body language, using the ears, eyes, nostrils, position of the head and neck, pawing with front hooves, cocking a hind leg as if to kick, and swishing the tail. Status in the band is reaffirmed by forcing others to move, particularly from favorite food, using body language. If the threat is unsuccessful, the more dominant horse will follow through with a bite or a kick.
- **Vocalization:** Vocalization is less common, including nickering, neighing (whinnying), snorting, and squealing.
- **Smell and Tactile Senses:** Smell and touch (nuzzling, grooming of each other in pairs) are other means of communication.

YOUNG HORSE BEHAVIOR

- **Play:** Foals and weanlings play mostly by themselves in the first 3 months of life. Interactive play peaks at 3 to 4 months of age. Friendships with particular horses will later develop.
- **Clacking:** Foals and weanlings defer to the authority of older, more dominant horses by clacking, a smiling and smacking action of the lips (Figure 4.1).

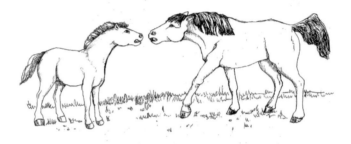

Figure 4.1 Immature horses defer to adult rank by smiling, clacking expression.

BREED BEHAVIOR

The temperament of horses depends much on their genetics. There are three general groups of horse breeds.

- **Hot Bloods:** The group believed to be the oldest are the hot bloods (Arabians, Barbs, and Thoroughbreds) which originated in hot climates and have been selectively bred for racing. Hot bloods are the most likely to be overreactive and hyperexcitable.
- **Warm Bloods:** Warm bloods (Quarter horses, Morgans, Andalusians) tend to be responsive and tractable, but when they react, their reactions are more explosive. They have been selectively bred for diverse forms of work involving light draft work or under-saddle tasks.
- **Cold Bloods:** Cold bloods (Clydesdales, Percherons, Friesians) are quiet and relatively unexcitable. Their breeding has been for their large size, quiet temperament, and ability to pull heavy loads.

SAFETY FIRST

Horses are frequently bred or purchased based on color or other physical attributes, yet owners want their horses to have good behavior which is not directly related to color or physical attributes. Behavior is a result of genetics, role modeling by well-behaved dams and other herd members, and by proper training. A good horse can be any color, or as often said "there is no bad color on a good horse."

HANDLER SAFETY

- **Learn Normal Behavior:** The best way to avoid injury from horses is to understand their normal behavior, anticipate their reactions in advance, and make the appropriate adjustments to avoid the situation or deal with it safely. Inherent dangers include the unpredictable nature of horses (i.e., their tendency to suddenly become frightened ("spook")) and to a lesser degree, their expression of normal aggression in certain situations.
    - **Situations That Stimulate the Flee Response:** Horses outweigh humans 5- to 10-fold with greater proportions of muscle and respiratory ability. Injury to themselves or to humans can be great due to the body size, strength, and speed of movement of horses.
    - **Normal Aggression:** Horses that are the most likely to injure a handler are stallions, nursing mares, or sick or injured horses. Normal aggression can be due to a natural role played in the herd, maternal protectiveness, or pain from injury or disease.
- **Avoid Incompetence and Negligence:**
    - **Incompetence:** Incompetence results in injuries to handlers who assume or claim a higher level of skill than the handler actually has.
    - **Negligence:** Forms of negligence are providing or using defective tack or other handling equipment, failure to assess surface or ground conditions that can cause a horse to fall, and failure to warn others of known dangers with a particular horse.
- **Provide Leadership:**
    - **Control Resources and Movement:** Horses have an intrinsic need for leadership in order to remain safe. Leadership is established by control of resources and movement. Handler and horse safety depend on the handler becoming the appropriate leader, and this must be done without scaring them.
    - **Avoid Anger or Excitement:** Anger or excitement is neither appropriate nor effective, and the horse should not be exhausted or excessively constrained.
    - **Show Affection at Appropriate Times:** Horses should be petted occasionally but only when they do something better than the last time they were asked for a response or action. Petting should be reserved for establishing or maintaining leadership, although petting can be appropriate for simple acts, such as the horse standing still when approached in a pasture.
    - **Allowing Rest:** Rest is a highly effective reward for proper actions by the horse.
    - **Food Treats:** The use of food as a reward is unreliable and inappropriate for training horses that are ridden or perform other work in variable environments and can destroy respect for a handler's personal space. Food has been used successfully by some trainers of horses to perform tricks in controlled environments. Use of food treats is counterproductive to establishing leadership.
    - **Develop Trust:** The goal for a relationship with a horse is for it to become the handler's working partner, not a pet. Good partnerships require mutual trust. Some horse handlers can manage horses without getting their trust, but the horse will remain untrustworthy and potentially dangerous, especially to other handlers.
- **Aggression:**
    - **Signs:** Expressions of attempted dominance aggression by a horse are pinning ears, dropping their head, swishing the tail, and hunching the back.
    - **Response to Aggression:** If the handler does not correct the behavior with appropriate timing and metered reaction, the horse will assume it has achieved a higher social rank than the handler. The appropriate response to aggression

Horses, Donkeys, and Mules 81

is to use a reasonable safe and timely means of getting the horse to move its feet as directed by the handler such as backing it up or moving its hindquarters laterally.

- **Effects of Environment:**
  - **Weather:** Changes in weather can make horses more difficult to handle.
    - **Wind:** Wind reduces their ability to smell and hear. It can also blow horse-scary objects like plastic bags around.
    - **Sudden Temperature Change:** A sudden return to more moderate temperatures will invigorate horses that were tired from heat and flies or horses that were well-rested hiding from cold winds.
  - **Unfamiliar Objects:** Unusual objects on their horizon will concern them such as a motorcyclist on the road, a moved trash can, or a veterinary truck parked in a new location. Horses kept for excessive periods in box stalls will be less attentive to the handler and more reactive when taken out to be handled.
  - **Distractions:** Irritation from flies can cause distraction, stomping, and kicking. A misbehaving horse will agitate others in the vicinity.
- **Promote Good Mental Health of Horses:** See Table 4.2.

Table 4.2   Promoting Good Mental Health of Horses for Easier Handling
• Provide opportunities to move freely
• Allow to forage at will
• Create times to see distant objects, hear new sounds, and feel changes in the wind
• Permit socialization with familiar horses
• Handle frequently in a consistent, fair manner.

- **Freedom of Movement:** Providing time at pasture with other horses improves a horse's ability to be handled by humans. When horses are kept in groups in pastures and pens, their shoes, especially hind shoes, should be removed to prevent serious injury from disciplinary kicks that might not otherwise be harmful from dominant horses.
- **Opportunity to Socialize:** Horses that are not allowed daily opportunities to socialize with other horses, run, roll, and graze tend to develop physiologic and mental problems.
  - **Physiologic Benefits:** Movement associated with socializing among horses is physiologically beneficial. Excessive confinement prevents normal muscular activity, venous and lymphatic circulation, and health and nutrition of joints. Stiffness, leg swelling, and lameness can result.
  - **Mental Benefits:** The opportunity to socialize with other horses is critical mental enrichment for maintaining proper behavior. Excessive confinement or isolation can cause or aggravate stereotypic behaviors, such as cribbing, weaving, and stall walking.
- **Consistency and Proper Timing:** For the best response from horses, a handler must possess confidence, firmness, patience, and kindness. Horses learn good habits quickly from pressure followed by properly timed release and being free enough to make a mistake and given appropriate correction within 3 seconds. After 3 seconds, the horse will not be able to make the connection between the action and correction.
- **Horse Manners:** Horses should be expected to maintain good manners.
  - **Stand Still:** Horses should stand still and pay attention to the handler when being handled.
  - **Respect Handler's Personal Space:** Horses should show no attempt at dominance over the handler such as nipping, shoving, or walking on the handler.

Horses should be expected to walk mannerly alongside the handler with no pulling, balking, or dragging along. They must respect the handler's personal space, which is to stay an arm's length away from the handler unless invited closer.

- **Early Socialization with Humans:** Socializing newborn foals (so-called "imprinting") is believed to affect the behavior of horses for the rest of their lives, but handling foals can be overdone. If attempting to socialize by imprinting, it is recommended to begin in the first 48 hours after foaling. Excessive handling of foals and not correctly handling weanlings, yearlings, and 2-year-olds can eventually endanger handlers.

  - **Method:** The mare should be caught first and held by an assistant with the mare against a wall or strong fence. The mare is rubbed and groomed for 10 to 15 minutes, followed by rubbing and handling all parts of the foal's body. Exposure to clipper noise and other stimuli it will encounter later in life is also recommended.
  - **Maternal Influence:** The effectiveness of foal handling can be negated if the mare is distressed and becomes agitated. Her actions will supersede the benefits of any rubbing of the foal by the handler.
  - **Adverse Effects on Training:** Excessive petting and scratching of horses between weaning and 2 years of age can teach a horse to move toward pressure while the basis of training is to teach horses to move away from pressure (i.e., a rein, rider's leg, or spur).

- **Body Language:** Most communications between horses and from horses to humans is by body language. The body language vocabulary is not large. They use ear, head, and neck position, movement, pawing, and tail swishing.

  - **Red Alert:** The essential body language for a handler of horses to know includes if the horse's head is up, its neck tense, the ears are forward, the eyes fixed on a perceived threat, it blows hard out the nostrils (snorts), and lifts its tail—this means red alert and it is ready to bolt.
  - **Ears:**
    - **Variable Meanings:** Ears held back moderately and head low can mean "I want you out of my space," but at grain feeding time, it often means "hurry up and give me food." When working, ears back means a sign of resolve to work hard and pay better auditory attention to the rider or handler.
    - **Threat of Aggression:** Pulling the ears back when aggressive, is a tighter flattening of the ears to protect them from being bitten. This does not enhance hearing.
    - **Nonaggressive:** Nonaggressive horses often turn their ears backward to focus their hearing on what is happening behind them. This is a typical ear position for horses when racing and the same posture used by stallions to drive herd members from behind the herd.
  - **Eyes:** Normally nearly all of the white of the eye of calm horses is not visible. Being able to see the white part of a horse's eye is a better indication of fear or aggression than the position of their ears.
  - **Hind Quarters and Tail:** Dancing or swaying on the rear feet and swishing the tail rapidly back and forth (if not being harassed by flies) means "I am dominant and my patience is gone." This is a signal the horse is ready to kick.
  - **Pawing:** Pawing the ground is a sign of impatience or frustration.
  - **Signs of Relaxation:** Relaxation body language can be licking lips, lowering head to wither's height, blinking eyes, or cocking a hind foot over onto the front of the hoof which means "oh, this is not as bad I as thought" or "been here, done that."

- **Respect of Handler Space:**
  - **Horses Should Respect Handler's Space:**
    - **Handler Personal Space:** Horses must be required to respect human personal space, an approximate 3 ft radius around a handler, unless invited closer.

      ○ **Moving a Horse out of Handler Space:** Horses instinctively push or lean toward pressure, but they must be taught to move away from pressure by tapping their shoulder or chest until they move out of a handler's space. Then, they should be immediately left alone until they invade a handler's space again.

      ○ **Avoid Attempts to Be Pinned:** Handlers should never allow a horse to pin them against a wall or other solid object. This is dangerous and a sign of dominance aggression with lack of respect for humans.

  ● **Handlers Should Remain Quickly Mobile:**

      ○ **Standing:** When necessary to work closely with a horse's body in a standing position, the handler should keep a hand on the horse to detect its movements and to push the handler's body away, if needed.

      ○ **Bending:** When working low on a horse's legs, a handler should not sit, kneel, or place a hand on the ground. The handler should crouch and remain on the toes so that the handler can immediately stand and move away quickly if the need arises.

● **Manage Bad Manners in Horses:**

  ● **Causes:** Wild horses digest food in small portions eaten throughout the day. They are designed to be continuously moving, traveling up to 50 miles per day to new grazing areas, occasionally socializing with other horses, and respecting their leaders. Most bad manners and vices in horses are the result of having developed a lack of respect for human dominance, excessive confinement, or a lack of socialization with other horses.

  ● **Nipping:**

      ○ **Purpose:** Nipping (pinching the skin) is to test dominance or to make a horse or human move.

      ○ **Association with Hand Feeding:** Nipping of humans almost always begins from being fed food treats by hand. Handing horses food treats gets them in the habit of associating hands and pockets with food. When the treats do not appear when it desires, the horse will invade the handler's personal space, do a body search with their nose and lips, and eventually nip the handler out of frustration.

  ● **Biting:**

      ○ **Intent:** A horse opening its mouth wide to grasp a handler's arm, shoulder, or neck is a highly aggressive and dangerous act. Among the injuries to handlers from horses, 3 to 4.5% are due to bites. A horse that attempts a grasping bite has no respect for humans.

      ○ **Resolution:** Most of these horses should be euthanized, humanely put to death, as they are a highly dangerous menace to handle and should not be bred. Stallions and some boss mares are most likely to aggressive bite and must be watched carefully.

  ● **Kicking:**

      ○ **Ability:** Horses can kick with the strength, speed, and accuracy to kill a mountain lion attempting to attack. Horses are agile and will kick with both hind legs with pinpoint accuracy when in great fear.

      ○ **Range:** The kick zone using both hind legs is about 6–9 feet. Horses cannot do a sweeping kick with one hind leg to the outside as well as cattle. However, they can hop forward raising both hind feet off the ground, twist their lumbar region and pelvis and kick one leg sideways at head height.

      ○ **Purpose:** One leg kicks to deter a nuisance may be used to discourage harassing dogs, other horses, and sometimes humans. Adult horses do not usually kick humans, except for when they are startled from behind or defensive due to fear of injury.

- ○ **Mitigating Risk:** Handlers should never approach a horse directly from behind. This is their blind spot and being startled can cause the horse to kick. Additional precautions when working near the hindquarters of horses are provided in Procedural Steps 4.1.

Procedural Steps 4.1	Precautions around the Hindquarters of Horses
1.	The horse should be spoken to as an announcement of a handler's presence from a distance when approaching at an angle from behind.
2.	When a handler walks behind a standing horse, the handler should walk closely enough to brush their body against its rump to prevent being at peak force range for a kick.
3.	The handler should keep the closest hand on its rump so the horse knows the position of the handler and the handler can feel any tension or shifting of weight in the horse.
4.	Alternatively, the handler should walk at least 10 feet behind the horse outside the kick zone.

- ○ **Disrespectful Positioning of Horses' Hindquarters:** A horse should not be allowed to turn its rump toward a handler. If this occurs in a stall, the handler should stay out of kick range and make a small movement and slight noise such as hitting a wall with a solid object that gradually escalates to more movement and louder noise to stimulate the horse to turn its rump away. The annoying movement and noise should cease the instant that the horse makes any effort to move its rump away from the handler and then repeat as necessary.
- ○ **Avoid Startling Sleeping Horses:** Horses can go into a light sleep while standing because of a unique stay apparatus that can lock their legs and keep them from collapsing. Care must be taken not to suddenly awaken a sleeping horse that is standing, or it may become startled and kick. The typical posture of standing sleep is head lowered, lower lip drooping, and tail motionless.
- ○ **Approach to a Painful Leg:** When working on an area of pain at the flank or back legs, it is best for a handler to run the hands over the normal area on the other side to allow the horse to adjust to the touch and then reach underneath from the normal side to the affected side to test the horse's sensitivity to the area of possible pain.
- **Striking or Pawing:** Striking or pawing with the front legs is a sign of impatience or a startle reaction. Horses should be trained as a yearling to stand tied for long periods to teach patience and prevent a habit of pawing.
  - ○ **Kick Chains:** If a horse develops a destructive and possibly injurious habit of pawing if restrained, kick chains should be considered. Kick chains are leather straps fitted around the pastern with a 1-foot stainless steel chain. The chain creates noise and bumps the leg without causing injury if the horse paws or kicks.
  - ○ **Kick Chain Precautions:** Kick chains do not cause harm to the horse if they are used only when the horse is in a stall. Kick chains should never be used on a horse that is in a pen or turned out in a pasture. Persistent use of kick chains is not necessary.
- **Dragging a Handler When Led:** When being led, a horse should not walk with its shoulder ahead of the handler's shoulder, but some will attempt to pull a handler forward. Correction requires repeated responses from the handler (Procedural Steps 4.2).

Procedural Steps 4.2	Response to Being Pulled or Dragged While Leading a Horse
1.	If a horse attempts to drag the handler, the horse's head should be pulled toward the handler while pushing the horse's hindquarters away.
2.	After turning the horse in tight circles and allowing the horse to calm down, the handler should lead the horse forward to give it a chance to behave.
3.	If it does not, the handler should repeat the circle and disengaging the hindquarters as many times as needed until the horse walks forward properly without dragging the handler.
4.	A chain shank on a lead can be tried on difficult cases.

- **Rearing:** A horse that rears when being led can be dangerous to handlers that overreact (Procedural Steps 4.3).

Procedural Steps 4.3	Managing a Horse That Rears
1.	A longer than usual lead with a stopper knot on the end should be used if rearing is anticipated.
2.	When a horse rears, the handler should give it more length of the lead rope and move away from range of the front hoofs because attempts to keep the horse down may result in it overcompensating and falling over backwards or pulling the handler in close enough to be hit by its hooves.
3.	While moving away, the handler should also move in a semicircle toward the horse's hip to make its hip begin to circle away from the handler when the horse comes down.
4.	Longeing it in small circles both directions immediately after it rears, can eliminate any thought of a reward by rearing and discourage it from rearing again.
5.	Jerking down on a lead rope as a misguided reprimand can cause the horse to rear again.

HORSE SAFETY

- **Handler Responsibility for Safety of Horses:** The safety of horses is entirely dependent on the handling ability of whoever handles them.
  - **Anticipate Flight Reactions:** Horses protect themselves instinctively by flight reactions. Their flight reaction occurs before thinking (i.e., run first, think later). Understanding how horses monitor for possible dangers and communicate with each other can be helpful in identifying and defusing potentially dangerous situations.
  - **Good Training Is Slow:** A form of flooding or mental exhaustion from persistent overstimulation works well for initial acceptance of the saddle and rider, but flooding does not cause lasting effects without daily, less intense, follow-up training periods. Slower, calmer, and shorter training periods are more effective; safer for horse and rider; and less stressful to young horses in the early stages of their training than flooding to exhaust them.
- **Senses for Safety:**
  - **Sight:** Horses rely to a large extent on their sight for safety. They have excellent peripheral distance vision and constantly scan the horizon, but they cannot see directly behind them. Handlers who remain watchful for dogs in the distance, blowing plastic bags, and other potentially horse-scary things have a safety advantage.

- **Hearing:** Horses' sense of hearing is acute and enhanced by highly mobile ears. Handlers who use a soothing voice inflection when horses wish to flee will be at a safety advantage. A handler trying to be too quiet or making excessively loud noises can cause horses to act nervously.
- **Smell:**
  - **Odors Are Associated with Danger or Social Status:** Horses monitor odors for danger and social status. Horse greet each other by smelling the breath of each other. Establishing a pecking order is begun at the first greeting.
  - **Avoid Initiating Social Interactions by Smell:** A handler should not allow strange horses to smell each other's breath while they are under his direct control. One horse may strike out when they begin the sorting of the level of their social status after smelling each other.
- **Touch:**
  - **Gentle Touching Evokes Trust:** When bonding with herd members and asserting social status within the herd, horses touch each other. Handlers can reinforce horses' respect and trust in the handler by grooming them and petting them after they perform a desired action or demonstrate a proper response. A handler's presence and touch should be associated with normal herd activities and relaxation, not just being worked or receiving medical treatments.
  - **Touch Sensitivity:** The sense of touch is well developed in horses. The touch of a fly on their skin will cause the skin to twitch to shake the fly off. Horses have a sensitive prehensile upper lip that can pick out grains of oats from corn and medication tablets from feed and can unopen latches on gates and doors.
  - **Rubbing versus Patting:** Patting a horse is not painful, and desensitization to pats are needed for horses kept in warm, humid climates since a handler may need to slap a horse to kill horseflies on its body for the protection of the horse and the handler. Horses quickly learn to not resent a non-injurious slap that protects it from painful bites. Desensitization to patting also prepares a horse for accidental pats or slaps while being tacked up, mounted, or dismounted.
- **Vocalizations:** Horses have a spectrum of vocalizations to communicate with each other to assist each other's safety.
  - **Nicker:** A nicker is used to acknowledge the near presence of a herd member. When calling out for the location of another herd member, a loud *neigh* or *whinny* is used.
  - **Clacking:** Clacking (snapping, tooth clapping or champing) is a chomping movement of the jaws with the corners of the mouth pulled back that signals submission. Clacking is used often by foals, weanlings, and yearlings to acknowledge the herd status of older, dominant members.
  - **Blow:** If a horse is feeling good and is excited, a deep breath and blow are used.
  - **Snort:** A snort is also used when excited, but it is an announcement that it is ready to run.
  - **Grunt or Groan:** Horses that feel they are working hard or harder than they desired will grunt or groan.
  - **Squeal:** A squeal is an aggressive noise used more often by mares to startle a potential opponent.
  - **Scream:** Screams are rare sounds of great fear such as in a barn fire.

RIDING SAFETY

For more information on horseback riding safety measures, see the companion textbook to this manual—Chastain, C. B., *Animal Handling and Physical Restraint*, Boca Raton, FL, CRC Press, 2018:233–242.

KEY ZOONOSES

(NOTE: Apparently ill animals should be handled by veterinary professionals or under their supervision. Precautionary measures against zoonoses from sick animals are more involved than those required when handling apparently healthy animals and vary widely. The discussion here is directed primarily at handling apparently healthy animals.)

Apparently healthy horses pose little risk of transmitting disease to healthy adult handlers who practice conventional personal hygiene. The risks of physical injury are greater than the risks of acquiring an infectious disease (Table 4.3).

SANITARY PRACTICES

A handler of horses should wear appropriate dress to protect against skin contamination with hair and skin scales or saliva, nasal, or other body secretions. Basic sanitary practices should be practiced, such as keeping hands away from eyes, nose, and mouth when handling horses and washing hands after handling them. Horse handlers should be vaccinated against tetanus every ten years and horses should be vaccinated annually against rabies and encephalitis viruses, including West Nile virus.

- **Control Arthropod Vectors:** Mosquito, tick, and fly control measures should be implemented.
  - **Mosquitoes:** Purposeless standing water should be eliminated. Water in stock tanks, pet bowls, and bird baths should be changed at least once per week. Handlers should wear mosquito repellent during mosquito seasons.
  - **Ticks:** Cutting or grazing pastures short will aid in controlling ticks.
  - **Flies:** Manure should be composted at least 150 ft from barns. Fly traps and sprays should be considered.
- **Control Rodents and Birds:**
  - **Prevent Entry:** Means of controlling rodents and birds should include sealing any holes more than 2 inch diameter in rooms with grain with steel wool.
    - o **Grain Storage:** Grain rooms should be constructed of gnaw- and peck-resistant materials. There should be less than 2-inch gaps between doors and thresholds and grain should be stored in sealed, rodent-proof bins. Grates on floor drains should have less than 2-inch gaps.
    - o **Hay Storage:** Hay and equipment should be stored on pallets so that rodent presence can be monitored. Lightly sprinkling flour on the floors can aid in tracking rodent activity.
    - o **Buildings:** One inch gravel, 6 inches deep, and 3 feet out from buildings can be an effective rodent barrier.
    - o **Livestock Drinking Water:** Sufficient water should be maintained in water troughs that birds cannot stand on the bottom and bathe in the drinking water.
  - **Deterrents and Depopulation:**
    - o **Birds:** Bird netting should be considered for use in rafters.
    - o **Rodents:** Rodent baits can be dangerous to children, dogs, cats, and birds. The rodenticide remaining in dead rodents can be poisonous to dogs or cats that consume them.
    - o **Deterrent Dogs and Cats:** Gentle, rabies-vaccinated barn cats or terrier dogs are usually good barn guardians against rodents, snakes, and undesirable birds. Rabies-vaccinated yard dogs weighing 40 lbs., or more, can be a deterrent to raccoons, skunks, foxes, and opossums.
- **Tack, Grooming Tools, and Bedding:** Grooming tools, halters, hay nets, waterers, and feeders should be thoroughly cleaned and, if impermeable, disinfected whenever they will be used for a new horse on the premises. Stall bedding should be discarded and stall walls, ceiling, and floor cleaned and disinfected for new horses. An effective disinfectant is 1 cup of household bleach in 5 gallons of water.

Table 4.3 Diseases Transmitted from Healthy-Appearing Horses to Healthy Adult Humans

Disease	Agent	Means of Transmission	Signs and Symptoms in Humans	Frequency in Animals	Risk Group*
Bites, Kicks and Crushing	—	Direct injury	Bite wounds to face, arms, and legs	All horses are capable of inflicting bites, kicks, and crushing injuries	3
Tetanus	*Clostridium tetani*	Indirect, puncture wounds that inoculate tetanus spores	Rigid muscle spasms that eventually paralyze respiratory muscles	Tetanus bacteria are very common in horse feces	3
Cryptosporidiosis	*Cryptosporidium* spp.	Direct, fecal-oral or indirect via contaminated water	Diarrhea	Uncommon	2
Leptospirosis	*Leptospira* spp.	Direct, urine and indirect from urine contaminated fomites	Flu-like illnesses and inflammation of the kidneys	Uncommon	3

*Risk Groups (National Institutes of Health and World Health Organization criteria. Centers for Disease Control and Prevention, Biosafety in Microbiological and Biomedical Laboratories, 5th edition, 2009.)
1. Agent not associated with disease in healthy adult humans.
2. Agent rarely causes serious disease and preventions or therapy possible.
3. Agent can cause serious or lethal disease and preventions or therapy possible.
4. Agent can cause serious or lethal disease and preventions or therapy are not usually available.

- **Prevent Transmission of Disease among Horses:** When handling horses from different origins, proper sanitation is required to prevent the spread of disease from carrier horses that have little to no signs of disease. Horses from different origins should preferably not be confined in the same barn or adjacent pens or pastures for three weeks. Special precautions are needed if sick horses are handled, and sick horses should be isolated from apparently normal horses.

APPROACHING, CATCHING, AND RELEASING

Approaches to horses have to be adjusted for the tameness and training level of the horse. Wild horses are captured differently than tame, domestic, or trained horses. Before attempting to capture a strange horse among other horses, the social structure in the herd should be observed and dominant horses removed first.

GENERAL CONSIDERATIONS
- **Training to Be Caught:** Problems with capturing horses can be minimized by handling exercises. Failure to do this results in most tame and trained horses having a flight distance of about 10 to 30 ft.
  - **Catch Routinely for No Other Reason:** Feeding in stalls for 15 to 30 minutes at least once per day will permit easier capture, grooming, and an inspection for health. Walking up to a horse while it is in a pen or pasture solely to pet it briefly for standing still and then walking way desensitizes horses to the fear of work or medical treatment after each approach.
  - **De-Stressing the Horse:**
    - **Calm Voice:** Calming techniques include using a calm voice when around the horse. Familiar unstressed voices aid in putting horses at ease.
    - **Handler Body Language:** Assuming a glancing gaze toward the horse's body and legs as well as a lowered chin, dropped shoulders, arms down, and hands near body posture is helpful in de-stressing a horse to be caught.
    - **Moderate Speed of Approach:** Approaching a horse too fast or too slow will negate other body language. The proper speed of approach has to be adapted to individual horses and is based on experience. If the handler tenses muscles, uses an unnatural tone of voice, or holds in breath, the horse will become ill at ease.
    - **Proximity to Calm Horses:** Being in close visual proximity to a preferred herdmate can be a calming influence, but in some cases, an undesirable distraction if the others do not behave. Blocking visual distractions by handling a horse in a stall or small pen with solid walls aids in adapting horses to focusing its attention on a handler and being handled.
- **Importance of Head Control and Haltering:** Control of the horse's head is paramount to controlling a horse and protecting both it and the handler. No horse should be handled or restrained without being able to control its head with the use of a head halter, or a rope around the upper part of its neck. Proper fitting of a halter permits two fingers under the crownpiece and the noseband.
- **Horses Are Claustrophobic and Explosive:** Some, especially quarter horses, may initially tolerate head restraint and then with explosive force, attempt escape, including flinging the head which can deliver a lethal blow to anyone nearby.
  - **Avoiding Injuries from the Head:** To reduce the risk, a handler's head should never be placed near the horse's head. If necessary to be near the head and keep the horse still, the handler should hold the cheekpiece of the halter with the elbow of the same arm against the horse's neck.

- ○ **Control the Hindquarters:** Control of the head permits control of the hindquarters which controls the horse.
- **Proper Application and Use of the Halter:**
  - **The Bear Hug Method—Recommended:** The safest method of putting a halter on a horse is the "bear hug" technique (Figure 4.2 and Procedural Steps 4.4).

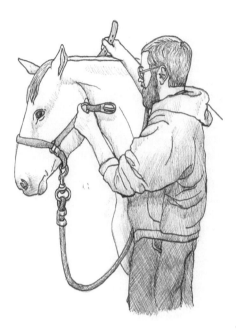

Figure 4.2   Proper "bear hug" haltering of a horse.

Procedural Steps 4.4	Application of a Halter (Bear Hug Technique)
1.	Attach a lead rope to the halter and never try to lead or restrain a horse holding only its halter.
2.	The handler should approach the horse's left shoulder (also called the *near side*; the right side is *far side*) at 45 degrees to the horse's neck and rub and scratch the shoulder.
3.	The lead rope is then put around the horse's neck just in front of the withers and then reach under its neck to capture the horse by the loop of lead rope around its neck.
4.	The loop should be moved to about the mid-neck area, and if necessary, the horse is repositioned in the stall or pen.
5.	The handler faces forward relative to the horse, releases the lead rope, and holds the halter buckle and strap in their left hand.
6.	The handler's right arm reaches over the horse's neck.
7.	The unbuckled crownpiece strap is transferred to the handler's right hand, which then allows the handler to restrict movement of the horse by a loop of the arms and the halter around its neck.
8.	The noseband of the halter is placed over the horse's nose with a scooping movement.
9.	The right hand brings the crownpiece over the neck just behind the ears and the halter is buckled, or tied if a rope halter.

- **The Underneath Method—Not Recommended:**
  - ○ **Short Handlers and Tall Horses:** Short handlers and tall horses make the recommended method of applying a halter more challenging. Because of this, some handlers use a reaching underneath method of putting a halter on. This method is not recommended.
  - ○ **Handler Positioned in Front of the Horse:** The underneath method involves the handler standing on the left side with the right shoulder under the upper part of the horse's neck. The noseband is placed over the nose. The crownpiece strap is held in the right hand and the buckle in the left hand and both arms are raised, one on each side of the horse's neck.
  - ○ **Risk of Handler Injury:** The crownpiece strap is flipped over the neck with the right hand and grasped with the left. The handler then steps to the left side and fastens the buckle. This method puts the handler at undue risk of being struck, run over, and hit by the horse's jaw.
  - ○ **Risk of Causing the Horse to Become Head Shy:** It also puts the horse at risk of having an ear slapped by a halter's crownpiece strap being flipped over its head.
- **Use of Halters in Pens and Pastures:**
  - ○ **Halters on Loose Horses Are Dangerous:** Halters should not be left on a horse in a pen or pasture because they can catch it on objects, leading to injury to the horse, and sometimes death. Foals, weanlings, and yearlings like to scratch their heads with a hind foot and may catch their foot in a halter or they will box with each other and can catch a foot in another's halter. Leather or webbed halters will also lead to skin problems if left on for days in warm weather.
  - ○ **Breakaway Halters:** If a halter is an absolute necessity on a pastured horse, a breakaway halter should be used.
  - ○ **Neck Straps:** If head control is needed on a horse that has not been trained to be captured, the use of horse ID neck straps are another option that is safer than halters on pastured horses. Neck straps should be fitted at the horse's throatlatch with a hand's width of space. Straps for pastured horses should have a breakaway fuse.
- **Temporary/Makeshift Halters:** The need to catch a horse is sometimes unanticipated and a temporary halter may be necessary.
  - ○ **Common Temporary Halter:** A temporary halter can be created with 15 ft of rope put around the horse's upper neck and tied with a bowline knot. A bight can then be put between the lower part of the neck loop and the horse's throat and then over the horse's nose (Figure 4.3).
  - ○ **Quick Release Halter:** A small loop (about 2 in diameter) is created near the end of a 15 ft rope and tied with a bowline knot. The rope with the small loop is placed around the horse's neck and then a bight is run through the small loop and then over the horse's nose. When the bight is released from the horse's nose, the loop around the horse's neck also releases, quickly freeing the horse (Figure 4.4).
  - ○ **Caution:** Temporary halters can slip off if a horse is allowed to play with slack in the lead rope. Never tie a horse with a temporary halter on. If it slips a quick release halter off its nose, it will also release the loop around its neck.
- **Walking behind Horses:**
  - **Reasons for Kicking:** Horses kick when they are startled, mistreated, or have had no previous handling. Horses that have been handled and not mistreated will only kick if startled or are kicking at other irritations (flies,

obnoxious dogs). Kicking at a nuisance is usually preceded by a lifted cocked leg (kick threat).

- **Kicking Is Usually Not Aggressive:** Kicking is primarily a defensive behavior. An aggressive horse is more likely to bite or strike.
- **Avoid Startling a Horse from Behind:** It is easy to startle a horse if approaching it directly from behind. Handlers should always talk to a horse or make other quiet noises, such as whistling, humming, singing, before approaching its hindquarters.
- **Monitor the Horse's Movement When near Its Hindquarters:** A hand should be kept on the rump as the handler moves around its rump. The handler should stay close enough to be brushing the rump with the side of the body as the handler goes around. If biting flies are present, it is wise for the handler to be prepared to block the tail with the other arm to prevent possible injury to the eye from the horse's swishing tail.

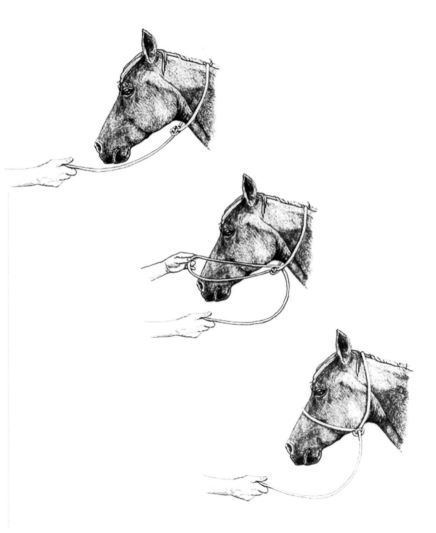

Figure 4.3 Common temporary halter.

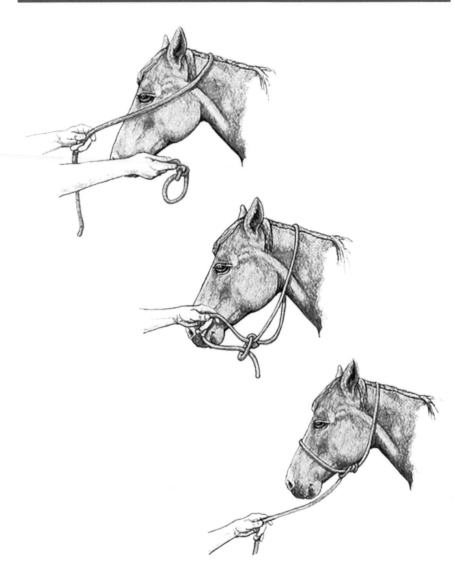

Figure 4.4   Quick release temporary halter.

CATCHING INSIDE PENS

- **Capture in a Pen:** See Procedural Steps 4.5.

Procedural Steps 4.5 Catching a Horse in a Pen	
1.	If the horse is alone in an enclosure and avoids being caught, the handler should walk briskly toward it staring it in the eye with an upright posture, shoulders held back, and arms down near the body.
2.	The moment the horse turns its head toward the handler, the handler should stop, look down, soften the posture, and turn at least 90 degrees away.
3.	Intermittent pauses and turning away are used to reward the horse for looking at the handler and not moving.

Procedural Steps 4.5	Catching a Horse in a Pen
4.	If it stands still, the handler can continue on slowly not looking directly at the horse and approaching it at a 45-degree angle to its shoulder.
5.	If the horse moves away, the handler should calmly persist and not allow the horse to stand still to eat.
6.	The handler should continue with a soft posture, eyes down, and indirect approach, if the horse's head is down.
7.	If it raises its head and moves away, the handler should go back to a brisk, direct, eyes forward, straight posture approach.
8.	The handler should pause and turn away briefly if the horse stops and maintains attention toward him.
9.	This same approach and pause are continued until the horse can be touched.
10.	After first touching the horse, the handler should walk a short distance away and give the horse a brief break to think about being touched.
11.	Then, the handler should approach the horse's left shoulder coming at 45 degrees from the front at a normal pace with confidence.
12.	The handler should lower the chin, and look at the horse's shoulder, not its eye, with shoulders relaxed and slightly drooped and arms at the sides.
13.	After briefly stroking its shoulder, the handler should stroke its shoulder with a hand and the end of the lead rope, and finally, put the lead rope around its lower neck.
14.	After the lead rope is looped completely around the horse's neck, it is moved toward the mid-upper neck to be able to pull its head around and move the hindquarters away, if needed.
15.	A halter can then be applied.

- **Hazardous Short Cuts:** Some handlers recommend training a hard-to-catch horse by keeping it in a small pen and using a breakaway halter with a short lead rope or with an extra-long lead rope that has to dragged but can be reached by the handler at a distance. However, this method risks the halter becoming caught on a structure. Trying to quickly snatch a short or drag lead on a difficult-to-catch horse is extremely hazardous.
- **Dangers of Using Food**
  - **Invasion of Personal Space:** Hand feeding horses or using food in a pen or pasture to capture a horse will teach the horse to invade a handler's personal space and become a dangerous nuisance.
  - **Mob Action:** It can be particularly dangerous to handlers if other horses are in the same pasture or pen.
  - **Not Always Available:** Treats are not always available when a handler needs to capture a horse. The reward should only be standing near the handler and being petted.

CATCHING INSIDE STALLS
- **Maintain Quiet Handling Environment:** All handlers should use good manners in a stable by avoiding loud noises or sudden quiet appearances that could startle a horse in a stall with another person.
- **Require the Horse to Face the Door:** The horse's attitude should first be assessed. If the horse has its rump directed toward the stall door, the handler should not enter until he can get the horse to turn around.

- **Never Allow Horse to Block the Exit:** Many horse stalls only have one exit, the stall door. Therefore, the stall door must always be open when inside a stall and a horse should never be allowed to get between the handler and the stall door.
- **Apply Halter and Lead Rope:** After the horse is facing the handler, the handler diagonally approaches the left shoulder, puts the lead rope around the horse's neck, and places the halter using the bear hug technique.
- **Exercise Safety with Stall Doors:** Doors should be sliding or open to the outside of the stall. When leading into or out of stalls the stall door should be fully open. Sliding latches or other protruding hardware should be fully retracted to prevent poking or scraping the handler or the horse.

CATCHING INSIDE PASTURES, PENS, AND CORRALS

- **Call or Entice into a Catch Pen:** Horses can be taught to respond to a whistle or call to come to a stall or pen for grain. The same whistle or call should be used every time that grain will be provided to them. A small catch pen adjacent to pastures where horses can be fed, caught, and individually released can improve safe handling of young or otherwise poorly trained groups of horses.
- **Catch with Favored Herdmates:** If a horse that needs to be caught has not been taught to come for feeding and is difficult to capture, it should be gathered with favored herdmates in a pen. The most willing horse to be caught should be captured first and tied outside the pen in a nearby location. The next most willing horse is caught, taken out, and tied, and so, on until all other horses are tied up outside or the one desired is willing to be caught beforehand.
- **Avoid Other Free Moving Horses:** Handlers should not work with a horse when other free horses can mill around the handler and the captured horse. If catching or returning a horse in a pasture or pen with other horses is unavoidable, the other horses may try to play or harass the caught horse or the horse to be released may attempt to escape and join the herd too soon. A second handler can provide interference, but if the handler is alone handling a horse grouped with other free horses, the handler should have a short whip or stick with a flag to control potential troublemakers.
- **Individual Capture:** See Procedural Steps 4.6.

Procedural Steps 4.6 Catching an Individual Horse in a Pasture	
1.	The handler should walk at normal speed with quiet determination directly toward the horse's shoulder.
2.	There should not be any efforts to hide the halter.
3.	As the horse moves away, the handler needs to apply pressure by continuing to walk toward the horse.
4.	Eventually the horse will stop and look toward the handler and at that instance, the handler must stop and turn away.
5.	After a 10-second rest, if the horse continues to stand still, the handler can walk a little slower in a zig-zag pattern toward the horse without looking directly at it.
6.	The handler should continue until close enough to rub the horse's forehead and approach its neck to put a lead rope around it.
7.	If the horse walks away at any point in the process, pressure should be applied by walking toward the horse and repeating the release of pressure at appropriate times until it permits capture.

- **Following Capture:**
  - **Encourage Relaxation:** After capturing the horse and haltering it, the handler should remain where the horse was caught and haltered while briefly grooming, scratching on its withers, and rubbing on its forehead and throat.
  - **Quietly Release:** The handler should then put the lead rope back around the horse's neck to control its movements, take the halter off, and then take the rope off its neck, and walk away before the horse moves. This catch and release should be repeated daily as long as necessary to disassociate the need to work or receive medication with being caught.

TRAPPING HORSES

- **Purpose and Method:** Feral horses have been trapped or moved using groups of trained handlers using steel tubular horse panels manufactured for small modular pens. The panels are 10 to 12 ft long, 5 ft tall, and weigh 50 to 80 lb.
- **Advantage:** Capturing horses by driving them into traps can be time efficient.
- **Disadvantages:**
  - **Flight Zone Stress:** Trapping untamed horses forces them to stay still while handlers invade their flight zone which is counterproductive to the basic training of horses. To learn to be calm around handlers, horses need to be able to move their feet and have some initial control of how far the handler is allowed to invade their flight zone until they learn the handler is a benevolent leader. That is the reason for round pen training.
  - **Injury Risks:** Pressing untamed horses into close confinement with steel tubular panels can be hazardous to the legs of horses that may kick, strike, or step through the panels and to untrained handlers who attempt to hold or move the panels against an untamed horse. Some trapping methods involve tying one end of a panel to another fence. If a gap of more than 3 inches is left between the panel and the fence, a horse can rear and trap a foot in the gap.
- **Limited Use:** Trapping or moving horses with tubular steel panels should be restricted to catching wild horses, performed by groups of trained handlers, and done with humane oversight by regulatory agencies.

RELEASING HORSES

How a captured horse is released affects how successful the next capture of it will be.

- **Proper Release in a Stall:** See Procedural Steps 4.7.

Procedural Steps 4.7 Releasing a Horse in a Stall	
1.	Release should be done only after the horse is calm and relaxed.
2.	The horse should be moved into a position facing the stall door with the handler between the door and the horse.
3.	The lead rope should be placed around the horse's neck for control during and after removing the halter.
4.	Control of the horse is maintained only with the lead rope around the neck while briefly petting it for standing still and talking to it in a soothing voice.
5.	The lead rope should be removed smoothly.
6.	After releasing a horse, the handler should always move away from the horse before the horse moves its feet.

- **Releasing a Horse into a Pen or Pastures:** When releasing a horse into a pen or pasture, it can get very playful just after release. The excitement may cause the horse to pull the handler or kick up as it leaves the handler.
  - **Preparation for Release:** The release should be when the handler has an immediate exit and in a manner that the horse has to change directions to go join their herdmates. If a catch pen is adjacent to the pasture, the horse should be released in the pen and then given access to the pasture.
  - **Go through and Then Face the Gate:** The horse should be led through the gate and into the pasture and turned back toward the gate. The handler needs to be positioned so that the handler may exit the gate as soon as releasing the horse and before the horse moves away.
  - **Never Reach through a Gate or Fence:** A handler should never attempt to release a horse by reaching over or through a gate or fence.
- **Releasing into a Herd:** Horses new to a herd can be bullied and put at risk of injury. Gradual controlled introductions are advised.
  - **Alleyways:** New horses should be introduced to established herd members in different pastures separated by an alleyway.
  - **Barred Grills between Stalls:** At other times, they should also be stalled next to each other with a barred grill between stalls.
  - **Introduce New Horses to Submissive Horses:** After the excitement of the new horse and the herd seeing, hearing, and smelling each other wears off, the new horse can be pastured or penned with the most submissive herd members. After acceptance by a portion of the herd, all horses can usually be kept together.
  - **Provide a Distraction:** Dominant herd members may still bully the new horse. Introducing them all to fresh pasture at the same time as introducing a new horse will ease the acceptance of the new member.

SPECIAL CAPTURES
- **Capture of Foals:**
  - **Two Handlers Required:** Capture of a foal requires two handlers.
    - ○ **Control the Mare First:** It is imperative to catch and control a nursing mare before attempting to capture its foal.
    - ○ **Back into a Stall Corner:** After catching the mare, it should be backed into a flat paneled corner that is strongly built. The handler of the mare should position the mare so that the foal can go between the mare and the wall to hide its face but not escape behind her.
  - **Approaching a Foal:** The foal handler should not try to pet the foal prior to getting it restrained.
    - ○ **Capturing a Foal:** After the mare is restrained and quiet, the foal handler should move at normal walking speed toward the foal and confine the foal with an arm in front of its chest and the other arm behind its rump (Figure 4.5). Whenever walking behind a foal, the handler should keep a side toward it to protect the abdomen and kneecaps from a kick. The tail should not be held if possible, since some foals will sit down when their tail is held.
    - ○ **Do Not Restrain Only the Foal's Neck:** A foal should never be held just around its neck. It will rapidly back up and either escape or cause injury.
    - ○ **Block Movement:** The handler should hold the foal as lightly as possible, and position it so that the foal is next to the mare in nursing position. The handler should never be between the foal and mare. The handler's arms should be used as barrier to excessive movement and not squeeze the foal.

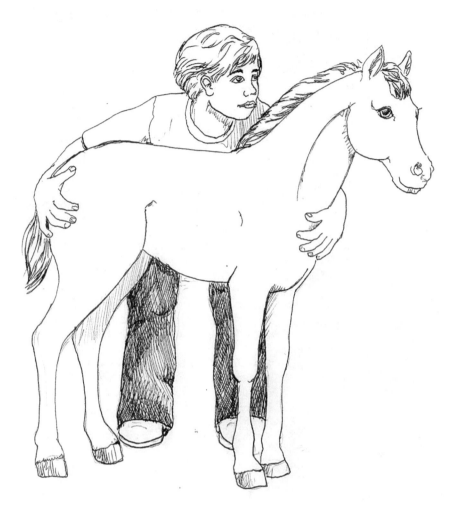

Figure 4.5   Restraint of foals is blocking of their movement, not squeezing them.

- ○ **Avoid Facial Injury:** When holding a foal, the handler should turn the head toward its rump to protect the handler's face in case the foal struggles and rears suddenly.
- ○ **Gates or Panels for Restraint:** A gate should not be used as a squeeze panel for restraint on foals or small horses if the gate does not have a solid panel on the lower half.
- **Large Foal Restraint:** Large foals may need to be held by two people. The front handler holds under the neck with a knee behind the foal's elbow and the back handler stands on the same side as the front handler and holds the base of the tail with a knee in its flank. The foal should not be lifted off its feet as this will add to fear and struggling.
- **Lateral Recumbent Restraint:**
  - ○ **Laying a Foal in Lateral Position:** If needed, a small foal can be laid down on its side by a handler standing by its side, bending its head away from the handler and toward its withers. The outside flank should be grasped and the foal gently slid down the handler's legs. Large foals or weanlings should be chemically restrained for lateral restraint.

- o **Maintaining Recumbency:** Lateral restraint can be maintained by a handler squatting with knee pressure on the foal's neck and reaching between the hind legs and pulling the tail through the hind legs and holding it. Placing a towel over its head and humming to it will increase its relaxation while down.
- **Capture of Stallions:**
  - **Inherent Danger:**
    - o **Social Deprivation:** Because of their potential value, stallions are often kept in separate enclosures and away from other horses. This, added to their strength, unflappable interest in mares in season, and desire to dominate other stallions, makes handling stallions more hazardous than handling mares and geldings.
    - o **Advanced Knowledge and Experience Are Needed:** The capture and restraint of stallions should not be attempted by novices. Only after a good degree of proficiency is reached by the handler in handling mares and geldings should the handling of stallions be attempted. No one, regardless of experience, should handle a stallion without another person within voice range.
  - **Carefully Selected Sire or Neglected Castration:**
    - o **Genetic Donor Potential Is Paramount:** The value of a stallion is in passing on genes that are desired to improve the quality of future horses. This supersedes the priority of any other use. Therefore, only stallions of exceptional quality that will be bred to high-quality mares should remain sexually intact.
    - o **Determination of Potential:** Determination of exceptional quality should be based on the unbiased opinions of others, not just the owner. After all, the foals produced will have to be appreciated by others to find future homes and proper care.
  - **Always Be Watchful:** Regardless of a stallion's prior handling and training, a handler in an enclosure with a stallion or restraining a stallion on a lead should always be conscious of the stallion's position and demeanor by keeping it in the handler's peripheral vision. A handler should never turn their back on a stallion when leaving its pen or stall.
  - **Remain Mindful of the Tendency to Bite or Strike:** Wild stallions control mares and challengers to their authority mostly by biting and striking. If agitated, they are much more likely to bite or strike handlers than mares and geldings are.
  - **Establish Leadership without a Challenge:** When entering a stallion pen, a handler should back the stallion away if it walks into the handler's personal space. When handling a stallion, the handler should stay at their shoulder or slightly behind it when possible for safety. This position provides the handler safety from being bitten or struck and better control of the stallion's hindquarters.
  - **Control of a Stallion When Breeding:**
    - o **Dedicated Breeding Location:** Handling of stallions is easier if breeding occurs in a dedicated shed or barn, training occurs in a separate arena, and turnout is a paddock not near the breeding or training sites.
    - o **Dedicated Halter and Lead:** Different halters and leads should be used for breeding and for training or exercise. Stallions will recognize the difference and become less excited when the non-breeding halter is used. An extra-long lead rope should be used to handle stallions when breeding because they have to rear up to breed.

HANDLING FOR ROUTINE CARE AND MANAGEMENT

When handling horses, dangerous objects and situations (junk, dogs, children) should be avoided in the handling area, and an assistant who does not pay constant attention to the horse should not be used.

BASIC EQUIPMENT AND FACILITIES

Handling equipment for horses that attach to the horse's body is called *tack*. Most tack is made of leather, but some is made of nylon or other synthetic materials. Stitching in tack can break and materials can wear out, particularly where leather bends sharply around metal rings and buckles.

- **Head Halters and Lead Ropes:** Halters and lead ropes are the most basic equipment needed to handle and restrain horses.
    - **Halters:**
        - **General Construction:** Halters are usually made of leather, rope, nylon, or polyester. Parts of a halter are the noseband which includes the nosepiece and chinpiece, connecting strap, throatlatch piece, cheekpiece, crownpiece, buckle or tie strings and loop, and tie ring or loop (Figure 4.6). Leather and synthetic strap halters have metal nose and cheek connectors.

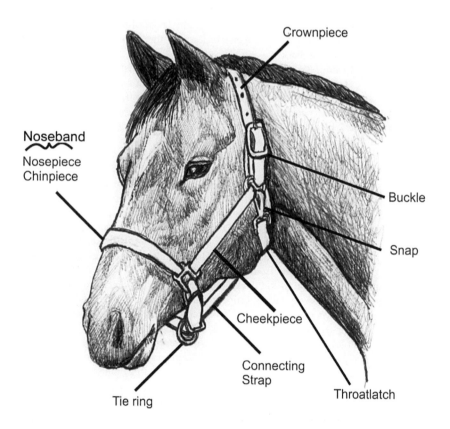

Figure 4.6 Parts of a halter.

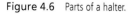

- **Leather:** Leather halters will break under pressure and cause little discomfort when pulled against. These characteristics promote disrespect for restraint in horses. The leather straps trap moisture and dirt underneath the halter that can cause skin problems.
- **Synthetic:** Nylon or polyester will not break, although their metal connectors can. They cause little discomfort when resisted against and trap less moisture and dirt than leather. If near a fire, a nylon halter can melt and become glued to the horse's skin.
- **Rope:** Rope halters do not have metal connectors and will not break. They will cause discomfort if pulled on and therefore evoke less resistance to restraint. Rope halters do not trap moisture or dirt.
- **Metal Connectors:** Leather or nylon strap halters have rings (connectors) that the nosepiece, chinstrap, cheekpieces, throatlatches, and crownpiece attach to. There are noseband, cheekpiece, and throatlatch rings and a single leading or tying ring on the lower aspect of the noseband. Attachments to the rings or the rings can break under moderate stress.
- **Breakaway Halters:** Horses should not be turned out in a pasture or pen with a halter on. If a pasture halter is considered absolutely necessary, a breakaway halter with Velcro attachments or a leather "fuse" (adjoining leather straps thinner than normal halter straps) joined by a Chicago screw should be used.
- **Halter Leads:**
  - **General Construction:** Lead ropes designed for only leading and tying horses are usually 9 to 12 feet in length. Longer, heavier lead ropes of 15 to 20 feet are used for longeing or leading other horses, such as pack horses from horseback.
  - **Cotton:** Twisted cotton lead ropes are the most comfortable for handlers. They are strong, provide good traction for gripping with the hand, and hold hitches well. Metal halter clips can be attached, but are not necessary for attachment to the halter since a double sheet bend hitch can be used.
  - **Braided Nylon:** Braided nylon is available in a variety of colors and a popular choice, but is slick and does not hold hitches as well. Metal halter clips are clamped on the end of nylon lead ropes. The metal clips or their attachment clamp on the rope is the weakest part of a nylon lead.
  - **Straps:** Lead straps with a chain shank and clip are sometimes used on difficult-to-handle horses, primarily racehorses and breeding stallions. The chain shank is clipped to a halter and then run through some of the halter rings to exert leverage and pressure on the nose, chin, or gums. Halters with round rings should be used if a chain shank will be used to reduce the chain from binding in the ring.
- **Riding and Driving Tack:** In addition to halters and leads, tack includes saddles, headgear, reins, harness, breast collars, cruppers, and martingales. Many horse handlers, especially veterinarians and veterinary technicians, may not use riding and driving tack, but it is important to know how others use tack on their horses in order to know how to inspect for improper use that could cause injury or safety problems. For more information on riding and driving tack, see the companion textbook to this manual—Chastain, C. B., *Animal Handling and Physical Restraint*, Boca Raton, FL, CRC Press, 2018:252–258.
- **Pens and Arenas:** Pens are usually small outdoor enclosures with loosened soil for better footing that may be used for longeing or training young horses. Arenas may be outdoors or under a roof and lined with fencing or not enclosed. Arenas typically also have loosened and dampened soil for safe footing when performing athletic maneuvers or in speed events.

TYING

- **Lead Tying:**
  - **Stout Tying Posts:** The risk that a horse may try to pull itself free from being tied must always be anticipated. Horses should only be tied to solid objects that can hold a typical 1,200 lb. horse pulling with all its strength and that does not rattle, clang, or make any other noise if pulled on. This excludes gates, fence rails, stall doors, and unhitched trailers as safe objects that a horse can be tied to.
  - **Unbreakable Halters and Leads:** If a horse pulls back and breaks the halter, lead, lead clip, or object it is tied to, it is much more likely to attempt pull-backs again in the future. Slippery nylon leads that do not hold a hitch well should not be used. Horses should not be routinely tied in a manner that incorporates a string to serve as a breakaway since permitting them to breakaway at their discretion encourages future pull-backs.
  - **Quick Release Hitch and Knife:** To create a safer environment for horses that may pull back when tied, leads should be tied with a quick release hitch to more easily free a horse in trouble, and a handler should always have a knife ready to cut the horse free, if needed, to prevent injury.
  - **Tie Withers Height, or Higher:** If a horse pulls back, it is more likely to become injured if tied too low or with too much lead between it and the hitch. A lead hitch should be tied at or just above withers height, about one arm length from the hitch (Figure 4.7).

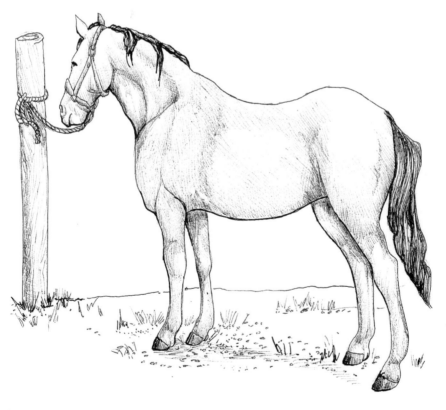

Figure 4.7 Proper lead tie.

- **Tie One Arm's Length Away:** Tying longer away than one arm's length can allow the horse's neck to get wrapped in the lead rope or the horse to step over the rope. Tying closer can cause many horses to feel claustrophobic and panic.
- **When Not to Tie:** The problem of pulling back usually begins by the horse being scared, pulling back, and escaping because of being tied to an insecure object or a halter or lead clip breaking. Therefore, a horse should not be tied and then introduced something potentially scary to horses. In situations potentially scary to horses, a handler or handler's assistant must hold the lead rope.
- **Safety Precautions around Tied Horses:**
  - **Never Go underneath the Lead of a Tied Horse:** Handlers should never duck under a tied lead rope. Horse cannot see under their jaw. This can startle even a quiet horse and cause a pull-back or catch the handler in a very dangerous position.
  - **Never Sit or Kneel next to a Tied Horse:** Handlers should always remain in a position that they can move away from a horse quickly. They should never sit or kneel with both knees on the ground next to a tied horse.
- **Discouraging Pull-Backs:**
  - **Long Lead:** Holding the end of a long lead rope that slips through a tie ring while a horse pulls back can prevent injury, as well as teach escape by pulling back does not happen. A Blocker tie ring is a metal ring with a curved metal bar in the middle that allows horses to pull back with varying degrees of resistance so that they gradually learn there is no escape by pulling back, but they do not get hurt in trying (Figure 4.8).

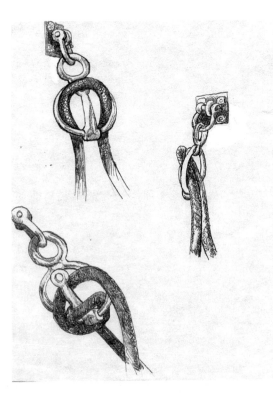

Figure 4.8   Blocker tie ring.

- ○ **Loop around the Chest:** An older method of preventing pull-backs involves putting a loop around the horse's chest with the honda underneath. The standing end of the rope is run between the front legs and then the halter. The horse is tied with a regular lead rope an arm's length way from the hitching ring, while the chest rope is tied a little closer to the hitching ring than the lead rope. If the horse attempts to pull back, pressure on the chest will inhibit most horses from pulling back, whereas feeling the pull on their head by a halter can make them panic.
  - ○ **Inner Tubes:** To discourage pull-backs, some trainers use rubber inner tubes from automobiles around a stout post to tie to with a nonbreakable halter and lead rope. These can injure a young horse's neck from recoil, or the inner tube can break. This method is not recommended.
- • **Unacceptable Tying:**
  - ○ **By Reins:** Horses must never be tied to a hitch ring or rail by their bridle reins. This can easily break the reins or cause the bit to do great harm to the horse's mouth and the incisor teeth. Horses should only be tied with a regular lead rope and halter or a neck loop with a non-slip knot (bowline).
  - ○ **By Chain Shank Leads:** Horses should never be tied with a chain shank lead. In addition to injuring the horse, the chain could break and become a lashing weapon.
  - ○ **In Conjunction with Head Restraint Tack:** All head restraint riding accessories (tiedowns, martingales) should be disconnected prior to leading or tying horses.
  - ○ **Closer Than 10 Feet from Another Horse or Unattended:** Tied horses should never be left alone or tied closer than 10 feet apart.
  - ○ **At the End of a Hitching Rail:** If tying to a rail, a horse should not be tied so close to the end of the rail that they can move to the other side of the rail.
  - ○ **To a Stall Door:** A horse should never be tied to any kind of stall door.
- • **Escape Artist ("Houdini") Horses:** Horses are inquisitive and are nimble with their lips, and many will teach themselves to untie hitches. The end of the lead rope should be dropped through a bight in the quick release hitch to prevent a pull on the end of the lead untying the hitch. A more secure tie is to use a bowline hitch.
- • **Cross-Tying:**
  - • **Advantages:** Cross-tying allows a groom to move 360 degrees around the horse easily (Figure 4.9). This is advantageous for grooming horses, but cross-ties have several potential disadvantages.
  - • **Disadvantages:** Horses have to be trained to tolerate cross-ties, because cross-tying allows little head freedom and horses can feel claustrophobic. If they panic, they are more likely to get free and learn to pull back for freedom or injure their neck or back than if tied more securely by a single lead rope. Furthermore, cross-ties are often not available in a safe location.
  - • **Method:**
    - ○ **Accustom Gradually:** Accustoming horses to cross-ties should be done gradually. A horse new to cross-ties should be allowed 1 to 2 feet of slack on each side and have close supervision. Gradually the slack is decreased on subsequent tying instances until the slack is only 6 to 8 inches on each side.
    - ○ **Create Proper Distance:** Cross-ties are usually 10 ft apart. They should not be more than 11 ft apart to prevent a horse from turning and getting twisted in the tie ropes.
    - ○ **Prevent Extended Back Up:** Cross-tying should be done where there is a wall close behind the horse so that the horse cannot back up too far.

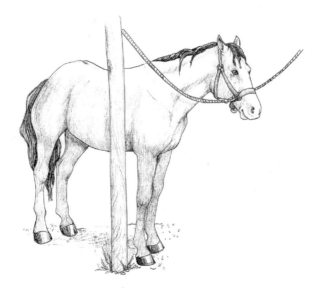

Figure 4.9   Cross-tying.

- o **Proper Wall Attachments:** The wall attachments should be 1 to 2 feet higher than the horse's head. The length of the ties should permit the horse to lower its head about 1 foot. Horses that need to lower their head more to clear their airway should not be tied by cross-ties.
- o **Proper Location:** Cross-tying is often done in barn aisles, but a separate area not used for pass through should be used for cross-tying. If a horse is cross-tied, another horse should never be led underneath one arm of the cross-tie to move through an aisle. The tied horse must be disconnected from a side, moved over in the aisle, and the other horse led by with its handler leading on the side that positions the handler between the horses.
- • **Breakaway Cross-Ties:**
  - o **Risk of Flipping Backward or Hung in Ties:** Agitated horses restrained by cross-ties can run forward and flip themselves over on their back, or lose their footing and fall with their head hanging from one or both cross-tie leads, if they are tied without breakaways. If a horse rears, it can get a leg over a cross-tie line and cause a fall on its side.
  - o **Use of a Breakaway:** Because of potential injuries with cross-ties, many handlers use string connections tied to the halter so that they will break easily if the horse tries to escape and will not leave a length of rope attached to the halter of a fleeing horse. Other options are using quick release snaps and commercial connectors at the wall end of the tie leads that break easily. This option can result in having broken metal connectors on the ends of cross-tie leads on a loose horse that are dangerous to the horse and handler.

RESTRAINT BY DISTRACTION

Distraction techniques work very well in most horses, but they must be applied with constant rhythmic stimulation. Patting the horse once and then holding the hand still instantly loses its effect. Persistent and rhythmic pats of varying intensity will distract a horse for long periods depending on what procedure requires the distraction technique.

- **Love Pats or Pinches:** Rhythmic flat hand pats or soft pinches work well as distractions, if used intermittently and with varying locations, rhythms, and intensity. Light rhythmic taps on a horse's forehead or behind an eye is often enough distraction to have a horse stand still for routine exams.
- **Eye Cover and Blindfolds:**
  - **Covering One Eye:** Short duration distraction can be achieved by petting the horse on the neck and then sliding the hand back and forth over the head eventually cupping the hand over an eye. The eye should not be reached for directly because this will scare most horses.
  - **Blindfolds:** Blindfolding horses using a small towel can calm many horses. Initial application also requires an approach-and-retreat sliding method with the blindfold cloth over the horse's neck and head. It can be held in place by tucking the cloth ends under the cheekpieces of the halter.
- **Front Leg Lift or Hobble:** Holding a horse's front leg up by using an assistant or one-leg hobble can cause most horses to stand still. If an examination or treatment is being performed, the front leg on the same side as the procedure should be lifted.
  - **Protect the Handler's Head:** If a handler holds a horse's front leg to assist someone, the handler should pick the foot up with their head toward the horse's rear, but after raising the leg, the handler should rotate their body to face forward with both hands holding the leg up.
  - **Inguinal Exam Restraint:** Lifting a left front leg with a left hand while facing the horse's side can enable a handler/examiner to palpate the inguinal area with the right hand, reducing the risk of a kick.
  - **Rear Legs:** The rear legs are never lifted up by hand as a means to restrain a horse's movements. A Scotch hobble created with a 15 ft cotton rope can restrain one hind leg, limiting movement and the ability to kick.

LIFTING FEET

- **Front Foot:** See Procedural Steps 4.8 and Figure 4.10.

Procedural Steps 4.8	Lifting a Front Foot
1.	The horse should first be standing square, that is, front and hind legs on each side equidistant, front legs parallel to each other, and hind legs parallel to each other.
2.	The handler then stands alongside the horse facing the horse's rump.
3.	Placement of the handler's foot should be at least 10 inches to the side of the horse's hoof to reduce the risk of being stepped on by the horse.
4.	The handler should slide the hand nearest to the horse down the back of the front leg to be picked up (Figure 4.10).
5.	If the foot is not offered to the handler by the horse at this stage, then the long hairs on the back of the fetlock are tugged, or the suspensory ligament or the chestnut is squeezed until the foot comes up.
6.	A handler should resist the temptation to push the horse's weight off the leg with the handler's shoulder as this will teach the horse to lean on a handler when holding the foot up.
7.	The foot should be held up primarily with a hand on the hoof wall since some horses are uncomfortable with being held at the pastern or coronary band.
8.	For the horse to be comfortable and not resist, the leg should be lifted straight up and not pulled to the outside.

Procedural Steps 4.8	Lifting a Front Foot
9.	Holding the horse's foot up for examination or cleaning can be done with one hand, but if both hands must be free to use hoof nippers or a rasp, the foot will need to be straddled and held between the handler's knees.
10.	If the horse struggles with its foot being held, the handler should maintain hold of the foot until the handler can place it down so that the horse does not think it escaped by struggling.
11.	If the horse leans on the leg being held up, the handler should drop it suddenly to teach the horse to stay balanced on three legs when the foot is being held up.

- **Rear Foot:** See Procedural Steps 4.9 and Figure 4.11.

Procedural Steps 4.9	Lifting a Hind Foot
1.	A hind foot should not be attempted to be picked up with one hand with the handler facing backward as this puts the handler at risk of being kicked without prior warning.
2.	The handler should start by standing next to the horse's flank with the handler's body touching the horse out of its kick zone.
3.	To pick up a left hind leg, the handler should face the right side of the rump with the left arm and hand on top of its rump.
4.	The handler then places a right hand on the horse's rump with the thumb up and slides it down the back of the rump, the upper leg, hock, and finally lower leg.
5.	When reaching for the left leg with the right hand, the handler's left hand remains on the horse's rump.
6.	Once the right hand reaches the lower aspect of the hind leg, if the foot is not offered by the horse, the hock can be pinched until the foot comes up or the leg can be pulled up toward the horse's abdomen into a flexed position.
7.	While holding the cannon bone up and the leg in flexed position, the handler moves backward and underneath the hock, resting the horse's left leg over the handler's left leg and inside the thigh.
8.	At the same time the left hand on top of the rump is slid down the rump and inside the leg with the handler's left elbow becoming positioned on the inside surface of the hock (Figure 4.11).
9.	If the horse struggles when holding a hind leg, it is important to hold onto the leg for the safety of the handler and to prevent the horse from learning to escape by struggling.
10.	Releasing the leg should be performed when the horse is quiet by reversing the procedure to pick it up.
11.	To release the left hind leg, the handler's left hand is slid up toward the horse's rump while the right hand grasps the cannon bone and flexes the leg, and the handler takes a step or two backward toward the horse's belly.
12.	The leg is lowered toward the ground with the right hand while the left hand is positioned on the horse's rump.

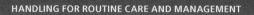

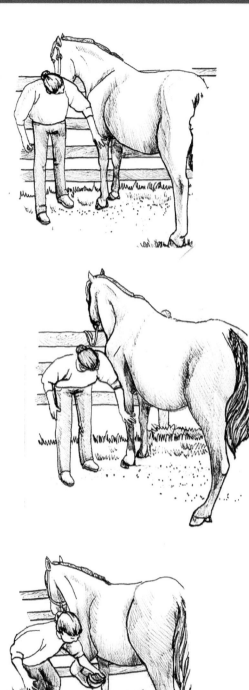

Figure 4.10 Lifting a front foot.

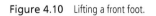

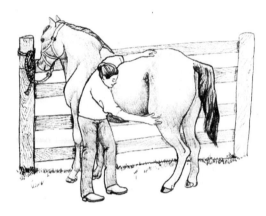

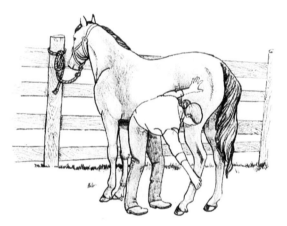

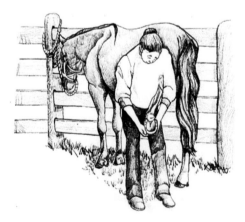

Figure 4.11   Picking up a hind leg.

MOVING HORSES

- **Leading:**
    - **Purpose:** Leading horses is good, mild exercise for horses, especially if done to cool off after strenuous exercise. Leading manners can also be ingrained during this exercise. Mechanical walkers are boring and do not provide the opportunity to teach proper manners when being led.
    - **Lead from the Near Side:** Horses are traditionally led on the handler's right side (horse's left or "near side"), but there are exceptions. When leading horses around people or horse-scary objects, the handler should stand or walk on the side that puts the handler between the horse and the people or object.
    - **The Horse's Head Should Be Even with Handler's Right Shoulder:** Leading a horse behind the handler with a long lead can allow a spooked horse to step or jump onto the handler. If the horse invades the handler's personal space, it should be calmly pushed over with the handler's right elbow. Yelling, staring at, or otherwise appearing annoyed with the horse will make the handler appear as an aggressive threat, opposed to just making the horse uncomfortable with a timely, elbow push.
    - **Handling of the Halter Lead:**
        - ○ **Method:** The lead rope should be held about 1 to 2 ft from the halter with the right hand when leading on the near (left) side of the horse. The remainder of the lead should be folded back and forth like an accordion in the left hand. It should never be looped around the hand or arm (Figure 4.12).

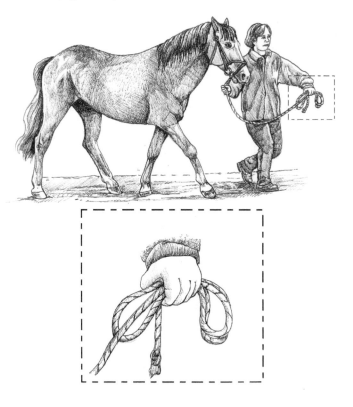

Figure 4.12   Proper leading of a horse and lead rope management.

- ○ **Caution:** A horse should never be restrained or led by holding onto the halter and not using a lead rope.
- **Horse Manners:** A halter-broke horse should move forward, turn, and stop when the handler does. If it does not, the handler should not face it and attempt to pull it forward.
- **Moving Forward:** Without facing the horse, the handler should pull it to the side or in a circle around the handler to get the horse's feet moving, then guide it to walk forward. A handler can also stand near a fence or wall and use a whip in the left hand to wave toward the horse's rump when it balks. This must be done while the handler continues to face forward and walk, not turning to watch the horse's hindquarters.
- **Backing:** Backing a horse with a lead rope can be difficult. On their own, horses do very little backing up since this requires them to move into an area in which their vision is blocked. Handlers should never stand directly in front of a horse and attempt to get it to back up due to the risk of being struck with a front hoof or getting run over.
- **Leading on Grades:** If leading a horse on a steep grade, the handler should always stay on the uphill side. If the horse spooks or resists, it could knock the handler down the slope or fall onto the handler.
- **Leading by Reins:** Horses trained for western riding should be able to be led by bridle reins regardless of the type of bit used. Horses routinely ridden with an English bridle with two sets of reins and bits should be lead only by the snaffle bit reins. The curb bit reins should be left on the neck and tucked under a run up stirrup strap.
- **Leading through Man-Doors or Man-Gates:**
  - ○ **One Horse at a Time:** A handler should never lead more than one horse if going through a man-door or man-gate. The door or gate must be completely open and fixed in a way that it will not swing while the handler or the horse passes through.
  - ○ **Prevent Crowding:** The handler should go through before the horse and not permit the horse to crowd him. If necessary, the horse should be backed up, if needed, to protect the handler's personal space.
  - ○ **Look Forward:** The handler must look forward and proceed with confidence so that the horse will follow. If the handler turns toward the horse or looks directly at the horse, it will not follow.
- **Assisting Another Handler with Same Side Restraint:**
  - ○ **Do Not Tie if Horse Scary Situations May Occur:** A horse should be held by a halter and lead rope, not tied, whenever potentially painful or horse-scary procedures may occur.
  - ○ **Assist from the Same Side:** The person holding a lead rope should nearly always remain on the same side as the person (veterinarian, farrier, etc.) working with the horse so if the horse jumps or shies, it moves to the side away from both handlers (Figure 4.13).
  - ○ **Exception:** When assisting someone who is working on the head or neck and sometimes a front leg, the restraining assistant will need to stand on the opposite side of the horse to prevent crowding and obstructing the other handler.
- **Chain Lead Shanks:** Difficult-to-lead horses should be properly trained or retrained to be led in a respectful way. When time does not permit retraining before it must be led, a chain shank may be needed rather than a lead rope to provide additional control. A chain lead shank should be used only when necessary and sparingly or its effectiveness is lost (Figure 4.14).
  - ○ **Never Use for Tying:** A horse should never be tied with a chain shank under its jaw, over its nose, or in its mouth.

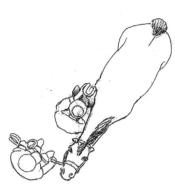

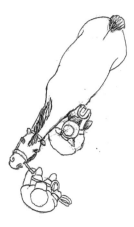

Figure 4.13 The handler controlling a lead rope must stay on the same side as the person performing a procedure on a horse.

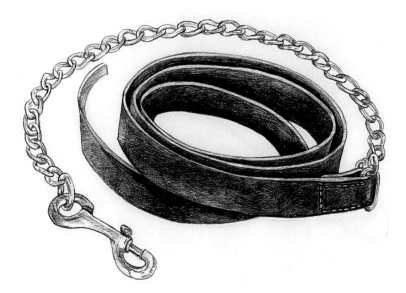

Figure 4.14 Chain lead shank.

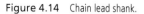

○ **Over the Nose, Non-Constricting:** A chain shank can be run through the left noseband ring, over the nose and out the right noseband ring and clipped back to itself. This method causes only mild discomfort since it does not constrict on the nose, as do the other methods.

○ **Over the Nose, Constricting:** A more forceful means of control is running the chain through the left noseband ring, then over the nose and through the right noseband ring and clipping it to the right cheek ring. This method is commonly used in leading stallions and young racehorses. Pressure on the chain encourages the horse to drop its nose and flex its neck (Figure 4.15).

○ **Under the Jaw—Advantages:** Additional control is gained by the chain being run through the left noseband ring, under the jaw, through the right noseband ring, and clipped on the right cheek ring (Figure 4.16). Clipping to the right noseband ring should not be done as it will twist the halter to the left when the lead is pulled on. Placement of the chain under the jaw may encourage desired forward movement in sluggish horses or raising of the head if shown in halter classes.

○ **Under the Jaw—Disadvantages:** Using a constricting chain shank under the jaw makes the horse throw its head up, and it is not recommended for saddle horses. When the strap or chain puts pressure on the lower jaw, the horse may rear or throw its head, injuring a rider.

○ **Gum Chain:** The most severe use of a chain shank is placing the chain in the horse's mouth, under the upper lip, and on the gums above the upper incisor teeth (Figure 4.17). This method, called a gum chain, is often used

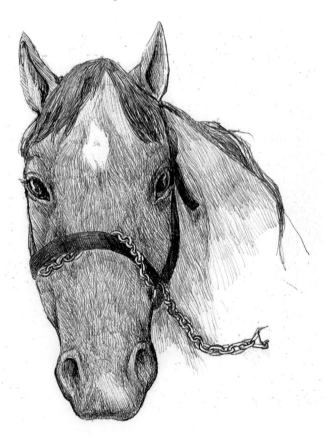

Figure 4.15   Chain shank over the nose.

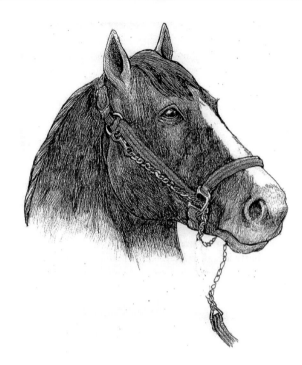

Figure 4.16   Chain shank under the nose.

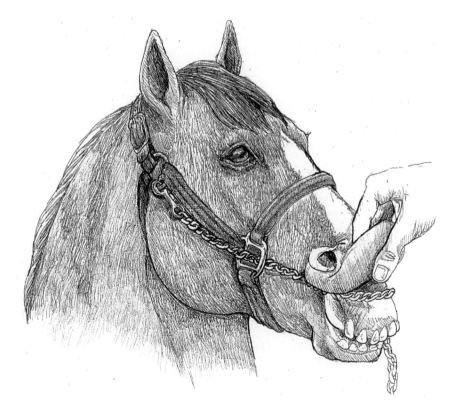

Figure 4.17   Gum chain.

in the horse racing industry on stallions, but this should be a last resort when normally handling horses as it frequently violates the rule of using the least pressure possible to get the desired result.

- ○ **Gum Chain Advantage:** This method permits a handler to control a horse while having another hand free to complete an examination or treatment procedure.
- ○ **Gum Chain Disadvantages:** There is no stepwise correction for correcting a horse misbehaving when using a gum chain and constant pressure is required for the chain to stay in place.
- ○ **War Bridles:** A loop of rope around the poll and through the mouth above the upper lip works like a gum chain. This is one form of crude head control referred to as a "war bridle." There are other rope restraints of the head or mouth in horses called war bridles.
- ○ **Never Create a Fixed Loop with a Chain Shank:** A chain shank should never be run through the halter tie ring and then snapped back to itself. A loop can be formed that the horse can catch on posts or other objects. If the horse lowers its head, it could step through the loop and trap its head down, causing a violent effort to get free.
- **Chifney Bit:** A Chifney bit (invented by a jockey, Samuel Chifney), also called a round bit or anti-rearing bit, is a restraint device for difficult-to-control horses.
  - ○ **Construction:** It typically has a straight portion that goes in the horse's mouth as a bit. The circular part goes over the horse's lower jaw and has three rings. The side rings are attached to the halter or a headstall with clips. The middle ring is an attachment for the lead rope clip.
  - ○ **Effect:** A pull down with the lead rope will put pressure on the roof of the mouth as well as the tongue.
- **Breeding Stallion Halters:** Leather halters designed for use on stallions during breeding or undisciplined horses are made of thicker leather and have round rings for use with a chain shank.
  - ○ **Purpose:** The increased weight of the halter is a signal for the stallion in preparation for breeding.
  - ○ **Leads:** Lead ropes should be longer for handling stallions for when they rear and the handler needs to move further away.
  - ○ **Safety Space When Leading a Stallion:** Breeding stallions should not be led closer than 20 ft from other horses.
- **Leading Foals**
  - ○ **Lead behind Mare:** Foals that have not been trained to lead should be moved by following its mare while it is being led.
  - ○ **Rump Rope:** A halter and lead rope assisted by a rope loop over the foal's rump can be tried if the mare is not available to be led.
  - ○ **Do Not Stand in Front:** A handler should never stand in front of a foal and pull on a lead rope. The foal may balk and then jump forward into the handler.
- **Longeing:**
  - **Proper Spelling:** Longeing (from Latin *longa* meaning "to lengthen") is often spelled phonetically and informally as lungeing or lunging.
  - **Purposes:**
    - ○ **Expend Excess Energy:** Longeing is an exercise that helps a horse stretch out and expend initial excess energy (*freshness*) before riding or working with the horse. Longeing should not be used to physically exhaust the horse.
    - ○ **Training:** Longeing a horse aids in training in response to handler body language and voice commands.

- ○ **Evaluate Soundness:** Other reasons for longeing include examination for lameness and mild exercise.
- **Method:**
  - ○ **Use Leg Protection on the Horse:** Splint boots, brushing boots, or leg wraps should be used on horses when they are longed to protect their legs during sudden turns. Longeing should be performed for less than 20 minutes if the horse is under 3 years old, due to stress on their legs caused by constant circling.
  - ○ **Free Longeing or Line Longeing:** Longeing can be done as free longeing in a round pen, or long line longeing on a 25–30 ft lead line (Figure 4.18). Short lines of 16 ft are safer for either handlers or horses that do not have much experience in longeing.
- **Round Pens:**
  - ○ **Size:** Round pens for free longeing should be 40–50 ft in diameter. If used for mounted training, a round pen should be at least 60 ft in diameter.
  - ○ **Solid Wall Construction:** Solid walls, 6 to 8 ft high that slant outward are much safer for the horse than modular steel pipe pens. Solid walls also eliminate visual distractions during training. The pen gate should only open to the inside and abut the post gate to prevent it from accidently opening to the outside if the horse bumps it.
  - ○ **Modular Steel Pipe Pens:** Because of all the openings between horizontal rails, modular steel pipe pens facilitate emergency escapes by the handler if attacked by a dominance-aggressive horse.
  - ○ **Allow Initial Acclimation:** Horses should be allowed 20 minutes alone in a round pen to acclimate to the surroundings before free longeing begins.
- **Line Longeing:**
  - ○ **Directing Movement:** When line longeing, the handler should point the direction for the horse to go with the hand holding the lead line and reinforce command by raising a whip in the other hand. To move the horse to the handler's left (counterclockwise), the lead line is held in the left hand, the left hand is raised to the 10 o'clock position, while a whip is held in the right hand. The lead line and whip must be switched if the direction of movement is changed to the handler's right (clockwise circles).
  - ○ **Response to Reluctance to Move:** If the horse is reluctant to move, the handler should raise the whip with the right hand. If raising the

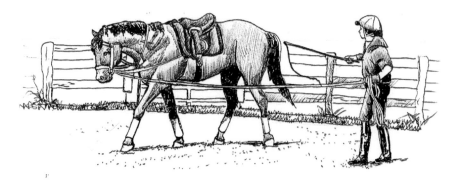

Figure 4.18 Longeing on a long line.

whip is insufficient to get the horse to move, the handler can escalate the pressure to move by slapping the whip on the ground. The whip is also used to psychologically push the horse away from the handler if it gets too close while circling by pointing toward the horse's near shoulder.

- **Changing Directions:** The horse should be asked to change pace and directions frequently. When longeing a horse in a regular halter, a change in the horse's direction just requires a switch in the hands in holding the lead line and whip while simultaneously stepping ahead to the horse's shoulder and slightly backward. When the horse changes directions in a fluid movement without heightened excitement, its attitude indicates a safer mental state to be ridden and that continuing to longe is unnecessary.
- **Safety Precautions While Longeing:** The handler must be careful to avoid coiling the lead line around a hand or arm or allowing it to wrap around one of the handler's legs. Talking with observers should not occur while longeing. Verbal communications should only be commands given to the horse.
- **Cooling Down:** After the horse has performed well, it should be stopped and allowed to relax. The horse should never be forced to run out of air from exertion or excitement as this can result in the horse panicking, becoming uncoordinated, or acting resentful.
- **Maintain Respect for Personal Space:** The horse should turn toward the handler during rest but not approach unless invited. If uninvited movement occurs that could invade the handler's personal space without invitation, the horse should be stopped and backed up.

- **Long Lines:** Long lines are two lines more than 8 ft long that run from a bridle through rings in a surcingle around the horse's chest or through stirrups on a western saddle.
  - **Purpose:** Long lines are used in preparing horses to go under saddle (i.e., be ridden), with proper responses to rein pressure. They are also used in the training of horses to pull carts or wagons and to perform tricks. The Spanish Riding School in Vienna, Austria uses long lines managed by a handler while assisted by a second handler with a whip to train their famous Lipizzan stallions.
  - **Method:** Long lines are first used with a horse in a round pen. The handler walks a safe distance behind the horse and directs its movements with the long lines.

- **Mechanical Hot Walkers:** Hot walkers are equipment that mechanically lead (lead or tie walkers) or push (panel walkers) horses in a circular path to cool the horse down after exercise or to provide mild daily exercise.
  - **Method:** Horses are usually walked in pairs and should be placed on opposite sides of the hot walkers. If used for exercise or rehabilitation, the duration should be 20 minutes, or less.
  - **Precautions:** Horses in a mechanized hot walker should be supervised at all times. Horses should never be ridden in a hot walker.

- **Moving Groups of Free Horses by Horseback:**
  - **Terms for Moving Horses:**
    - **Wrangling:** A group of saddle horses is called a *remuda* (from Spanish word *remudar*, meaning "to exchange") or *cavvy* (Spanish word *cavvietta*, meaning a ranch's "herd of horses"). The western term for herding horses is *wrangling* from the Spanish word *caverango*, meaning "herder of saddle horses."

○ **Jingling:** *Jingling* is another term for herding horses when one or two dominant mares have a shiny bell tied around their neck to enable handlers to locate them in environmental conditions with poor visibility.

- **Method:**
  ○ **Risks:** Moving groups of free horses while on horseback can be dangerous. Two riders, wranglers, are typically used to move horses. The wranglers' horses need to be accustomed to being in groups of horses and not bothered by other horses moving away from them.
  ○ **Following a Familiar Horse:** Experienced herds will follow a lead wrangler's horse while the second wrangler follows behind to move stragglers a little faster.
  ○ **Herding:** Horses unaccustomed to being wrangled have to be moved by both wranglers behind and to the sides of the herd moving them quietly by invading the herd's flight zone.
  ○ **Wrangler Horse:** A horse has to be trained to be a wrangler's horse and not every saddle horse can become one. A wrangling horse has to move at the desired speed of the rider in all circumstances and move away from the herd at the rider's will. Older, more dominant, horses are usually used for wrangling and are warmed up under saddle long enough each time to focus on the rider before approaching a horse herd to be moved.

ENVIRONMENTAL PROTECTION

- **Fly Masks:** Domestic horse confinement exacerbates fly problems, many which are attracted to eye moisture. Horses have the largest eyes of any land animal and are highly susceptible to irritation from flies and eye injuries (Figure 4.19).
  - **Uses:** Fly masks are used to protect the horse's eyes from irritation by flies. They are also used to protect the eyes from flying debris when traveling in stock trailers and to protect eyes from UV light damage. Fly masks should not be left on overnight.
  - **Fitting:** See-through, insect barrier face masks for horses should be clean with soft points of contact with the skin. There should be darts or rounded inserts to prevent the mask from touching the eyes and eyelashes. Proper fitting allows a finger to fit under the mask at all contact points.
  - **Desensitize to Attachment Noise:** Attachments are usually hook and loop (Velcro). The horse must be desensitized to the ripping sound of detaching hook and loop attachments before it can be expected to wear a fly mask.
  - **Keep Clean:** Before each use, the mask should be checked for dirt in the mesh to be cleaned and for damage from prior use. A second mask should be worn while the first one is drying from being cleaned. Wet masks should not be worn.
- **Blanketing:**
  - **Prevent Winter Hair Coats:** Horse blankets (not to be confused with saddle blankets) are often used to prevent show horses from growing a winter coat. They can be used to keep horses warm in cold weather, but if healthy horses are allowed to acclimate to colder weather, blankets are generally unnecessary. However, once blankets are used for a couple of weeks, they will reduce a horse's ability to adapt to cold weather and will necessitate continued blanketing.
  - **Disadvantages:** Blankets have the disadvantages of causing rub injuries and facilitating infection, restricting movement, entrapping legs, and causing overheating and chilling.

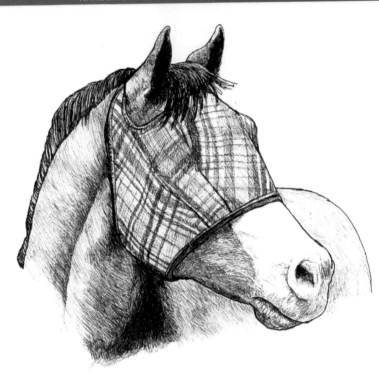

Figure 4.19   Equine fly mask.

- **Advantages and Indications:** Blankets may be needed for sick or elderly horses, on horses riding in stock trailers in cold weather, or on horses that have been clipped. Blankets should be considered for any horse if temperatures go below 0°F. Lightweight blankets with tight mesh may be used for control of fly bites.
- **Body Clipped Horses:** Body clipping may be necessary in horses that do hard work in winter and sweat. Clipping aids in drying the horse, and blankets are needed to keep them warm when not working.
- **Applying a Blanket and Removing a Blanket:**
  - ○ **Halter and Lead:** A halter and lead rope should be on the horse in advance of putting blankets on or off, or during adjustments.
  - ○ **Cinches:** Blankets have two cinches: a front and back cinch. The front cinch should always be fastened first going on and unfastened last coming off.
  - ○ **Static Electricity:** Caution is needed when horses with long hair coats and synthetic fiber blankets are being adjusted or taken off because static electricity may startle the horse.
- **Blanket Cut and Insulation:**
  - ○ **Cuts:** Horse blankets can be "standard cut" for stock horses or "European cut" for horses with narrow shoulders.
  - ○ **Open or Closed Front:** They may have an "open front" which is closed by buckles or snaps or "closed front" which has to be lifted over the horse's head. Closed front blankets can be put on quicker and are stronger but are not as adjustable. Some horses may not adjust to having the front placed over their head.
  - ○ **Denier Number:** Insulating fiber strength is measured in Denier. Higher Denier numbers reflect coarser fibers and greater strength.

HANDLING FOR ROUTINE MEDICAL PROCEDURES

Most handling and restraint of horses can be and should be done without tranquilization, sedation, hypnosis, or anesthesia. However, some handling and restraint procedures should be restricted to veterinary medical professionals due to the potential danger to the animal or handler. These require special skills, equipment, or facilities, and possibly adjunct chemical restraint or complete immobilization by chemical restraint.

RESTRAINT OF INDIVIDUAL HORSES OR PORTIONS OF THEIR BODY

- **Whole Body:**
  - **Stocks and Stall Corners:**
    - ○ **Description:** Stocks are standing stalls for examination and treatment of horses (Figure 4.20). The dimensions for average horses are 36 inches wide, 84 inches high, and 88 inches long. Horses are led into the stocks from the back gate and when done, they are led forward out the front gate (Figure 4.21).

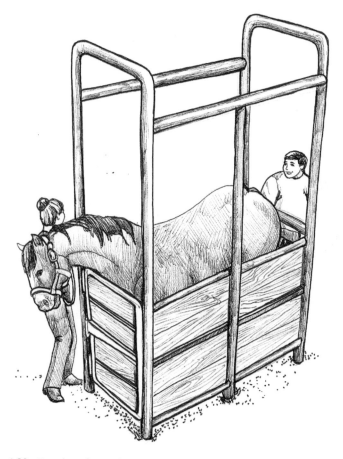

Figure 4.20   Horse in stocks restraint.

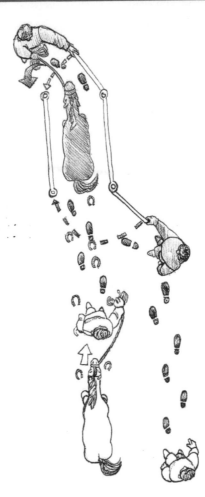

Figure 4.21 Leading a horse through stocks.

- o **Caution:** Stocks are the safest method of physically restraining horses. Forward, backward, and side-to-side movement is restricted while in stocks, but the safety of horse stocks should not be overestimated. Horses can rear and strike over the front gate and they can kick over the back gate, if not further restrained.
- o **Nursing Mares with Foals:** If mares with nursing foals must be restrained in stocks, the stock should have a small pen attached to the front of the stocks, so the mare and foal can be face to face until the mare can rejoin the foal.
- o **Entering the Stock:** To move a horse into a stock, the horse is led into the stock with both gates open, as if going through it. After the handler walks through and passes the front gate, in a calm and quiet manner the front gate is closed first and then an assistant closes the hind gate. After the hind gate is fastened, the horse's lead rope can be tied.
- o **Improper Entrances to Stocks:** A horse should not be driven into a stock from behind with a front gate closed, or with the handler attempting to lead the horse from outside of the stock.

    ○ **Proper Supervision in the Stock:** A halter and lead rope should always be left on the horse. A handler must never approach a horse in a stock while in its blind spot (directly behind it) and startle the horse. A handler or assistant should remain with the horse at all times while it is in stocks.

    ○ **Stall Corner as a Stock Substitute:** If stocks are not available, a horse can be backed into a flat-walled, strongly built corner with a ceiling that is high enough that it will not hit its head if it rears. The corners of most box stalls are sufficient. Having the horse's rump in the corner prevents backing and avoidance with right or left movement of its rump.

    ○ **Control in a Stall Corner:** When restraining a horse with its rump in the corner of a stall, the handler should face the horse standing at 45 degrees to a shoulder to psychologically inhibit forward movement and reinforce control with voice, halter and lead, and distraction techniques.

    ○ **Hay or Straw Bales as a Stock Substitute:** If a procedure must be done on or near the horse's rump, such as rectal palpation, makeshift stocks can be made of hay or straw bales for protection of the handler.

● **Casting Assist to Chemical Restraint:**

    ○ **Description:** Casting is laying a large animal down on its sternum or side. Horses are too large and strong to be safely cast without moderate to deep chemical restraint. However, supplementary physical restraint can provide greater control of how horses become recumbent than occurs from chemical restraint alone.

    ○ **Handlers Required:** Casting of horses requires at least three handlers. One handler controls the head with a halter and lead rope. The other two handlers manage the long lines.

    ○ **Laying the Horse Down:** See Procedural Steps 4.10.

Procedural Steps 4.10	Laying a Horse Down with Casting Ropes
1.	Create a neck collar with a bowline on the bight in the middle of 70 ft of rope.
2.	Place the collar on the neck with the knot on the lower part of the collar and in front of the horse's breast.
3.	Run the long lines between the front legs to the hind pasterns and through leg straps with metal rings.
4.	Bring the lines back on the outside of the shoulders and underneath the rope collar.
5.	After the horse is sedated enough to want to lie down, one handler standing in front of the horse pulls a hind leg about 6 inches off the ground.
6.	The other handler wraps a long line around the horse's hip and stands 90 degrees to horse on the same side as the front handler.
7.	As the horse lays down, both hind legs are pulled up toward the abdomen, wrapped with figure 8s and half hitches with the long lines to keep the legs in flexion, and finally tied to the neck collar.
8.	The front legs can be hobbled and a rope connected to the hobbles, run over the withers, the front pasterns pulled up to the horse's chest, and tied to itself.
9.	The horse's head should be placed on thick padding and restrained by the lead rope handler resting on its neck and holding the halter.

- **Head and Mouth Restraints:**
  - **Tongue Hold Restraint:** A cursory examination of the mouth can be performed by grasping the tongue through the bars of the mouth (diastema). One hand is placed on the bridge of the nose while the other, palm down, reaches in the bars of the mouth to grasp the tongue and then pull it to the side.
  - **Full Mouth Speculums:**
    - **Sedation Required:** Examination of the mouth of sedated horses can be aided by a hinged speculum that is placed and cranked open. Full mouth speculums should only be used when a horse is chemically restrained due the risks of injury to the horse and handler.
    - **Types:** The McPherson (Hausmann) speculum pries the mouth open by pushing the upper and lower incisors apart and locks in place with ratchets. The PowerFloat speculum is fixated by screw knobs.
  - **Cradles:** Cradles are collars of parallel wooden rods tied with cord that can wrap around the horse's neck to prevent a horse from chewing its front legs and some of the rear parts of its body (Figure 4.22). A cradle can also be a deterrent to cribbing and prevent biting and tugging on blankets. Although it permits grazing, it must be removed for the horse to eat from an elevated feed bunk.
  - **Side Sticks:** A side stick is a pole attached to the halter and a surcingle (strap around the chest) which prevents a horse from reaching back to chew any of the back parts of its body, but it can reach the distal aspects of its front legs. Side sticks do not interfere with eating or drinking.

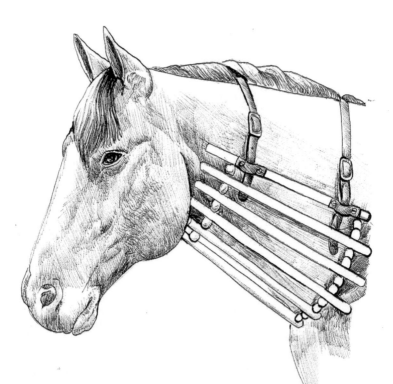

Figure 4.22   Neck cradle.

- **Grazing Muzzle:**
  - **Grazing Control:** Grazing muzzles are used to prevent horses from eating bedding or too much lush grass or from choking on food pellets. They have mesh openings that allow very limited amounts of grass to be grazed. Muzzles can allow overweight horses to get pasture exercise and socialization with other horses while being on a restricted diet.
  - **Construction:** A grazing muzzle should be lightweight, provide for air circulation, fit well, and have a breakaway safety mechanism for release if it is caught on a fence or other stationary objects.
  - **Fit:** The fit should allow one inch from the bottom of the muzzle to the lips and 3 to 4 fingers' width on the side of the muzzle.
  - **Remove Twice per Day:** A grazing muzzle should be removed for an hour twice per day to ensure that the horse drinks and can lick salt. They can drink with it on but some horses will not.
- **Cribbing Muzzle:**
  - **Cribbing Description:** The initial cause of cribbing is controversial, but regardless of the inciting cause, it is aggravated by boredom. When a horse cribs, it grabs a stationary horizontal object with its incisors usually immediately after eating grain, flexes its neck, and leans back while grunting and sucks air into its throat.
  - **Control of Cribbing:** Grazing muzzles may also prevent cribbing. Some stables attempt to eliminate all horizontal objects that horses could crib on. Surgery to prevent cribbing is no longer recommended.
  - **Efficacy of Grazing or Cribbing Muzzles:** A common problem with the efficacy of grazing and cribbing muzzles is intermittent use. To be effective, they must be used every time the horse has access to grass or to a horizontal object that it can crib on, respectively.
- **Cribbing Collar:**
  - **Description:** A cribbing collar goes around the ears and throat causing discomfort when the horse pulls down and back with its mouth. Some collars emit a low voltage electric shock when the horse cribs.
  - **Controversy:** There is debate as to whether horses should be physically prohibited from cribbing since this is blocking an emotional, perhaps physiological need to crib and physical restraint may make the desire to crib worse.
  - **Risk:** Since there is risk of a horse in a pasture getting the collar caught on fencing or other objects, at least one attachment should be breakaway. If something startles the horse and it raises it head too high, the strap on some collars can press on the trachea and carotid arteries causing the horse to stagger or faint.
  - **Alternative or Adjunct Management of Cribbing Horses:** Horses that crib should be on pasture with other horses for distraction and confined with electric fencing that they cannot crib on.
- **Bib:** An equine bib is a leather flap that attaches to a halter that is used to prevent chewing of wounds or blankets. It must be removed to allow the horse to eat. Drinking is possible with the bib in place, but the horse may not attempt it and must be monitored for attempts to drink.
- **Neck Straps:**
  - **Purpose:** Neck straps are similar to dog collars and are fitted to be worn on the upper neck. The strap's purposes are for identification and minimal restraint. They are primarily used to identify individual broodmares.
  - **Safety When on Pasture:** Neck straps are less prone to being caught by bolts, limbs, etc. than halters on pastured horses.

- o **Not a Restraint:** A horse should not be led by a neck strap. Straps should be breakaway for the safety of the horse at turnout and the safety of the handler who tries to use the strap for more than minimal restraint.
- **Tail Restraint:**
  - **Attach Tail Tie Only to the Horse's Body:** Horses' tails may be tied with a quick release sheet bend and then to its neck with a bowline knot. The tail should never be tied to anything other than the horse's body.
  - **Tail Tying Method:** To grasp and tie the tail, the right-handed handler stands next to the horse's left hip and slides the right hand over the horse's rump and reaches around with the right hand to grasp and pull the tail toward the handler, rather than standing in the kick zone. A sheet bend (tail tie) is begun by laying the rope perpendicular across the tail hair and folding the tail over the rope, not by wrapping the rope around the tail hair.
- **Placement of Rectal Thermometers:** Rectal temperatures are routinely taken on horses with minimal head restraint (Procedural Steps 4.11).

Procedural Steps 4.11	Handling a Horse for Placement of a Rectal Thermometer
1.	Using a halter and lead rope, an assistant should hold the horse or if the horse is well tamed, it can be tied by the lead rope.
2.	The horse should be positioned near a wall or strong fence.
3.	The handler should walk next to the left side of the horse and stand with their body touching the left flank with the left hand on top of the horse's rump.
4.	The handler grasps the base of the tail with the left hand and slightly lifts the tail.
5.	While holding a lubricated thermometer in the right hand, the handler leans toward the horse's anus.
6.	The right hand should be slid over the left hip toward the anus to prevent startling the horse.
7.	The thermometer is then placed in the rectum.

WORKING WITH A DOWNED HORSE

- **Handler Safety:**
  - **Ideal Rescues:** Ideal rescue operations on downed horses are performed by trained personnel with optimum equipment for safety of the horse and the personnel assisting with the rescue. Ideal methods are available from Technical Large Animal Emergency Rescue, www.TLAER.org.
  - **Best-under-the-Circumstances Rescues:** Trained personnel for horse rescues are not plentiful or able to respond quickly enough in many instances. A local veterinarian should always be called since the horse will probably require chemical restraint and medical care. Plus, the owner or others with a strong emotional attachment may be unable to make objective decisions during the rescue attempt.
- **Restraint of a Recumbent Horse:**
  - **Attempts to Stand:** A recumbent horse rises on its front legs first. Control of front legs is most critical to preventing a horse from rising at an undesired time. A horse laying on its side must lift its head, lay on its sternum, and extend its front legs to rise.
  - **Control of the Head Prevents Ability to Rise:** Kneeling on the horse's neck or holding the nose up and pulled toward its withers will prevent a recumbent horse from regaining its feet. Another person should maintain a strap or rope to the person leaning over the horse to pull the handler away, if the horse

thrashes before it is restrained. All procedures done on a downed horse should be done with the handler standing behind its back, not on the legs' side in range of being struck.

- **Prevent Injury to the Horse's Eye or Facial Nerve:** When a horse is laying on its side, it can injure its down eye or its facial nerve if its head is not cushioned or its head flexed upward and held in that position.

- **Cast in a Stall:**
  - **Description of Being Cast:** Some horses, particularly younger ones, will sometimes attempt to roll in their stall. When they do, there is a risk of being cast in a stall (i.e., rolling three-fourths of the way to fully over next to a wall and becoming entrapped with their legs folded against a wall) (Figure 4.23).
  - **Risks, if Cast:** When cast, a horse cannot push itself back over or away from the wall, and they will panic, thrashing with their legs and head. Remaining in this position can be deadly for the horse.
  - **Initial Response:**
    - **Summon Help:** To rescue a horse that is cast in a stall, the handler should call for assistance while also appearing calm to the horse. The handler should talk to the horse to be sure the horse knows of the handler's presence.
    - **Avoid Thrashing Head and Legs:** As soon as an assistant is present, the handler should position themselves near the lower part of the horse's neck while not getting near the horse's legs or trying to step or reach over the horse.
  - **Pull Away from Wall:** The safest method of moving the horse is to place a rope loop around its neck, work the loop toward the upper part of the horse's neck, and then pull the neck away from the wall and toward the middle of the stall until the horse can get its legs underneath its body. In the absence of a rope, the mane in the mid-neck area can be pulled to move the horse. Pulling the horse by a halter and lead rope to reposition a cast horse could injure its neck.
  - **Avoid Horse's Attempts to Stand:** Care must be taken by the handler not to get stepped on or pinned against the wall by the horse as it attempts to stand.
  - **Alternative Rescue Method:** An alternative method involves putting long lines or ropes on the horse's legs to pull the horse toward the handler. This method is not recommended.
  - **Monitor the Horse for Post-Cast Complications:** Afterwards the horse should be observed for an hour after standing for signs of colic that could result from being cast or swellings in the legs from injuries that may have occurred.

- **Lifting a Trapped or Injured Horse:**
  - **Web Slings and Mechanical Hoists:** It is best to lift horses with straps designed for slinging a horse. New, improved hoist slings for horses have been designed in the last 20 years.
  - **Rope Sling and Block and Tackle:**
    - **Emergency Alternative:** If a sling harness and trained personnel are not available in time to save a horse in a ditch, well, or other life-threatening situations, it may be able to be lifted with a block and tackle and 3/4-inch rope. A halter, lead rope, blindfold, and a rope sling should first be applied to the horse.
    - **Control the Head:** The halter and lead rope should be applied first. If a halter and lead rope are not available, a temporary one can be made with a rope by a neck loop tied with a bowline knot and then a bight through the neck loop and over the nose. A blindfold should be applied next, preferably with padding over the eyes using a jacket, towels, or a woman's bra.
    - **Create the Sling:** A rope sling can be made using 50–70 ft of 2 inch or thicker nylon rope by making a collar in the middle of the rope using a

bowline on a bight. The collar is placed on the horse's neck with the bowline on a bight on the front of the horse's chest. The rope ends are passed under the front legs, up and under the neck loop collar, crossed over the back, run under the hind legs (from front to back) without crossing the ropes under the horse.

- ○ **Create a Hoist Attachment:** The ropes should be brought up the back of the legs near the base of tail, under the crossed ropes on the middle of the back and under the collar. The ends are bent back behind the crossed ropes and tied with a quick release knot. The hook on the traveling block of the block and tackle is attached to the back ropes just behind the withers.
- ○ **Pad the Ropes under the Legs:** Towels or clothing should be placed under the leg ropes for padding.
- ○ **Control Head Movement during Lift:** Lifting should be slow while someone restricts large movements of the head by holding onto the halter's lead rope.
- ○ **Rope Guides:** In some situations, a metal rod bent in a C-shape with the end bent back to bunt the leading edge and attach the rope to the other end may be needed to thread the rope under the legs. Blunted hooks on poles should be used to retrieve ropes near the horse's legs or feet.

- • **Moving Downed Horses on Glides:**
  - • **Description:** Glides (also called "slides" or "skids") are sheets of slick plastic that a downed horse is placed on and moved by sliding the sheet (Figure 4.24).
  - • **Method:**
    - ○ **Assistants Required:** The horse is pulled onto the glide after "sawing" or "flossing" restraint straps under its body and around its chest and flank. One person must maintain control of the head with a halter and lead rope while several others pull the horse, back-first with the straps around its body, onto the glide.
    - ○ **Chemical Restraint:** The degree of restraint to maintain the horse on the glide varies, but often requires chemical restraint, a padded face mask to protect its eyes and facial nerve, hobbles, and straps over the torso.
    - ○ **Assisting Glides:** Assisting glides may be needed to cover rough surfaces to allow the glide to slide more easily.
  - • **Emergency Alternatives:** In emergencies, if a glide is not available, a heavy tubular steel gate at least 8 feet long can be used as a glide or travois to move a downed horse over rough ground.

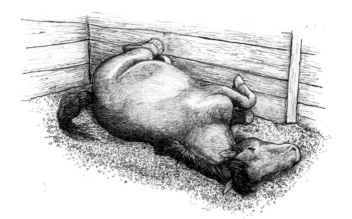

Figure 4.23 Horse cast in a stall.

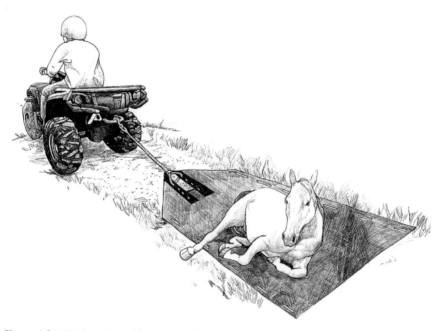

Figure 4.24 Moving a downed horse on a glide.

INJECTIONS AND VENIPUNCTURE

- **Access to Veins:**
  - **Veins for Venipuncture:** The jugular vein in the neck is almost always used to access the bloodstream in horses. The cephalic vein in the foreleg, transverse facial vein near the eye, saphenous vein, and lateral thoracic vein are dangerous to use in an un-sedated adult horse. The medial saphenous vein can be accessed in a foal, if the foal is held in lateral recumbency.
  - **Restraint:** A halter with a lead rope is usually sufficient restraint for venipuncture. The handler may use mild distraction techniques when needed. The phlebotomist occludes the vein and collects the blood without further assistance.
- **Injections:**
  - **Intramuscular:**
    - **Most Common Location:** Most injections in horses are intramuscular (IM) and done in the neck (lateral cervical) area. The preferred lateral cervical location in adult horses is a triangle that has the borders of one hand's width above the jugular vein, one hand's width in front of the shoulder, and one hand's width below the crest of the neck (Figure 4.25).
    - **Helpful Distraction:** Gentle pinches of the skin near where the injection will be given are preparation for horses immediately prior to inserting the needle into the muscle after which the syringe is attached to the needle.
    - **Alternative Sites:** Less commonly, injections might be given into the pectoral, triceps, gluteal, or semitendinosus/semimembranosus (thigh) muscles. Injections into the thigh or gluteal muscles should be performed by the handler pressing their body against a side of the horse and leaning around or over the horse to make the injections on the opposite side than the one where the handler is standing.
    - **Nursing Foals:** Intramuscular injections should not be given into the neck muscles of nursing foals. Resulting soreness may prevent it from nursing. The thigh muscles should be used for IM injections in nursing foals.

Horses, Donkeys, and Mules 129

- **Subcutaneous:** Subcutaneous (SC) injections are poorly absorbed in horses and can result in severe reactions. They are very rarely administered in this species. The lateral cervical area is used when SC injections are indicated.
- **Intravenous:** Intravenous injections in un-sedated horses are nearly always given in the jugular vein.

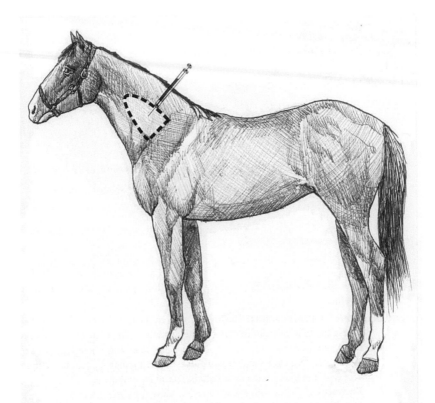

Figure 4.25   Preferred site for IM injection in horses.

ADMINISTRATION OF ORAL AND OPHTHALMIC MEDICATIONS

- **Oral:**
    - **Disguised Medications:** Although giving oral medications to horses is usually not difficult, it is helpful if the medication or its vehicle tastes pleasant to the horse.
        - **Crushed Tablets in a Treat:** Tablets can be crushed with a mortar and pestle, small plastic pill crusher, or a medication-dedicated coffee grinder. Crushed medication may be added to a paste of applesauce, corn syrup, molasses and brown sugar, banana, cherries, shredded carrots, peppermint, pudding, peanut butter, or yogurt to improve palatability.
        - **Hiding in Grain or Alfalfa Pellets:** Palatable medications can often be added to the horse's grain or a treat such as a small amount of alfalfa pellets to successfully administer the medication.
    - **Oral Syringe:**
        - **Mouth Should Be Empty:** Before giving a paste by oral syringe, there should be no grass or hay in the mouth, which could enable the horse to mix it with the paste and spit it out.

- ○ **Proper Placement in Mouth:** If hiding the medication in food is not possible or tolerated, an oral syringe may be used to administer a paste or liquid medication. The paste should not be administered into the cheek pouch. Instead, it should be placed in the interdental space ("bars of the mouth") and injected on top of the tongue.
- ○ **Method:** See Procedural Steps 4.12.

Procedural Steps 4.12	Use of an Oral Syringe
1.	In most cases the oral medication is administered with a syringe from the horse's left side.
2.	The oral syringe is held in the right hand.
3.	The handler should put their left fingers on the halter's noseband and thumb in the corner of the horse's mouth while standing close to the horse's shoulder and bending the horse's nose toward the handler.
4.	The back of the right hand is pressed against the horse's cheek and the hand rotated to place the syringe into the left bars of the mouth beneath the thumb of the left hand.
5.	After inserting the tip of the oral syringe into the mouth, the syringe plunger is pushed slowly to deliver the medication.

- **Stomach Tube:** Administration of large volumes of oral fluids requires the passage of a stomach tube, which is done through a nasal passage. The horse is restrained with a halter, lead rope, and long-handled nose twitch for the passage of the nasal tube.
- **Balling Guns:** A metal balling gun to deliver tablets (boluses) should never be used on a horse due to the risk of injury to the horse or handler.
- **Ophthalmic:**
  - **Incidence of Eye Problems in Horses:** Horses have the largest eyes of any land animal. The size of their eyes alone puts them at high risk of injuries.
  - **Resistance to Administration of Ophthalmic Medications:** Like all animals, horses are protective of painful eyes. Even if they stand still for an exam and treatment, they have very strong palpebral muscles which clamp the eye fissure shut.
  - **Method:** See Procedural Steps 4.13 and Figure 4.26.

Procedural Steps 4.13	Routine Administration of Ophthalmic Medications
1.	An assistant stands next to the horse's neck and restrains the horse with a halter and lead rope.
2.	The treatment administrator handler stands in front of the horse and to treat the left eye, places the horse's lower jaw on the handler's left shoulder.
3.	The handler's left arm is placed over the horse's face and the left hand is placed on the horse's left upper eyelid (Figure 4.26).
4.	While holding the medication tube or bottle in the handler's right hand between the thumb and forefinger, the third and fourth fingers of the right hand can gently pull the lower eyelid down to administer the medication in the eye.

- **Treatment of Highly Compliant Horses:** Treatment with dropper bottles or ointment tubes can be attempted by stabilizing the heel of the hand holding the medication on the horse's skull above the affected eye. The handler's other hand pulls the lower lid down to open the palpebral fissure and drop the medication onto the eye or inner surface of the lower lid. Most horses will either move away or clamp their eyelid shut with this approach.

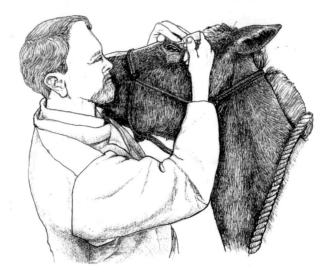

Figure 4.26   Head restraint for administration of ophthalmic medication.

- **Alternative Method:** Another method of administering ophthalmic ointment is to wear a sterile glove and place ointment on the gloved index finger. The handler's ungloved hand is used to open the palpebral fissure while the gloved finger scrapes the ointment onto the inside surface of the lower lid.
- **Avoid Trapping Hand in Halter:** When ophthalmic medications are administered, the treatment hand should be stabilized against the horse's head and move with movements of the horse's head. This should be done with constant pressure rather than the more hazardous method of running a hand under a halter to stabilize the hand.
- **Subpalpebral or Nasolacrimal Tubes:** Reliable frequent administration of ophthalmic medications to horses often requires sedation and surgical placement of a subpalpebral or nasolacrimal tube.

SPECIAL EQUIPMENT

TWITCHES
- **Purpose:** Twitches are distraction techniques applied to the neck or nose of horses. Twitches are used as restraint for passing stomach tubes, standing castrations, treating wounds, and farrier work.
- **Proper Use:** Twitches cause a temporary diversionary stimulus while other procedures are done on a horse that otherwise would not tolerate the procedure. Twitches can injure tissue if applied too long (more than 10 to 15 minutes), and they should be applied effectively on first attempt. Gently rubbing the skin where the twitch was applied after its removal will improve recirculation of blood in the area and provide a kind release for the horse to remember.
- **Inappropriate Uses:** Twitches should not be used to try to control a distressed horse that is thrashing, when the area to be twitched has been previously injured, or as a means of discipline and training of horses. Twitches should never be used on a foal due to the risk of inflicting pain and injury.

- **Questionable Role of Endorphins:**
  - **Theory of Euphoria:** Conventional opinion, on weak evidence, is that twitches work by the release of endorphins which are internally produced morphine-like substances. Human long-distance runners' brains produce endorphins during running which causes euphoric sensation and addictive behavior associated with running. Conversely, horses usually become resentful and anxious about a nose twitch being used repeatedly.
  - **Modulation of Discomfort:** Endorphins are released to modulate the discomfort and speed the recovery of having a twitch applied. Horses that have had nose twitches used, particularly if used aggressively or for too long, are likely to strike with a forefoot when a handler works near its head. When a nose twitch is used, the horse becomes motionless and submissive to protect its lip from the possibility of being torn, risking the horse's survival.
- **Types:**
  - **Long-Handled Nose Twitch:**
    - ○ **Construction:** The long-handled nose twitch, made from hickory wood, is most commonly used to twitch the nose (upper lip), but it should be used as infrequently as possible and for the shortest possible time. Long-handled twitches are about 30 inches with a rope or cord, leather, or chain loop which creates the clamping effect on the upper lip (Figure 4.27). Rope or cord twitches are preferable.
    - ○ **Method:** See Procedural Steps 4.14, plus Figure 4.28 and Figure 4.29.

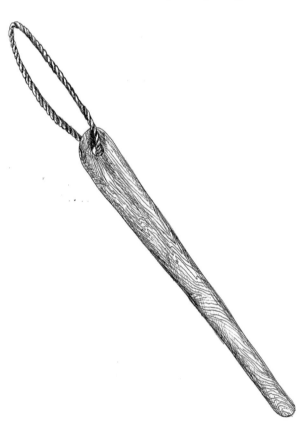

Figure 4.27   Long handled twitch.

Procedural Steps 4.14	Application of a Nose Twitch
1.	The handler should not stand in front of the horse since there is a risk of the horse striking out with a front leg.
2.	The horse should be in stocks or standing with its right side next to a solid wall or fence.
3.	The handler stands on the left side of the horse and holds the twitch handle with the right hand about 1 ft from the twitch loop, grasps the cheekpiece of the halter, and pulls the head to the left.
4.	The handler places the twitch's loop over the left hand with the little finger outside to prevent the loop from sliding over the wrist (Figure 4.28).
5.	The horse's upper lip is grasped between the thumb and three fingers of the left hand and the loop is slid over the fingers onto the lip.
6.	While keeping the fingers holding the lip out of the way, the handle is twisted clockwise with the right hand which also continues to hold the lead rope (Figure 4.29).
7.	The left hand assists in keeping the rope from wrapping around the twitch handle.
8.	The handler should slowly rock or jiggle the twitch handle to continue the distraction.
9.	Within 5 minutes the twitch should be removed by grasping the lip, untwisting the twitch, and removing it in a controlled manner (not pulled off) while desensitizing the horse by rubbing its nose and petting its neck.
10.	Neither twisting the loop on nor off should be done rapidly.

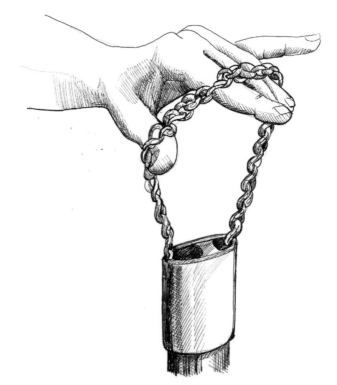

Figure 4.28   Hand position to apply a long-handled nose twitch.

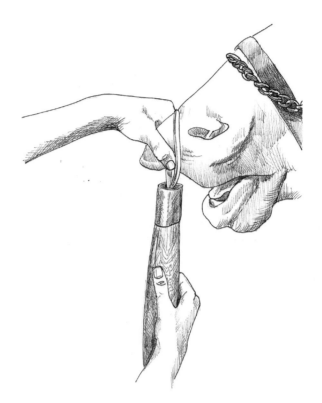

Figure 4.29 Applying the nose twitch.

- **One Hand Nose Twitch:**
  - **Bare Hand:** A nose twitch can be performed using a bare hand. The upper lip is squeezed between the thumb and the index and middle fingers. This is effective only for a few minutes.
  - **Small Rope Loop and a Rod:** A leveraged twitch can be improvised with a small loop of rope and a stick. This can be maintained longer than just using a bare hand. The application is the same as with a long-handled twitch.
- **Skin Twitch:** A skin twitch (the "Gypsy Hold") consists of grasping a fold of skin on the neck just in front of a shoulder. The fold of skin should be rolled over the fingers so it can be held in a tight fist and slowly rocked or jiggled.
- **"Humane" or Kendal Twitch:** The "humane" or Kendal twitch is a small hinged clamp that is curved to prevent an excessive pinching effect and is placed on the horse's upper lip (Figure 4.30 and Figure 4.31).
  - **Dangerous:** The humane twitch is no more or less humane than other twitches that are applied correctly. It is intended to be clipped to the halter to free the hands of the handler. However, the twitch can be knocked off by the horse allowing the twitch to become a swinging menace to the horse and handlers.
  - **Safer Use:** It is much safer if used by an assistant who continues to keep hold of the twitch as long as it is applied, but this may not be possible if the horse rears or is tall in stature and elevates its head. Like other twitches, jiggling or rocking motions will prolong the distraction effect. However, the humane twitch is more likely to slip off the nose than a long-handled twitch with a rope or cord.

- **Wilform Twitch:** The Wilform twitch is a metal square with a screw and a bar that acts as a vice (Figure 4.32). It has no bars sticking out to the side as does the Kendal twitch. Due to the leverage of the screw, it can be applied too tightly and if not applied tightly enough, it can be slung off by the horse as a highly dangerous metal missile.
- **Ear Twitches:** A horse's ear should never be held in a manner that might inflict pain.
  - ○ **Description:** An ear twitch is when the ear is roughly pulled on by a hand or a long-handled twitch, or even bitten by a handler. Twitching an ear can damage the horse's ear cartilage, blood supply, or nerves. In some states in the U.S., ear twitching is illegal.
  - ○ **Negates Good Training:** Good horsemen spend hundreds of hours desensitizing horses to having their ears handled. This can be ruined in one application of an ear twitch.
  - ○ **Potentially Lethal to Handlers and Horses:** Ear twitching can cause a horse to sling its head, strike, or rear. The pain can make the horse head shy and a danger to anyone who tries to halter or bridle the horse in the future. If the horse becomes disfigured, useless, and unsafe, it may have to be put to death.

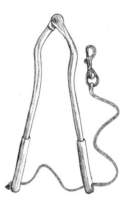

Figure 4.30 Kendal twitch.

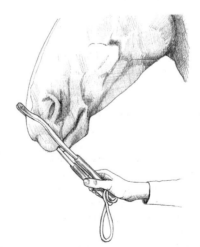

Figure 4.31 Kendal twitch applied to upper lip.

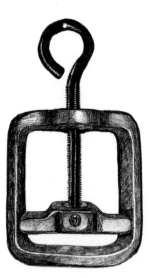

Figure 4.32 Wilform nose twitch.

HOBBLES

Hobbles can be useful in restricting a horse's movement. However, hobbles should not be used on horses with a history of neuromuscular problems, those that are sedated, or if a painful procedure may be required. A handler who puts any type of hobbles on a horse should remain near enough to immediately provide reassurance and aid to a horse that might struggle violently.

- **Front Leg Hobbles:**
  - **Require Gradual Training:** Front leg hobbles will often calm a horse that is trained to accept them to many stimuli that might otherwise bother them. However, using front leg hobbles on a horse for the first time in an emergency can cause them to panic and lead to injury. Hobble training should be done gradually.
  - **Water Risk:** Horses should be allowed to drink water before being hobbled. Hobbled horses that try to drink from ponds, lakes, or streams can trip and drown.
  - **To Teach Patience and Discipline:** Front leg hobbles are also used to teach patience and discipline. They can teach the horse not to panic if the legs become entrapped in wire or with rope.
  - **To Restrict Movement:**
    - **Restricted Leg Movement:** Front leg hobbles are also used to prevent a horse from traveling far when turned loose (Figure 4.33). They may be used for short periods when a rider must be dismounted and cannot tie the horse to a suitable object, or used for longer periods to allow grazing. However, some horses can learn to do a modified lope with hobbles on.
    - **Overnight Hobbles:** When multiple horses are hobbled for overnight, one horse should be tied, saddled, and fed grain so it can be used to retrieve escaped horses. The lead horse in the group should also wear a neck strap with a bell to locate a group if they escape.
  - **Tom Fool Knot:** It has been suggested that the Tom Fool knot can be used as hobbles for horses.
    - **Description:** The Tom Fool knot is essentially two bights through a loop in a rope and is similar to the Handcuff knot.

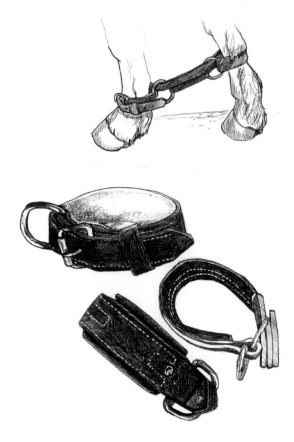

Figure 4.33   Front leg hobbles limit movement and permit grazing.

  o **Impracticality:** The Tom Fool knot cannot be applied to a horse's legs without picking each foot up. The knot jams the legs against each other, making it hard for the horse to maintain its balance if it attempts to move.
  o **Possible Use:** It may have value in restraining the legs of a recumbent, anesthetized horse.
- **One Leg Hobble ("Rarey Strap"):**
  - **Description:** A one leg hobble ties a front leg in flexion. It can be used to restrain difficult horses for procedures that they would otherwise not tolerate. The one leg hobble was made popular in the 1800s by an American horseman, John Rarey.
  - **Struggling Potential:** If not trained in advance for a front leg hobble, the hobble should be applied on soft footing and the horse's movements should be controlled at a distance by the lead rope and halter. Struggling may result for a relatively short period before resolution to the restraint occurs.
  - **Disadvantage:** Horses with a one leg hobble applied can still rear and pivot on the hindquarters which can be dangerous to handlers.
- **Picket (Staking or Pegging) Hobble:**
  - **Description:** A horse that has been trained for hobbles can be staked with a hobble strap on one leg to allow grazing without a fence. A single leg leather hobble with an attached metal ring, stake lead rope, and swivel snaps on the stake and permits safe grazing within the radius of the stake lead rope. The

stake should be well anchored in the ground but visible above the ground and without sharp points.

- **Hind or Front Leg:** Either a front leg or a hind leg can be hobbled, but hobbling a hind leg is safer for the horse. If the horse should spook and jump and is staked with a hobble on a front leg, it could be tripped and fall.

- **Side Hobbles:**
  - **Description:** Two straps connected by a line are placed around a front leg and hind leg on the same side of the body.
  - **Purpose:** Side hobbles are used to discourage kicking or as a transition to training for front leg hobbles. They permit more freedom while grazing but do not allow a horse to lope.
  - **Australian Hobbles:** Australian hobbles are the use of two side hobbles attached diagonally to the front and hind legs forming an "X" beneath the horse.

- **Breeding Hobbles:**
  - **Purpose:** Some horse breeders use hobbles on the hocks of mares when breeding to prevent kicking of the stallion.
  - **Description:** Breeding hobbles can be created by using a folded rope with a bowline on the bight knot to form a collar. The long lines are run between the front legs to strap and ring hobbles over the hocks and then back along the shoulders to the collar. The ends of the long lines are tied to the collar with quick release hitches.
  - **Risk:** Breeding hobbles may protect the stallion from being kicked, but the hobbles can also create a new danger if the stallion gets one of his forelegs caught in the hobble rope.

- **Scotch Hobbles:** Scotch hobbles are used to inhibit kicking (Figure 4.34).
  - **Description:** A Scotch hobble is created with a 18-foot long soft rope. A non-sliding neck loop is made with a bowline knot. The working end of the rope is run from the neck loop to a hobble strap with metal rings on one hind leg pastern and then back through the neck loop. The movement of the pastern can then be restrained or the high leg lifted slightly (2 inches) toward the horse's belly to prevent kicking.
  - **Avoid Rope Burns:** The rope that goes to the pastern should not be run around the pastern because rope burns could result.
    - **Leather or Nylon Straps with Metal Rings:** The end of the rope should be run through the metal rings of a leather or nylon foot strap (hobble) from the inside aspect of the hind leg to the outside.
    - **Improvised Pastern Strap:** A makeshift pastern hobble can be made with 3 to 4 feet of rope tied by the ends with a sheet bend to form a circular rope. The rope is folded and placed on the back of the pastern and each end pulled forward. The bights on each side provide a channel for the rope from the neck to slide and not burn the back of the pastern.
  - **Supplement to Chemical Restraint:**
    - **Description:** Scotch hobbles may be used to supplement chemical restraint for veterinary procedures. It is used to pull a hind leg up slightly and restrain it from kicking while a horse is anesthetized.
    - **Method:** As the horse is anesthetized and the head is controlled with a halter and lead rope, the hobble rope is used to pull the hind leg up and lay the horse down in a more controlled manner. It is continued to be used for leg control when the horse is laying on its side for castration or other veterinary procedures on the abdomen or groin. A Scotch hobble should not be used to lay a horse down that has not been chemically sedated, because struggling can release myoglobin from muscular injury and can damage the horse's kidneys.

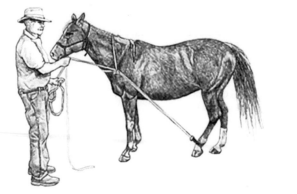

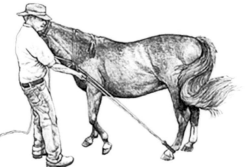

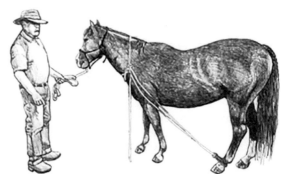

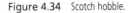

Figure 4.34 Scotch hobble.

FEED BAG (MORRAL)

- **Description:** A feed bag, also called a *morral* (Spanish, meaning "bag"), is a canvas bag with grain in it that is strapped over the horse's muzzle (Figure 4.35). The morral eliminates wasting of grain and makes horses easier to catch.
- **Use Must Be Supervised:** A horse being fed with a morral should be supervised to reduce the risk of catching the morral on a fence or other structure, and it should not have access to water until the morral is removed. If a horse attempts to drink with a morral on, the bag could fill with water and possibly cause drowning or aspiration pneumonia.

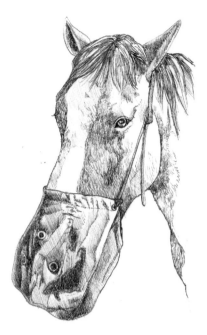

Figure 4.35   Feed bag for feeding grain.

TRANSPORTING HORSES

GROUND TRANSPORT

- **Dangers:** Loading and unloading horses from a trailer is one of the most potentially dangerous activities of a horse handler. Much of the danger can be removed by early training of the horse, routine practice, thorough preparation of the trailer and towing equipment, and careful driving.
- **Trailers and Vans:**
  - **Basic Transport Requirements:**
    - **Sufficient Size:** Trailers and vans should be road worthy and of sufficient size for the horses to be hauled. Most trailers are 7 feet tall from floor to ceiling which will accommodate horses up to 16 hands in height. Taller horses require taller trailers.
    - **Good Ventilation:** Ventilation is important even in winter. Closed trailers should have at least one overhead vent per horse.
    - **Non-Injurious Interior:** There should be no protrusions or sharp edges inside the trailer or van. Flooring should be non-slip.
  - **Basic Training and Refreshed Training:**
    - **Need for Training:** Many horses are trailered for the first time when being taken to a veterinary clinic or hospital because of illness or injury. This is too late. Forcing the horse into a trailer or a horse van is a setback for training the horse to load properly and is an unsafe situation for handlers.
    - **Basic Training:** Before horses can be loaded and unloaded from a trailer, they need to be able to walk on a wooden platform to experience stepping up, hearing the hollow sound made on a plank floor, and backing up and stepping down.

- **Loading:**
  - **Preparation of the Trailer:** See Table 4.4.

Table 4.4	Preparation of a Horse Trailer Prior to Hauling
•	Horses should be loaded last, after everything else has been loaded
•	The trailer needs to be attached to the tow vehicle and tires chocked so that it is immoveable prior to the horse loading
•	The trailer's interior should be as bright as possible, using lights, windows, and light-colored paint
•	Trailer gates/doors should be tied back or otherwise secured so that they cannot be blown open or closed by wind
•	In warm weather, the driver should check for wasp nests in trailer corners, wheel wells, behind bumpers, in storage compartments, windows, and the trailer tongue
•	Any old feed that may have been left from a previous trip must be cleaned up in case it has become moldy
•	Interior surfaces should be inspected visually and by touch for sharp, rough, or pointed areas.

  - **General Styles in Horse Trailers:**
    - ○ **Enclosed:** Adequate ventilation and temperature control can be a problem, particularly at stops. More protection against extremes in weather is provided. Unseasoned horses can be reluctant to load in trailers that appear more confining.
    - ○ **Stock:** Stock trailers permit greater ventilation, visibility of outside surroundings, and natural lighting. Horses with little to no experience in loading into trailers are more likely to accept entering a stock trailer. There is less protection against weather extremes than in enclosed trailers.
    - ○ **Step-Up Horse Entry:** Step-up entries are sufficient for small trailers.
    - ○ **Ramp Horse Entry:** Large trailers may have a much higher flooring level and require ramps for loading. Ramps should not have more than a 25-degree grade of incline.
  - **Remove Distractions:** Distractions, especially dogs, should be removed from the loading area.
  - **Never Tranquilize or Sedate:** A horse should never be tranquilized or sedated before hauling due to risk of it being injured by an inability to keep its balance.
  - **Leading the Horse to Load:**
    - ○ **Lead Ropes:** A cotton or leather lead rope is best for trailering. Nylon lead ropes can burn the hands if the horse rushes backwards.
    - ○ **Train to Send the Horse In:** Horses should be trained to load without being led in. The handler should never stand in a trailer in front of a horse and attempt to get it to load due to the risk it could jump into the handler.
    - ○ **Ensure the Handler's Exit:** The handler should never be positioned with the horse between him and the only exit while loading. There should be direct access to a front exit, the handler should stand on the other side of a divider, or the horse should be taught to be sent in rather than led into the trailer. The lead rope should be tied by reaching into the trailer from outside or there should be direct access to a front exit.
  - **Encouraging the Horse to Load:**
    - ○ **Avoid Making the Horse Feel Entrapped:** Some handlers run a lead rope around a tie ring or other stationary structure inside the trailer and will attempt to pull the horse toward the trailer and hold it, then pull it closer and hold it, and continue until the horse loads. However, pulling and holding can intensify a horse's fear of trailer loading.

- ○ **Approach and Retreat:** A better method involves allowing a horse to move its feet by longeing it near the trailer. The handler sends the horse on the longe line toward the trailer. The handler then lowers their energy, allowing the horse to become more relaxed whenever it investigates the trailer and remains still.
- ○ **Continue in Short Increments:** Approach and retreat is repeated until the horse willingly enters and stays still in the trailer. This is a training process that should be done in short increments over several days, when needed.
- ○ **Inside the Trailer Should Be a Safe Refuge:** No reprimands, such as sharp jerks on the lead rope, should ever occur in a trailer. Nothing that might cause fear or pain should ever occur in a trailer.
- ○ **Avoid Food Rewards:** Food rewards are not recommended. Food treats are not always available when horses need to be loaded. In emergencies such as barn fires, food may not be readily available.
- **Appropriate Distribution of Weight in Trailers:**
  - ○ **Straight Load, One Horse, Left Side:** With straight load trailers, the most weight should be distributed on the left side of the trailer for stability (i.e., a single horse goes on the left side, or if there are two horses, the heaviest goes on the left side). Having most of the weight on the side closest to the center of the road reduces the risk of the trailer tipping during left turns into a lane that is slanted to the road's shoulder. It also can ease getting a trailer back onto the road if the right tires drop off the pavement.
  - ○ **Slant Load:** Slant load trailers eliminate much of the instability of straight load trailers, shorten the length of trailers, and allow horses to better maintain their balance when the trailer goes around curves. There is more room in the back stall of slant load trailers, so the largest horse should be loaded last.
- **Loading Untrained Horses:** In medical or environmental emergencies, untrained horses may need to be loaded in trailers without delay.
  - ○ **Encourage Movement:** Horses not trained for trailer loading can be encouraged by a lariat loop around their rear, a person waving their arms or a broom behind them, or slapping the ground with a longeing whip. However, just making noise by rhythmically slapping leather chaps or making some other flapping sound is often more effective.
  - ○ **Follow a Seasoned Horse:** Watching and following a seasoned horse that loads well aids loading horses new to trailers. This should be done during the handling of nursing foals by following their mother into a trailer.
  - ○ **Shoving Methods:** Use of a rump rope or two handlers grasping each other's wrists behind the horse's rump to force loading can increase the risk of the horse rearing. If using a rope around the horse's rump, about two-thirds of the pressure to move should be applied to the rump rope and one-third to the halter's lead rope. Long ropes can be tied to each side of a trailer and crossed behind horse and held by two assistants to aid loading a reluctant horse.
  - ○ **Risks of Shoving:** If these techniques are used, the handler with the lead rope should use an extra-long lead rope for safety if the horse rears. Two handlers grasping each other's wrists prevents rope burns to the horse and sideways evasions to loading.
  - ○ **Blindfolds or Backing:** Use of a blindfold or backing the horse into the trailer increases the risk of the horse jumping into or onto the handler.
- **Butt Chains or Bars:** After the horse enters the trailer, the butt bar or chain should be secured before tying the halter lead. The handler who secures the bar or chain should not stand directly behind the horse in case the horse suddenly tries a hasty exit.

- **Tying in Trailers:** Past the age of weaning, halter-broke horses in trailers should be haltered and tied. Tying horses should be done through a window from the outside or from an interior location with a barrier separating the horse from the handler after they are loaded.   A cotton lead rope should be used for tying in a trailer.
  - o **Release in Accidents:** A breakaway halter or tie ring that permits sliding (Blocker tie ring) should be used to inhibit the horse from lowering its head during a normal trip but still permits it to free its head if in a trailer accident.
  - o **Tie Loose Enough for Proper Balancing:** Tying in a trailer should be loose enough that horses may brace themselves against the back or side of a trailer to keep their balance during travel and short enough to prevent them from stepping over the lead rope and becoming entangled.
  - o **Tie Loose Enough to Be Able to Clear Airways:** For trips lasting more than 3 hours, a horse must be able to lower its head. Respiratory secretions are not properly cleared if horses cannot lower their head below the height of their withers within 6 hours. Accumulated mucus and other secretions can then become media for bacterial growth.
  - o **Horses Not Halter-Broke:** Foals or other horses that have not been halter-broke should not be tied. The untied horse should be blocked off with a divider or gate and a trained and seasoned horse tied in the back of the trailer.
- **Protective Travel Wear for Horses:**
  - o **Types:** See Table 4.5.

Table 4.5	Protective Travel Wear for Horses
•	Leg wraps
•	Bell boots
•	Head bumpers
•	Tail wraps
•	Blankets.

  - o **Disadvantages:** Some horses will not tolerate travel apparel, particularly leg wraps. They may persistently stomp their feet, and risking developing bowed tendons. Protective wear can also get too hot in warm weather.
  - o **Potential Advantages:** If in a turnover accident, horses fight to regain a standing position. Injuries often occur to the head and legs in the effort to stand and may be reduced if a horse is wearing protective wear.
- **Remove Tack:** Horses should not be hauled while wearing tack. In addition to the damage that can occur to the saddle, the saddle and saddle blanket can increase the risk of the horse overheating and having more serious injuries in a vehicular accident.
- **Nursing Foals:** Nursing foals should always travel with their dam. If other horses will travel with mare and foal, the mare and foal should be in a compartment separated from other horses.
- **Traveling:**
  - **Plan the Route:** Prior to traveling, a driver hauling horses should plan a route, check the weather, and ensure proper paperwork is at hand.
  - **Driver Preparations and Practices:**
    - o **Practice Towing and Backing:** In preparation for hauling horses, drivers should practice towing and backing the trailer.

- ○ **Remain Alert:** Drivers must stay alert and avoid driving if tired, injured, or on medications that adversely affect their ability to remain alert or decrease their reaction time. Distractions, such as the use of cell phones, should be strictly avoided while towing a horse trailer.
- ○ **Use Slow Starts, Turns, and Stops:** Proper driving while hauling horses in a trailer takes practice, otherwise a horse can be thrown off its feet with fast starts, sudden turns, or quick stops. To test a driver's skills, a bucket of water can be placed in an empty trailer that will be hauled to determine if a driver can pull a trailer without spilling the water bucket.
- ○ **Double the Safe Distance between Vehicles:** Drivers must always remember that extra room is needed to stop when hauling a trailer with horses. The normal distance between the towing vehicle and a vehicle ahead of it should be doubled when hauling a horse trailer. Safe driving becomes even more important when hauling horses in adverse weather conditions.
- ○ **Danger in Smoking While Driving:** Smoking materials should never be thrown from the towing vehicle. Lit cigarettes or matches can be sucked into the horse trailer and cause a trailer fire.
- **Check Horses and Trailer:**
  - ○ **First 2 Hours of Travel:** A brief stop to check all horses and the exterior of the trailer should be done after the first 2 hours of travel.
  - ○ **Rechecks and Rest Every 4 Hours:** Every 4 hours the horses should have at least 30 minutes of trailer rest at a stop. Trailering is particularly tiring on horses since they stand the entire time, balancing and bracing with the start, stops, and sways of the trailer. Drivers should keep their own rest stops as short as possible while the horses are still trailered.
  - ○ **Overnight Rest after 8 Hours:** At least one night of rest should be provided after each 8 hours of trailering. Signs of discomfort in the horses can include restlessness, sweating or trembling, or laying down.
- **Rest Stops:**
  - ○ **Half-Hour Rests:** Stops should occur at least every 4 hours for 30 minutes to allow horses to rest from balancing, drink, and if possible, eat grass.
  - ○ **Encourage Drinking:** Some horses will not drink water that is not from their home. Adding peppermint oil to the horse's water at home and later to water from other sources may induce them to drink water that is not from home. Colic can occur because of reluctance to drink adequately during travel.
  - ○ **Encourage Urination:** Stallions and geldings stretch backwards and spread their hind legs to urinate and many will not urinate in a trailer. Stops every 200 miles or 4 hours may be necessary to prevent urine retention. It is important to stop in places away from traffic where the horse can walk around, graze, urinate, and defecate before resuming travel.
- **Flooring:**
  - ○ **Mats:** Floor mats increase traction, reduce noise, and road heat. For short distance trips, only the rubber mats are sufficient.
  - ○ **Loose Bedding:** Bedding on top of the mats is desirable for longer (more than 2 hours) trips when horses are more likely to urinate in the trailer. Because bedding can reduce the air quality, only low-dust pine or large-flake shavings should be used.
  - ○ **Stall Dividers and Flooring:** Trailer stall dividers should not go to the floor so an adult horse has more room to balance itself. However, if there is a possibility of a foal going under or being thrown underneath a divider, the bottom of the divider should be blocked.

- **Providing Feed:** No feed is needed during short trips of less than 3 hours. Feeding should be done 3 or more hours prior to travel and grass hay provided every 2 to 4 hours to maintain normal gastrointestinal activity. Dust is reduced if fed in a trailer with a manger and wetted hay cubes are used.
- **Blanketing:** Blankets should be avoided in most cases to reduce the risk of overheating. However, in cold weather, the trailer should still be well ventilated. This may necessitate blanketing horses, especially in stock (open) trailers.
- **Eye Protection:** If hauling in a stock trailer or a horse trailer with windows that will be open for ventilation in warm weather, horses should wear fly masks to protect their eyes from flying insects and debris in the trailer, particularly loose bedding materials.
- **Stops for Emergencies:**
  - **Unloading:** If a stop for an emergency becomes necessary, horses should not be unloaded next to a highway. An off-road area away from the highway should be sought and unloading done only if necessary.
  - **Use Emergency Flashers:** Emergency flashers should be turned on. If pulling off the roadway is not an option, flares or flashing lights should be placed 20, 50, 100, 200, and 300 feet behind the trailer. If flares or lights are not available, other people should be enlisted to alert motorists.
  - **Limited Power of Attorney Document:** A Limited Power of Attorney for Animal Health Care document should be kept in the towing vehicle to direct emergency responders who have legal authority to make decisions on treatment of the horses if the owner is injured in an accident while pulling horses in a trailer. Free forms are available at www.usrider.org. USRider is an equestrian motor plan that provides roadside assistance and towing services for the vehicle and horses.
- **Unloading:**
  - **Untie the Lead Rope:**
    - **Untie First:** The lead rope should be untied before releasing the butt bar or chain or opening the back door of the trailer.
    - **Untie without Entering the Trailer Stall:** Untying a horse while in its trailer stall is dangerous and should be avoided whenever possible. Untying horses in stock trailers can be done from outside the trailer. Other trailers may allow the handler to get to the tie ring from a window, a front compartment, or an empty stall adjacent to the horse to be untied.
  - **Train to Wait for Permission to Unload:** Horses should be trained to wait a short period after being untied until they are given permission to come out.
    - **Untie, Wait, and Back When Permitted:** After the horse is untied, the handler should open and secure the back door against wind gusts and then release the butt bar or chain. The handler then goes into the trailer to pet the horse briefly for standing still and then asks it to quietly back up.
    - **Risks:** If the horse rushes back and is still tied, a handler could get caught in the thrashing. Rushing back is unacceptable and indicates the need for more training in loading and unloading for the horse.
  - **After Unloading:** After the horse is unloaded, care should be taken if tying to the trailer. Ties near door latches that may catch a lead rope or wheel wells where a pawing hoof might get caught should be avoided.
- **Trailer Check, Maintenance, and Towing:**
  - **Proper Trailer and Towing Vehicle:** Safer trailering requires proper trailer and towing vehicle selection and maintenance.
    - **Vehicle Towing Capacity:** Towing weights should not exceed 85% of the towing vehicle's maximum towing capacity.

- ○ **Towing Packages:** The vehicle should have a factory-equipped or after-factory-added towing package. Towing packages typically include over-sized battery, high output alternator, wiring harness for the trailer, heavier brakes and suspension, transmission oil cooler, oversized radiator, high-capacity water pump, and an axle ratio that is geared for towing. Over-sized extendable side mirrors are also helpful.
- **Annual Inspection:** Most states do not require yearly safety inspections of horse trailers, but an annual inspection should include the wiring, brakes, and emergency breakaway cable, pin, and control box (Table 4.6).

Table 4.6	Annual Inspections of Horse Trailers
•	**Wheel Bearings**—Wheel bearings should be repacked annually or every 12,000 miles
•	**Emergency Breakaway System**—Horse trailers are required to have a battery-operated emergency breakaway system to activate the trailer brakes if the trailer comes uncoupled from the truck during travel
•	**Flooring**—Wood floorboards should be checked for rot and aluminum floorboards checked for weakening from oxidation
•	**Tire Tread**—Tires should have at least 1/4 inch of tread, but trailer tires should be replaced at six years, regardless of the extent of wear
•	**Tire Load Rating**—The load rating for most trailers is at least "D," that is, an 8-ply tire designed ST (stiff sidewalls) to prevent sway and carry heavy loads
•	**Brake Adjustment**—Drum brakes should be adjusted every 5,000 miles.

- **Pre-Trip Maintenance Checklist for Horse Trailers:** A maintenance checklist should be reviewed prior to each trip (Table 4.7).

Table 4.7	Checklist Prior to Hauling Horses
•	Check tire tread, tire pressures, vehicle and trailer lights, brakes, and floor of the trailer.
•	Check interior for sharp edges, protruding nuts or bolts, wasp or rodent nests, and spoiled feed.
•	Open vents, but do not open drop down windows if horses could stick their head out during travel.
•	Clean and inspect flooring after each haul.
•	Inspect all fluid levels in towing vehicle.
•	Lubricate the trailer ball and check it for tightness and check coupler on trailer for proper operation and an effective locking mechanism.
•	After hooking up the trailer, make sure the hitch is properly attached and locked in place, the safety chains are crossed underneath the hitch and attached to the towing vehicle properly, and the break-away emergency stop cable is attached.
•	Pull the trailer empty and check the brakes on the towing vehicle and the trailer.
•	Load emergency materials for people and horses: first aid kits, A-B-C rated fire extinguisher, blankets, and drinking water.
•	Load emergency tools: flashlight and spare batteries, jumper cables, duct tape, extra halters and lead ropes, spare vehicle bulbs and fuses, crowbar, pliers, screwdrivers, wrenches, hammer, traction devices in winter, properly inflated truck and trailer spare tires, vehicle jacks, lug-nut wrenches, three emergency reflective triangles, and four tire chocks.
•	Load hygiene tools: broom, shovel, manure fork, bucket, and sponges.
•	Secure all tack and supplies to prevent slipping, sliding, or rolling around during travel.
•	Carry legal and emergency paperwork: registration papers and titles for the truck and trailer, emergency veterinary contact information, Limited Power of Attorney for Animal Health Care document, veterinary health certificates (Certificate of Veterinary Inspection) if crossing state lines, Coggins test papers, and if needed, a brand inspection certificate.

- **Trailer Turnover Accident:**
    - **Be Calm to Calm Horses:** If confronted with a trailer turnover accident with entrapped live horses, the handler should approach the trailer slowly to minimize the risk of inciting struggling.
    - **Set up a Perimeter Containment:** A perimeter containment should be created in case a horse becomes free.
    - **Carefully Free the Horse's Head:** If a horse cannot stand because its head is tied fast, tape a knife to a pole to cut the lead rope. Do not climb or reach into the trailer.
- **Pickup Beds:**
    - **Feasibility for Hauling:** Most domestic ranch and farm animals can be transported in appropriately prepared pickup beds, including horses. Pickup beds can be floored with mats to improve footing and outfitted with a rack on all four sides that are withers height or higher. Seasoned ranch horses can be trained to jump into pickup beds.
    - **Advantages:** Transporting them in a pickup bed avoids the expense of a trailer, the time involved in hooking and unhooking a trailer, and the difficulty of backing and parking a trailer.
    - **Disadvantages:** There is risk of the vehicle being top-heavy, increasing the possibility of tip-over. Eye injuries may occur, especially if the horse is not tied to face backward to the cab or does not wear a fly mask. Plus, there is no overhead shelter from sun, rain, and hail.

AIR TRAVEL

- **Occurrence:** Horses have been transported in airplanes for more than 70 years. Travel containers are similar to a small box stall. The horse is usually cross-tied.
- **Pre-Flight Preparation:** At least 5 hours should be allowed for a horse to rest before it is loaded onto an air transport plane. Grain should not be fed immediately before, during, or immediately after flying.
- **In-Flight Attendant:** A handler needs to stay with the horses during takeoff, turbulence, and landings. There should be at least one groom for every three horses.
- **Water and Hay:** Hay should be available and water offered every 1 to 2 hours.
- **Halter Only:** The horses should wear only a halter. Leg wraps are avoided since they can come loose during flight and are unsafe to reapply while in flight. Blankets, boots, and head bumpers can cause the horse to overheat.
- **Allow Sufficient Rest:** At least one night of rest should be provided after each 2 hours of air travel.
- **No Chemical Restraint:** Tranquilization or sedation is inadvisable since it could affect the horse's ability to balance itself during flight.

DONKEYS, MULES, AND HINNIES

Donkeys have served as beasts of burden for humans for about 5,000 years. They have been used for riding, pulling wagons and carts, and guarding livestock, especially sheep from canine predators. Donkeys bred to horses produce the hybrids mules and hinnies. There is unique terminology for the gender and species of donkeys and mules (Table 4.8).

Table 4.8	Gender and Species Terminology for Donkeys and Mules	
•	**Jack**—MALE DONKEY (ALSO CALLED AN *ass*)	
•	**Jenny**—FEMALE DONKEY	
•	**Mule**—OFFSPRING OF A JACK AND MARE	
•	**John**—MALE MULE OR HINNY	
•	**Molly**—FEMALE MULE OR HINNY	
•	**Hinny**—OFFSPRING OF A STALLION AND A JENNY	
•	**Burro**—DONKEY IN SPANISH.	

DONKEYS

- **Natural Behavior:**
  - **Social Structure and Reaction to Danger:** Donkeys evolved in rocky, arid, semi-desert conditions which required the ability to defend themselves from predators since they were unlikely to outrun them. Food was scarce and large groups could not find enough food in one location. Their social structure became based on family units rather than herds.
    - **Family Unit:** The family unit is typically a jenny, foal, and yearling protected by a dominant jack. Less dominant males usually form bachelor groups.
    - **Strong Bond with Favored Herdmate:** Within families and bachelor groups, a donkey will form strong bonds with just one or two other donkeys and become very distressed if separated from their preferred herdmate. If they do not have a donkey herdmate, they will bond with a horse or pony which, if removed from the pasture for training or work, will cause the donkey to become distressed.
    - **Reactions to Danger:** A donkey's ability to flee from danger is less than that of horses, so donkeys are less flighty (less likely to easily startle and run) and more fighty (they are more likely to attack or freeze in place, if threatened). They will bray loudly to either communicate with scattered members of the family unit foraging for food or to deter a predator. Mules retain most of these donkey characteristics.
    - **Aversion to Dogs:** Donkeys have a natural aversion to dogs. Desensitization to dogs usually requires a longer period than in horses.
  - **Protective of Territory:** Donkeys become very territorial and are intolerant of new animals in their environment or smaller animals such as dogs, cats, sheep, and chickens if not desensitized to them.
  - **Tolerant:** Because of their calm disposition, jennies have been used to teach foals to be led by a halter and lead rope and to develop patience in being handled.
  - **Variations in Size:** Minis are under 36 inches in height at the withers. Standards are 36 to 54 inches, and Mammoths are taller than 54 inches. Each can carry up to 25% of its weight in combined tack, supplies, and rider.
- **Approaching and Catching:**
  - **Benefits of Early Training:** Capturing a donkey that has had frequent handling when it was young is usually easy. Most will approach a handler, and others will stand still when moved to a corner.
  - **Move with Herdmate:** Separating a donkey from a herd is very difficult because they usually have a special buddy and do not like separation. It is best to move the herd to the desired location, capture the donkey wanted, and then

move the herd back. If the buddy has been identified, it should be kept with the desired donkey, if possible.

- **Neck Collars:** Breakaway neck collars are convenient means of capture and restraint with less risk than halters of catching on pasture hazards.

- **Handling for Routine Care and Management:**
  - **Routine Restraint:**
    - **Use Minimum Required Restraint:** As with other animals, as little restraint as possible should be used with donkeys. It is good to talk to and pet donkeys, but a handler should avoid stroking their eyes, ears, and flanks which they may resent.
    - **Halters:** Halters for ponies or horses can be used on donkeys, but many donkeys do not like their ears touched, so their ears should be avoided when haltering. Handlers should unfasten the crownpiece strap, position it behind the ears, and refasten. The crownpiece should not be pulled over ears.
    - **Head Hug and Chin Hold:** The chin hold consists of placing a thumb into the bars of the mouth and grasping its chin (Figures 4.36 and 4.37). A halter or loop of rope around the donkey's neck should also be present and held with the other hand, rather than grasping an ear. If the donkey backs up to escape the hold, the handler should go with it and guide it using the chin hold as a rudder to position its rump into a corner of a stall or pen.
    - **Avoid Nose Twitches:** Nose twitches are not well tolerated and donkeys will often strike out with a foreleg.
  - **Leading and Tying:**
    - **Leading with a Lead Rope:** Donkeys that are frequently handled may be led with a halter and lead rope as with a horse. Those that do not lead by a halter and lead rope can be driven by the handler being on the donkey's left side and reaching over the donkey's flank to tap the donkey's right flank with a hand or a stick (Figure 4.38).
    - **Lead Plus Rump Shove:** If three people are available to move the donkey, one can lead while the other two use a tied loop to assist with the rump.
    - **Two Handler Carry:** Untrained donkeys may be small enough for two handlers to cradle in their arms and carry short distances (Figure 4.39).
    - **Tie by Lead Rope:** Donkeys are tied by their lead rope in the same manner as horses, but tie rings must be placed lower than that for horses. The donkey should be tied at its withers height, or a little above. Donkeys are not as claustrophobic as horses and can be tied closer than horses to a tie ring.
  - **Riding, Guiding, and Driving:**
    - **Carrying Weight Capacity:** Adult donkeys can carry people who weigh up to about 100 lb.
    - **Required Riding Tack:** They have a much different conformation of their back and thorax than that of horses and ponies. Therefore, saddles must be made specifically for donkeys because pony saddles will not fit properly. Due to the shape of their chest, the saddle should be fitted with a crupper, a strap that attaches the back of the saddle to the base of the tail to prevent the saddle from sliding forward.
    - **Directing Movement:** Depending on the style of training received, saddle donkeys can be guided by taps with a stick on the sides of their neck or by a bridle with a snaffle bit and reins.
    - **Pulling Capacity:** On level ground, a donkey can pull up to 300 lb. when trained with long reins, a proper harness, and light cart.
  - **Lifting a Foot:** Handlers must not lift the feet as high as is typical of holding horses' feet. Instead, donkey feet should be held lower for their comfort, not above the handler's knee. If they are older and could have arthritis, their feet should be lifted as low as feasible.

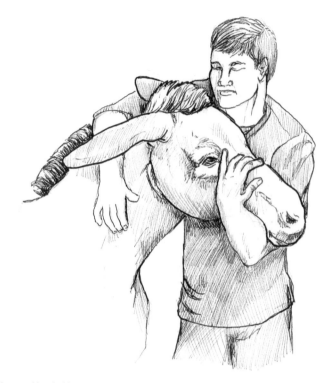

Figure 4.36　Head hug hold.

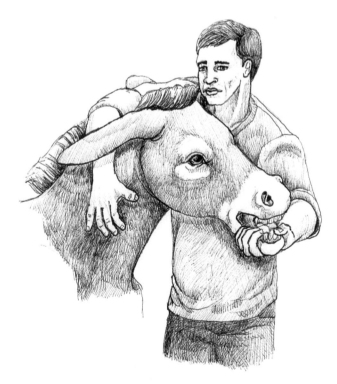

Figure 4.37　Chin hold.

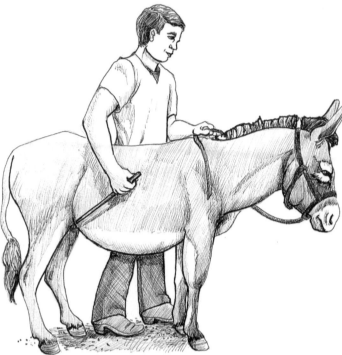

Figure 4.38   Driving a donkey by tapping with a stick.

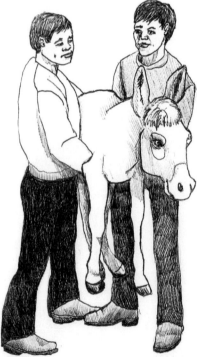

Figure 4.39   Small, untrained donkeys may be carried by two handlers.

MULES AND HINNIES

- **Comparison of Mules and Hinnies:** See Table 4.9.

Table 4.9 Comparisons of Mules and Hinnies

	Mules	Hinnies
Parents	Male donkey, female horse	Female donkey, male horse
Overall Size	Horse size	Smaller than average horse
Color	More similar to donkey	More similar to horse
Behavior	Somewhat similar to a horse	More similar to donkey
Popularity	More common due to easier breeding and larger size	Less common

- **Mules:**
  - **Behavior:**
    - **Independent:** Mules are more independent than horses, but like donkeys, they will not entrust as much leadership to humans as horses do. Mules will defer to human leadership, but they are less submissive than horses. They are less herd bound and less inclined to spook and bolt.
    - **Intolerant to Rough Handling:** Mules are less prone to forgive rough handling than horses. Difficulty in handling mules may be from bad experiences the mule had earlier in life. A mule will remember specific individuals who have been unkind to them.
  - **Physical Characteristics:** Mules have exceptional strength, endurance, and donkey-like, hard feet that are small for their size and designed for rocks and desert conditions. The manes of mules are roached (cut short) because the mane is stiff and sticks up getting in the way of a pulling collar. They are less athletic in turning and running than horses.
- **Hinnies:** Hinnies have a more horse-like appearance than mules. However, they tend to have more behavioral characteristics of a donkey since they are imprinted by their jenny mother around donkeys, compared to mules being raised by their mare mother around horses.
- **Handling Mules and Hinnies:** Mules and hinnies are handled similarly to horses.
  - **Packing:** Horses and mules can be used for packing but require differently shaped pack side bars than donkeys. The average pack weight for a horse is 175 lb., for a mule 225 lb., and for a donkey 200 lb.
  - **Riding:** Mules and hinnies can also be used for riding. They have thicker withers than horses which cause saddles to slide forward easily, requiring the use of breeching or a crupper, and a breast collar.

BIBLIOGRAPHY

1. Birke L, Hockenhull J, Creighton E, et al. Horses' responses to variation in human approach. Appl Anim Behav Sci 2011;134:56–63.
2. Christensen JW, Ladewig J, Sondergaard E, et al. Effects of individual versus group stabling on social behavior in domestic stallions. Appl Anim Behav Sci 2002;75:233–248.
3. Heather Smith Thomas. Storey's Guide to Training Horses. Storey Publishing, North Adams, MA, 2003.
4. Hill C. Horse Handling and Grooming. Storey Publishing, North Adams, MA, 1997.
5. Lagerweij E, Neils PC, Wiegant VM, et al. The twitch in horses: A variant of acupuncture. Science 1984;225:1172–1174.

6. Mackenzie SA. Equine Safety. Delmar, Albany, NY, 1998.
7. McGreevy P. Equine Behavior: A Guide for Veterinarians and Equine Scientists. 2nd edition. Saunders, New York, 2012.
8. McLean AN. The positive aspects of correct negative reinforcement. Anthrozoos 2005;18:245–254.
9. McMiken DF. Ancient origins of horsemanship. Equine Vet J 1990;22:73–78.
10. Miller RM. Handling Equine Patients. Robert M. Miller Communications, Truckee, CA, 2010.
11. Moyer E. Horse Safety. Bow Tie Press, Laguna Hills, CA, 2008.
12. Payne E, Boot M, Starling M, et al. Evidence of horsemanship and dogmanship and their application in veterinary contexts. Vet J 2015;204:247–254.
13. Reeder D, Miller S, Wilfong D, et al. AAEVT's Equine Manual for Veterinary Technicians. Wiley-Blackwell, Ames, IA, 2009.
14. Sarrafchi A, Blokhuis HJ. Equine stereotypic behaviors: Causation, occurrence, and prevention. J Vet Behav 2013;8:386–394.
15. WorkSafe. Riding Horses on Farms. WorkSafe New Zealand. https://www.worksafe.govt.nz/topic-and-industry/agriculture/working-with-animals/horses/riding-horses-on-farms-gpg/, 2017.

5

CATTLE

DOI: 10.1201/9781003110910-5

Cattle have been domesticated and handled by humans for approximately 8,000 to 10,000 years, beginning in the Middle East and North Africa. The U.S. leads the world in beef production followed by Brazil and the European Union. It is second in the world to India in milk production and dairy processing. Age and gender terms are provided in Table 5.1.

Table 5.1 Age and Gender Terminology for Cattle	
•	**Bull**—ADULT, SEXUALLY INTACT MALE
•	**Steer**—CASTRATED MALE
•	**Ox**—STEER USED FOR PULLING WAGONS
•	**Cow**—ADULT, SEXUALLY INTACT FEMALE
•	**Dry Dairy Cow**—NOT CURRENTLY PRODUCING MILK
•	**Freshen Dairy Cow**—RECENTLY CALVED AND PRODUCING MILK
•	**Heifer**—YOUNG FEMALE COW THAT HAS NOT YET HAD A CALF
•	**Calf**—IMMATURE BULL OR COW.

NATURAL BEHAVIOR OF CATTLE

INHERENT HERD BEHAVIOR

- **Groupings:** Cattle are highly social animals that will form herds whenever possible. Within a herd, three groups tend to develop: female, male, and mixed gender.
  - **Females:** Female groups contain about ten cows, possibly with some young males.
  - **Males:** Male groups are smaller and composed of young males. Older males tend to remain alone when not breeding.
  - **Mixed Gender:** Mixed gender groups form during breeding seasons and contain approximately 15 animals.
  - **Calves:** By 7 weeks of age, calves will sleep in groups.
- **Herd Hierarchy:**
  - **Categories:** Social hierarchy categories within a herd of cattle include leaders, dominants, and submissives (also called subdominants and timids). When a herd moves the leaders lead, followed by the dominants, and trailed by the submissives. Roles as leaders, dominants, and submissives can shift somewhat among some herd members depending on the activity.
  - **Attaining and Maintaining Social Rank:**
    - o **Cows:** In general, the social rank of a cow is well established by 2 years of age and maintained by threat posturing followed by butting when the correct social response does not promptly occur.
    - o **Bulls:** Young bulls play fight to develop tactics and test strength. They gradually become more aggressive and territorial.
    - o **Attaining Rank:** Higher social rank is based on horn size, age, and weight.
  - **Social Roles:**
    - o **Bulls:** The herd bull is the most dominant herd member. The bull does not participate much in herd discipline, except in controlling young bachelor bulls. Other than breeding, its primary objective is to keep the herd separate from other herds.
    - o **Cows:** An older, heavier cow with large horns is more likely dominant than smaller, younger cows, or those with shorter or no horns. Cows

determine their rank in a group by shoving, and each is an individual with a different level of desire to test their rank.

○ **Dominance versus Aggression:** The most dominant individuals are usually not the most aggressive. Dominant adults tend to break up fights among younger herd members. Dominant members maintain a larger personal space than submissives.

○ **Leaders:** Leader cows stay on the periphery of the herd at the edge of their *social distance*, which is the maximum distance that cows will stray from the bulk of the herd. Leaders are inquisitive and initiate movement of the herd. They are also the most likely to approach a handler first and are licked by other cattle more often than other herd members.

SPECIAL SENSES

- **Smell:** Although recognition of herd members is visual, auditory, and olfactory, the sense of smell is more important to cattle than sight or sound for identifying herd members. It is primarily by smell that cows and their calves recognize each other.
- **Visual:** Most communication among cattle is visual by body posture.
- **Auditory:** The "moo" is used in demanding attention from others. A call (also called the hoot or roar) is higher pitched and occurs in a series of short bursts. This is even more demanding and often indicates distress.

DAILY ACTIVITY

- **Grazing:** Cattle graze by apprehending grass with their tongue for 4 to 9 hours per day, mostly in the early morning and late evening. When grazing, cattle spread out more than when moving or resting. Dominants move the greatest distance away from possible threats.
- **Resting and Ruminating:** During midday, cattle seek shade to rest and ruminate. Lying down comprises half of the daytime hours.

DEPRIVATION OF NATURAL BEHAVIOR

Some management practices for cattle do not permit natural behavior.

- **Feedlots:** Feedlots became popular in the 1950s and 1960s to speed weight gains and reduce time to market.
  - **Description:** Feedlots are highly concentrated, unnatural environments for fattening cattle for 75 to 200, or more days. Grazing is eliminated and replaced by multiple feedings of grain and high-energy roughage.
  - **Growth Supplements:** Feedlot cattle are typically treated with antibiotics to prevent liver abscesses that occur from highly concentrated diets, and hormones to stimulate muscle growth. A beta-agonist may be fed to reduce the development of fat, although it can cause anxiety and loss of hooves during hot weather.
- **Veal Production:** Veal is tender meat from dairy bull calves that are 16 to 20 weeks of age. Veal calves in the U.S. may be kept in individual tether stalls and unable to turn around so that they remain cleaner until slaughter. Group housing of veal calves is mandated in Europe.
- **Concentrated Feed Operations:**
  - **Advantages:** Feedlots and veal calf isolation have some advantages over pasture feeding, such as labor economy, inexperienced animal handler safety, protection from predators, and rapid weight gains. However, weight gain can occur without good handling of livestock, so this is not a valid indication of good management.

- **Disadvantages:** The behavior of cattle in feedlots is significantly different from their natural behavior. The risk of cattle fighting, being injured, becoming lame, having bloat, and diarrhea is higher in concentrated animal feeding operations than in pasture management operations.

SAFETY FIRST

Despite their long domestication, cattle are still the most likely farm animals to injure people who handle them (Table 5.2).

Table 5.2	Keys to Safer Handling of Cattle
•	Accustom them to handler presence and handling facilities prior to the need to handle them for other purposes
•	Respect their ability to injure handlers
•	Recognize difference in breed, gender, and seasonal aggressiveness
•	Beware increased self-defensiveness in isolated herd members
•	Herd them quietly and slowly using calmly applied pressure and release on their flight zone
•	Cull overly aggressive individuals.

HANDLER SAFETY

Risks to cattle handlers include being knocked down, trampled, crushed against a wall or fence, stepped on, butted, gored with a horn, kicked, and hit by a tail. Cattle have no upper incisors, just a dental pad, and do not bite. It is important to use the minimal amount of pressure and restraint required to move, sort, or administer treatment.

- **Cause of Handler Injuries:**
  - **Flight and Fight:** Unlike with horses, flight is not an effective means of defense for cattle. Cattle are more inclined to stop and fight.
  - **Improper Handling and Carelessness:** Most injuries to handlers are the result of improper handling or carelessness. Reducing the risk of handler injury requires preventing unnecessary agitation in cattle, preventing improperly maintained containment and handling facilities, and recognizing signs of the desire of some cattle to exhibit aggression.
- **Basic Prevention of Injuries:**
  - **Cull Based on Bad Behavior:** Genetic selection of calm cattle is prudent. Overly aggressive individuals should be culled.
  - **Train Calves Early:** Walking among calves in their first 3 months of life and gentle handling will pay dividends in being able to work with them later as they age. It is good husbandry to socialize calves to humans within a distance that permits cattle movement without undue stress and allows screening inspections for disease or injury. A flight distance no greater than 15 feet should be a goal.
  - **Use Low Stress Handling:** Good handlers move cattle with patience and give them limited options where to go and some time to think about it. If stressful procedures are necessary, they should not be performed by the routine handlers and should be done as gently as practical.
- **Cattle Defenses and Offenses:**
  - **Butting:** If restrained, cattle will thrash their heads to the side to butt. Adequate head restraint of cattle during handling is critical.

- **Kicking:** Cattle kick one leg at a time with a sweep to the outside and down (*cow kick*). Calves may kick with both hind legs at once. A danger zone from a kick backward is within 8 feet from the base of the tail.
- **Slap with a Tail:** A cow's tail is heavy and can inflict pain to any part of the handler's body it hits. A tail can also cause serious injury to eyes.
- **Trampling:** Cattle do not care where they step and will make no attempt to avoid stepping on handlers' feet or running over a downed person.
- **Defensive Aggression:** Bulls, cows with nursing calves, injured cattle, or previously mistreated cattle may charge a handler with an attempt to butt and crush. This is expected inherent defensive aggression by cattle.
- **Dominant Aggression:** Individual bulls or cows that have dominant aggressive behaviors which endanger other cattle or handlers should be culled. One-third of the farm fatalities involving cattle in the Midwestern U.S. are caused by cattle that have exhibited dominant aggressive behavior in the past.

- **Breed Variations:** Temperament of cattle is affected by type and breeds.
  - **Dairy Cattle:** Dairy cattle are selected primarily for their ability to produce milk, not their behavior.
  - **Beef Cattle:** Beef cattle are selected for mothering ability and are more prone to maternal aggression. Beef cows are typically more difficult to handle than dairy cattle because beef cattle are not selectively bred for their ability to be handled, and they are handled little. When they are handled, it is usually for frightening and uncomfortable or painful procedures.
    - **Asian Cattle (Brahman):** Among beef cattle, Brahman are more excitable, sullen, and aggressive than European cattle breeds. Brahman or Brahman crosses (Santa Gertrudis) are more likely to lie down in an alley if stressed. They are also more difficult to sort because they more strongly resist being isolated.
    - **European Breeds:** Large European mainland beef breeds (Charolais, Limonsin, or Simmental) are more excitable than British breeds (Black Angus, Red Angus, or Hereford). All these differences are generalizations that can vary widely among individual cattle and can be markedly altered by good or bad handling.
  - **Dominance among Breeds:** There are also general differences in dominance aggression between members of breeds. Angus and Brahmans are usually dominant to Herefords and Shorthorns. Ayrshires are dominant to Holsteins which are dominant to Jerseys.
- **Gender Variations:**
  - **Bulls:**
    - **Young Bulls:** When bulls are yearlings, they are aggressively playful. As they age beyond 2 years, they can become territorial and more dangerous, particularly during a breeding season if pastured with other bulls.
    - **Adult Bulls:** Bulls are unpredictable and can be exceedingly dangerous. Territorial aggression is demonstrated by pawing, bellowing, tossing their head, and standing broadside to the intruder. Bulls require special handling (Table 5.3).

Table 5.3	Reducing Bull Handling Risks
•	Never try to make a pet of a young bull
•	Never handle a bull alone
•	Bulls should not be raised alone
•	Move them regularly to reduce the risk of territorial aggression and have a companion, at least one steer or dry cow

(Continued)

	Table 5.3 (Continued)
•	Groups of bulls can be maintained without serious fighting if rotation grazing is used, but new members or groups should not be added
•	Moving bulls should not be done by a handler on foot and is best done if moved along with a small group of steers or cows
•	A long, strong stick should be at hand, and an emergency escape route should be identified in advance of need
•	Handlers should be careful of approaching any group of cattle since a bull could be mingling with them and overlooked until it becomes aggressive
•	If moving bulls into a pen, they should be moved at a trot until well inside or they may stop inside the gate and begin fighting because their individual zone has been invaded by competitors
•	Handlers should not attempt to interfere with bulls that are fighting
•	Bulls that will be handled often should have a nose ring and when being led, their heads should be held up by the nose lead
•	Well-trained dogs can be helpful in distracting or herding bulls.

- **Cows:** Cows with calves can be dangerous.
  - **Catching a Nursing Calf:** When catching a calf with the mother nearby, the calf should be kept between the handler and the cow, and the handler should hold the calf's mouth shut. A long, stout stick should be at hand as an emergency deterrent to the cow.
  - **Moving Cows with Calves:** If moving cows with calves, the handler should start the move slowly, allowing time for each cow and calf to find one another. Herding dogs should not be used to move cows with calves.
- **Handling Facilities Risks to Humans:** Cattle handling facilities have at least a holding pen, a crowding tub, a narrow alley, and a chute with a headgate.
  - **Facility Maintenance:** In each area, all surfaces should be free of sharp or rough edges. Nails should be hammered in flat and bolts that are too long should be sawn off.
  - **Proper Attire:** Loose-fitting clothes and rolled-up long sleeves that can get caught on fences and restraint equipment should be avoided.
  - **Catwalk Construction:** Catwalks and walkways more than 2 feet high should have handrails. Catwalks should be 18 inches wide and 36 to 42 inches below the top of the fencing, which is slightly higher than waist height when standing on the catwalk. All catwalk floors and stairs should be non-slip.
  - **Avoid Trapping Arms in Handling Facilities:** Cattle should never be handled between rails of an alleyway due to the risk of head injury or fractured hands and arms.
  - **Handling Facilities and Children:** Children should not be allowed around livestock yards due to danger from the animals and their handling facilities.
- **Exit Strategies and Fending off Attacks:** Cattle handlers must always have a predetermined, feasible emergency exit from a pen or pasture.
  - **Common Escape Route:** The most common emergency exit for cattle handlers is to scramble over or under a fence. The need for a rapid escape is most likely if handling a bull, cow with a calf, or otherwise aggressive cow. Possible escapes in a pasture other than fences can be climbing nearby trees or farm or ranch equipment.
  - **Signs of Impending Attack:** Usually cattle display advance signs of pending attack or group panic.
    - **Head Position:** When cattle are not grazing but relaxed, they hold their head at shoulder height. A head held higher than their shoulders is a sign of fear.

- ○ **Steady Stare:** A steady stare can be a sign of aggression. More definite signs of aggression are slinging of the head or a lowered head with a fixed stare.
- ○ **Broadside Display:** A bull that paws the ground with a broadside display is body language for impending charge.
- ○ **Bellow or Growl:** Bulls will make grumbling sounds if irritated.
- **Response to Possible Attack:**
  - ○ **Stand Erect with Arms Raised to the Side:** The proper response by a handler to signs of aggression is to stand erect, face toward the cow or bull, spread both arms out, and stare at it. Most will move away. Unlike horses that will jump to the side without looking, cattle first look in the direction they plan to move.
  - ○ **Do Not Try to Outrun:** Cattle can outrun a human. Handlers must not try to escape by outrunning an aggressive cow or bull. If a cow showing signs of aggression does not eventually retreat, the handler should continue to stare at it and walk slowly backward. The handler should seek a safe location and later cull the cow from the herd.
  - ○ **Seek a Barrier:** If reaching the other side of a fence from an aggressive bull or cow is not feasible, seek a barrier such as a tree, truck, large hay bale, or other large stationary object to prevent a direct charge.
  - ○ **Move away in 90-Degree Diagonal Paths:** If challenged by a bull, the handler should turn their side to it and walk away sideways or backward. If running to a fence or tree seems possible, the run should be in a zig-zag pattern. There should be no attempt to run in a straight line away from a charging bull or cow.
  - ○ **If Charged, Force the Bull to Turn Frequently:** An evasion action can be to run at a right angle to a charge and force the bull to turn in circles. If in a pen with a bull, a handler is already within their flight zone and a charge may occur without prior indication.
  - ○ **If Down, Crawl or Roll:** If a handler is knocked down by a cow or bull, the handler should not try to stand, nor lay still. It is safer to crawl or roll to safety.
  - ○ **Do Not Handle Bulls Alone:** Handlers should not work a bull alone. Another handler should be present to distract the bull, if the primary handler is trapped or down.
  - ○ **Carry a Big Stick:** If the possibility of aggressive cattle is expected, the handler should carry a 5 or 6 ft stick with a diameter about the size of a baseball bat handle. Just holding a stick up increases the handler's profile size and height which makes the handler appear more dominant.
  - ○ **Whips:** With sufficient practice, stockwhips can be made to make a loud crack that will encourage cattle to move or discourage a challenge to a handler's personal space. However, proper use of a stockwhip is a learned skill. Without sufficient experience in their use, stockwhips can be dangerous to handlers, especially the risk of eye injuries.
  - ○ **Imminent Danger:** Sticks and whips should not be used to strike a cow, except when a handler believes a charge is imminent or has begun and no escape or barrier protection is available. The blow should be to the nose. Serious damage to the cow or bull is unlikely, while striking the animal may save the handler's life.

CATTLE SAFETY

- **Abuse from Handling Ignorance or Economic Gain:** Corporate livestock production, with multi-tiered management, increases the chances that animal handlers may not have sufficient experience and training to handle cattle well or that they have become desensitized to procedures that are abusive.

- **American Meat Institute Foundation Audits of Good Management Practices:** Assessments of the welfare of cattle in meat plants have been advocated by Temple Grandin, livestock welfare advocate. These include how many cattle are limping, the percentage of cattle that vocalize during handling (no more than 3/100 head), running into gates or fences (1/100 or less), and percentage that fall down (no more than 1/100 head).
  - **Acts of Abuse:** Acts of abuse include dragging a live cow with a chain, running cattle on top of each other on purpose, prodding cattle in sensitive parts of their body, slamming gates on cattle on purpose, and beating a cow.
  - **Application of Critical Point Criteria:** Plants that supply McDonalds, Wendy's, and Burger King food chains must be audited for compliance with the critical care criteria. Family-owned cattle and pig farms are not audited although cattle abuse can also occur on some of them.
- **Handling Facilities Risks to Cattle:** Cattle handling facilities can have physical hazards to cattle or be a psychological barrier that causes them to balk. Facilities should be reviewed for hazard potentials before working cattle (Table 5.4).

Table 5.4	Inspection of Cattle Handling Facilities
•	Handlers should drive in protruding nails, saw off bolts that are too long, replace rotten lumber, lubricate gates, and pad clanging steel parts
•	Floors should be uncluttered, sloping to provide drainage, and roughened to provide traction
•	The floor of forcing pens and alleyways should be concrete
•	Fences and gates must be strong enough to hold crowded, pushing cattle
•	Chutes and alleyways should be solid-walled and wide enough for cattle to move forward easily without being able to turn around
•	Handlers should eliminate distractions in the work area, such as clutter, water puddles, shadows, dangling chains, people in flight zones, and hissing and loud noises
•	Blood on the ground or floor can cause cattle to balk and must be cleaned up
•	Gates should be padded with rubber stops to reduce noise
•	The yard design should have cattle moving away from the yard entrance to holding pens but going toward the entrance when in forcing pens and alleyways
•	Movement should be on the same level or uphill
•	Good drainage is important to reduce cattle-distracting pools of water
•	The bottom half of steel pens should be paneled to prevent legs from being caught
•	Yard pens should be long and narrow to aid one person in moving cattle
•	Funnel-shaped entrances into alleyways should be constructed to exit a crowding pen.

- **Handling Methods Adverse to Cattle Care and Safety:** Unfavorable handling of cattle results in decreased weight gains, performance, and resistance to disease as well as causing bruising and injuries. Common handling procedures that cause stress include disbudding/dehorning, vaccinations, castration, weaning, pregnancy checks, dipping, and drenching.
  - **Loud Noises:** Yelling agitates cattle. Handlers should speak at a normal volume with a low tone of voice. Talking to an animal in a calm manner can reduce fear in animals and agitation in the handler.
  - **Isolation from Other Cattle:** Individual animals worked alone are easily stressed and panicked. An escaped animal should never be chased. After herding a cow into an enclosure, a handler should allow 30 minutes for it to calm down before trying to draw it back to a familiar group.

- **Electric Prods:** Electric prods are painful and will panic cattle into injuring themselves or other cattle. Plastic paddles, flags, and streamers should be used rather than electric prods to move or turn cattle (Figure 5.1).
- **Rushing the Gathering Process:** When moving cows with calves, handlers should begin slowly to allow the grazing cows to gather their calves. Cows will hide young calves and graze away from them, returning about every 4 hours to nurse. Rushing a gathering process will result in cows abandoning their calves.

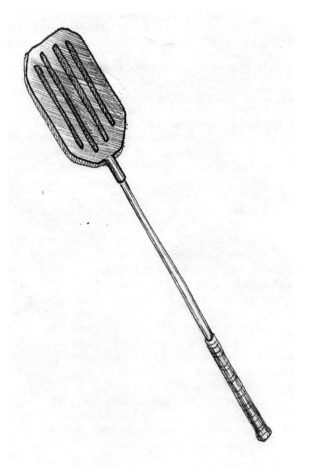

Figure 5.1   Plastic paddle for moving cattle.

- **Balking:**
  - **Causes:** Situations that cause cattle to refuse to move (*balk*) can cause cattle to injure themselves as well as cause inefficiency in their handling. Common causes for balking are seeing commotion or hearing loud noises at the end of the alleyway, seeing a dead end in an alleyway, people in the way of cattle movement, anything that flaps, strange smells, shadows and drains, anything that contrasts with the general appearance of ground or flooring, and moving into glaring sunlight.
  - **Preventing Balking:** See Table 5.5.

Table 5.5	Prevention of Balking
•	Use a chute with a headgate that faces a holding pen with resting cattle
•	Use small pens and work small groups at a time
•	Use the same flooring throughout forcing pen and alleyway
•	Have a floor or ground surface that is level or a rising incline
•	Provide a direction of movement into bright, but not blinding, sunlight
•	Use curved alleyways with solid walls that allow cattle to view two body lengths ahead
•	Pad steel working equipment to reduce noise
•	Reduce the width of the crowding pen.

- **Failure to Desensitize to Handling Environment:**
  - **Desensitize with Food and Water:** Feeding and providing water to cattle in holding pens without working them will help to desensitize them to the fear of being confined and being around handling facilities.
  - **Allow Rest before Working:** The handler should close the gate after cattle are in a pen and let them stand for an hour. Then, the handler should let them out without handling them. Later, the cattle should be released by opening up the crowding pen and alleyway, and letting them progress through the squeeze chute and headgate without catching them.
  - **Benefits of Desensitization:** Familiarization to working facilities without stress will facilitate efficient movement, lower the stress, and improve the safety of handling cattle for needed procedures.
- **Confinement of Dairy Cattle:** Commercial dairy cattle have been selectively bred for milk production without sufficient concern for some other genetic qualities. Their range of movement during a day has been confined, and they are often confined part of the day on concrete. These, and other factors, contribute to a higher susceptibility for lameness in dairy cattle in large-scale operations than in beef cattle on pasture.
- **Docking Tails:** Docking tails is an amputation of up to two-thirds of tail length that is performed on some dairy cattle to reduce a soiled tail from contaminating milk, handlers, and equipment. Tails are also occasionally docked in feedlot cattle to prevent tails from being stepped on in close confinement.
  - **Adverse Effects:** The adverse effects of tail docking in cattle can include inability to avoid biting insects, associated abnormal avoidance behaviors, stump infections, and neuromas.
  - **Controversy:** Although prophylactic tail docking is opposed by the National Milk Producers Federation, the National Mastitis Council, and the American Veterinary Medical Association, tail docking persists in many U.S. states. It is illegal in at least three states and five European countries. McDonald's Corporation has announced that they will not purchase dairy products from groups that practice tail docking.

KEY ZOONOSES
(NOTE: Apparently ill animals should be handled by veterinary professionals or under their supervision. Precautionary measures against zoonoses from sick animals are more involved than those required when handling apparently healthy animals and vary widely. The discussion here is directed primarily at handling apparently healthy animals.)

Apparently healthy cattle pose little risk of transmitting disease to healthy adult handlers who practice conventional personal hygiene. The risks of physical injury are greater than the risks of acquiring an infectious disease (Table 5.6).

Table 5.6 Diseases Transmitted from Healthy-Appearing Cattle to Healthy Adult Humans

Disease	Agent	Means of Transmission	Signs and Symptoms in Humans	Frequency in Animals	Risk Group*
Crushing, Butting, and Kicks	—	Direct injury	Crushing, butting, or kick injuries which can be permanently disabling or lethal	All cattle can inflict serious injuries. Injuries from adult cattle can be fatal.	3
Cryptosporidiosis	Cryptosporidium spp.	Direct, fecal-oral. Indirect from contaminated water	Diarrhea	Common, particularly in dairy calves	2
Colibacillosis	Escherichia coli, 0157:H7	Direct, fecal-oral	Bloody diarrhea, kidney failure, death	Common	3
Brucellosis	Brucella abortus	Direct—secretions, especially placental fluid	Undulant fever, muscle aches, and lethargy	Very low, due to U.S. federal eradication program	3
Q Fever	Coxiella burnetii	Direct with body secretions, particularly milk or placental fluids. Indirect from inhalation of contaminated dust.	Flu-like signs and atypical pneumonia	Moderate in cow-calf operations	2
Leptospirosis	Leptospira spp.	Direct from exposure to urine. Indirect from urine-contaminated water.	Kidney infection	Common in some locations and varies with vaccinations	3
Listeriosis	Listeria monocytogenes	Direct from fecal-oral transmission, but most from ingestion of contaminated beef or dairy products.	Septicemia, atypical pneumonia, and encephalitis	The incidence in cattle and other farm animals may be as high as 52%	3

*Risk Groups (National Institutes of Health and World Health Organization criteria. Centers for Disease Control and Prevention, Biosafety in Microbiological and Biomedical Laboratories, 5th edition, 2009.)
1. Agent not associated with disease in healthy adult humans.
2. Agent rarely causes serious disease and preventions or therapy possible.
3. Agent can cause serious or lethal disease and preventions or therapy possible.
4. Agent can cause serious or lethal disease and preventions or therapy are not usually available.

SANITARY PRACTICES

Sanitary practices when working with cattle are important to prevent transmission of disease from cattle to handlers or to other cattle (Table 5.7).

Table 5.7 Sanitary Practices for Handling Cattle
• Wear appropriate dress to protect against skin contamination with hair and skin scales or saliva, urine, and other body secretions
• Ticks on cattle should be controlled with acaricidal pour-ons, ear tags, or dips
• Keep hands away from eyes, nose, and mouth when handling cattle and wash hands in warm soapy water afterwards
• No one should eat or drink in an animal handling area
• Handling equipment (oral speculums, stomach tubes, dehorning instruments, grooming instruments, balling guns, endoscopes, ultrasound probes, and thermometers) should be cleaned and disinfected before used on cattle from another origin which may be immunologically naive to diseases that a previous group may have carried
• Chutes, alleyways, and concrete flooring should also be cleaned and disinfected
• Sick cattle should be isolated from apparently normal cattle
• New herd members should be quarantined for at least 2 weeks to reduce the risk of transmitting a disease that new animals could be incubating
• Animals, especially calves, should be kept in a clean, dry enclosure
• If handling cattle with diarrhea, handlers should wear gloves and a face shield
• Rubber or plastic gloves should be worn when assisting with calving
• Cattle should be vaccinated for leptospirosis, and exposure to wildlife, especially rodents, should be controlled.

APPROACHING AND CATCHING

CATCHING CATTLE

- **Reasons to Catch:** The degree and frequency of catching and handling cattle varies greatly, as do the reasons.
    - **Dairy Compared to Beef Cattle Reasons:** Freshened dairy cattle are handled twice every day for milking, but beef cattle are usually handled just twice a year.
    - **Calves:**
        - ○ **Twice per Year Collection:** All calves are castrated, vaccinated, and ear tagged in the spring. In the fall, the entire herd is vaccinated and calves are given boosters 2 to 3 weeks later.
        - ○ **Horned Breeds:** Disbudding of horned cattle is performed at 2 to 6 weeks of age with appropriate pain management. Dehorning is performed on older cattle as soon as possible after 6 weeks of age.
        - ○ **Castrations:** Castration should be performed within the first weeks of birth. Castration may be done on weaned calves but should be done in conjunction with local anesthetics.

- **Individual Cow Reasons:** Individual cows may have to be restrained and handled at other times to treat illnesses or injuries, check for pregnancy, or artificially inseminate.
- **Preparations to Catch:**
    - **Facilities Inspection:** Prior to catching cattle, an inspection of all fences, gates, alleyways, and restraint chutes used for catching should be conducted. Weakened points in the facilities should be repaired and distractions to the movement of cattle removed. The facilities should have been previously cleaned and disinfected, appropriate to the type of facilities.
    - **Visual Inspection of Cattle:** The cattle to be caught should be visually inspected prior to catching them. Lameness, labored respirations, lack of appetite, depressed attitude, or other abnormal signs could indicate a need for special handling or rescheduled handling.
- **Most Common Method of Catching Cattle:** The most common approach to catching cattle is to herd them quietly toward or along an enclosure and into an alleyway that goes toward a squeeze chute with a headgate. This should be done without a lot of excitement using a soothing voice. The herd's collective flight zone should be approached at 45 degrees from behind, moving toward a shoulder of one of the dominant cattle in the center of the herd.

CAPTURE AND RESTRAINT OF CALVES

Weaned calves must be handled gently in order to have gentle adult cattle later. Mother cows can be maternally aggressive and should always be removed from the calves before handling the calves. Therefore, handlers should always work in pairs when sorting and catching calves.

- **Capturing a Calf:**
    - **By Hand:** Small calves can be caught by hand if herded with its mother into a pen and then the mother is sorted into another small pen.
    - **Leg Crook:** Small calves may be caught in large pens with a leg crook on a long pole.
    - **By Lariat:** Branding, castration, and disbudding of calves can be efficiently done by roping calves if handlers are skilled in using a lariat.
- **Moving a Calf:** Small calves, under 50 lb., can be moved by putting an arm in front of their chest and the other arm around their rump. They are then picked up and carried, or they are walked forward while blocking backward or side movements. Larger calves must be herded in ways similar to adult cattle.
- **Standing Restraint for Venipuncture:** To perform a venipuncture on a calf, it is backed into a corner by the handler. The handler straddles its neck facing the calf's nose. Access to the jugular vein with both hands can be gained by bending over and pushing the calf's head to the side and holding it with the handler's elbow. This leaves both hands free to perform the venipuncture.
- **Flanking a Calf:** Flanking a calf up to 200 lb. can be useful in treating the umbilicus (navel) or for tattooing, branding, ear tagging, or castration.
    - **Small Calves:** Small calves can be laid down on their side in the same manner as putting a dog in lateral restraint by reaching over the calf's neck and the flank and grasping the front and hind leg closest to the handler's legs (Figure 5.2). The calf is lifted up and its legs rotated away from the handler while letting its body slide down the handler's legs. It is held on its side using the handler's forearm on its neck and holding onto its lower front and rear legs.

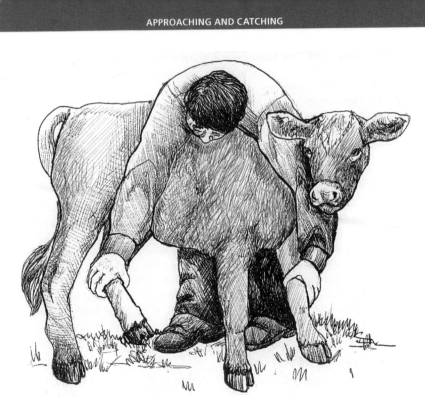

Figure 5.2   Flanking a small calf.

- **Large Calves:** See Procedural Steps 5.1.

Procedural Steps 5.1	Flanking a Large Calf
1.	For larger calves, the handler should stand next to the calf's left side with the left arm under its neck.
2.	The right hand grasps its right flank skin and the left hand is moved and reaches over the calf's back to grasp the right foreleg at its knee.
3.	The handler's right knee is pushed into the calf's left flank.
4.	The calf is lifted in timing with its attempt to jump out of the grasp and its feet rotated away from the handler.
5.	The calf is continued to be held as it slides down the handler's right leg.
6.	To continue to hold a calf down, a handler places a knee on its neck while bending over and holding the upper foreleg.

- **Tying a Flanked Calf with a Pigging String:**
  - ○ **Grasp a Front Leg:** With a downed calf on its left side, a handler straddles the calf's rump in a kneeling position and the right knee is placed behind the calf's hocks. The left hand holds the calf's right front leg, and the right hand is prepared to tie the legs.
  - ○ **Wrap the Three Legs:** To tie the legs, the upper front leg is held in backward extension and a constricting loop on a short cord (pigging string) is placed on the leg. Both hind legs are picked up while pulling the foreleg back. The pigging string is used to make wraps around all three legs and half hitches to tie the three legs together.
  - ○ **Caution:** Both front legs are not tied due to the risk of impairing respiration.

- **Tying a Flanked Calf with a Loop over the Neck:** Another method of tying a downed calf is to use a rope about twice as long as the calf.
  - ○ **Hind Legs Immobilized:** Both hind legs are tied with an end of the rope using half hitches. The middle part of the rope is crossed beneath the calf and placed over the calf's neck. If adjusted correctly, both hind legs should be pulled forward and prevent the calf from rising to its feet.
  - ○ **Castrations:** Castration can be performed with the calf in this position.
  - **Restraint of Large Calves:** Larger calves laid on their side may need to be restrained by two people. One person restrains the head with a knee on the calf's neck while holding the uppermost foreleg in flexed position. The second handler holds and stretches the upper hind leg while sitting behind the calf and bracing a foot against the back of the calf's other thigh. When releasing the calf, the handler restraining the hind legs should release first.
- **Packing Groups of Calves:** Calves can be crowded into alleyways as the only restraint for procedures that require minimal restraint, such as vaccinations and pour-on insecticides. Calves can also be *drenched* (given liquid medications) moving through the group from front to back. Treated individuals are marked with livestock paint crayons to prevent double treatment or missing a treatment.

HANDLING FOR ROUTINE CARE AND MANAGEMENT

TRAINING CATTLE TO BE HANDLED

All cattle should be habituated to being handled by humans with short practice exercises less than 30 minutes for reasons of safety of humans and cattle and for reasons of maintaining optimum productivity in the production of beef or milk. As with other species, whenever a handler is around cattle, the handler is training them for good or bad future responses whether or not they realize it. Handling needs to be consistent among all handlers and from one handling to the next.

- **General Considerations for Training:** When handled often, cattle can be moved by hand motions, body language, and verbal directions (Table 5.8).

Table 5.8 Basics of Training Cattle to Be Handled	
•	Walking among cattle when they are weanling calves with no purpose other than to have them adjust to a handler's presence makes a great difference in how they can be handled later
•	If dogs or horses may be used to handle cattle, they should be led as a handler walks among the cattle
•	When mingling with cattle, the handler should wear the same hat, call them with the same call, talk or sing to them in the same way, and otherwise act in the same manner
•	Direct stares, which could be perceived by cattle as a predator stare, should be avoided
•	Mingling among the cattle by handlers will assist in assessing individual cow behavior
•	The handler should stand with their side toward the cattle and arms by their side to minimize their appearance until the cattle become more adjusted to their presence
•	When a handler moves, it should be with natural movements with the arms and shoulders at a normal pace.

- **Training in a Holding Pen:**
  - **Allow Time to Settle:** Training is accomplished by putting a small group of calves or untrained cows in a holding pen and allowing them to settle for 20 minutes.

- **Slowly Press the Collective Point of Balance:** The handler slowly moves them around the inside of the pen's perimeter by briefly invading their flight zone at about 45 to 60 degrees behind their collective point of balance. Only the edge of the flight zone is worked. Invading the flight zone will cause cattle to run, scatter, or fight.
- **Allow Rest as a Reward:** The handler should occasionally stop the cattle in a corner and allow them to rest for a couple of minutes. After the brief rest, they are moved again and stopped in another corner. This exercise is done for up to 30 minutes.
- **Repeat Training Exercise on a Regular Basis:** Movement should be practiced both directions and should be repeated daily for at least three days. Refresher moving exercises should be done monthly for at least three consecutive days. A primary goal of the exercises is to move the cattle with them remaining at a walk.
- **Use One Handler and One Person to Work Gates:** More than two handlers in a pen at the same time is confusing to the cattle. One handler moves the cattle and the other works the gates.
- **Moving by Horseback:** If cattle will be moved by horseback handlers, practice cattle moving exercises on horseback similar to walking handler exercises should be done. If horseback handlers move cattle, there should be no walking handlers in the pen due to the likelihood of those on foot being trampled.
- **Dairy Cows:**
  - **Dairy Heifers Must Be Trained to Be Herded:** Dairy cows have calves in order to become freshened, but since the milk production is for human consumption, heifer calves are moved in the first day of birth to hutches with small pens.
    - **Market Calves:** Surplus or market calves are sold at 2 weeks of age.
    - **Veal Calves:** Some bull calves may be kept for veal production. They will remain in individual pens or stalls until sent to slaughter by 20 weeks of age.
    - **Replacement Heifers:** Replacement heifers remain in individual pens for the first 8 weeks of life and are fed a commercial milk replacer. They learn to approach handlers for food and mental enrichment and may become aggressive which can be problematic when they become older and must be herded. Therefore, young heifers need to be grouped by 9 weeks with other calves and taught to be herded.
  - **Milking Parlors:** Introduction of heifers to a milking parlor should be quiet and gentle. Food should be provided.
    - **First Handling of Udder:** If there is an objection to the first handling of the udder (which should be brief and gentle), a tail jack, chest twitch, or flank rope or clamp can be used until the heifer tolerates the handling. The release from restraint should be delayed until after the heifer quietly accepts the food, being in the parlor, and receiving gentle handling. Release from restraint should be gradual and blended with exhibiting calmer behavior.
    - **Rectal Palpation Should Not Be Performed in the Milking Parlor:** Palpation for insemination or pregnancy diagnosis should not be done in milking parlors. Nothing should occur in a milking parlor that might cause a heifer to avoid going into the parlor in the future.

BASIC HANDLING AND RESTRAINT EQUIPMENT AND FACILITIES

- **Location, Flow Assessment, Lighting, and Maintenance:**
  - **Location and Fencing:** A handling and restraining site should be along a central fence line to aid in moving cattle toward working facilities at a point that is well-drained and reasonably dry. Fences near and in the working facilities need to be higher and stronger than pasture fencing.

- **Video Assessment of Flow:** Balking in alleyways and chutes can be more carefully investigated by making a video at cattle height while walking through the cattle passages. The movie can be evaluated for noises, changes in flooring, visibility of handlers, glare of light, and other reasons for discouraging the movement of cattle.
- **Lighting:**
  - **Bright and Diffuse:** Lighting should be bright, diffuse lighting that does not glare into the cattle's eyes. Translucent plastic panels permit diffuse light that eliminates shadows.
  - **Subdued Colors:** Dull, subdued colors should be used on painted areas.
  - **Directed Lighting:** Lighting should become brighter toward the restraint stanchion or headgate. However, cattle should not be expected to move into glaring sunlight that will impair their vision and raise suspicions of the unknown.
- **Constant Maintenance:** The facility should be designed and maintained in a condition that eliminates gouges and cuts (bolt ends cut off, nails pounded in, sharp or jagged metal edges repaired) and is functional and relatively quiet (fence gates, drop down gates, and squeeze chutes lubricated and padded).
- **Basic Components:** Basic handling facilities for cattle include collecting pens, crowding pens, working alleyway, squeeze chute and headgate, and loading/unloading chutes (Figure 5.3). Alleyways, crowding pens, squeeze chutes, and loading ramps should have solid sides to block cattle's peripheral vision.

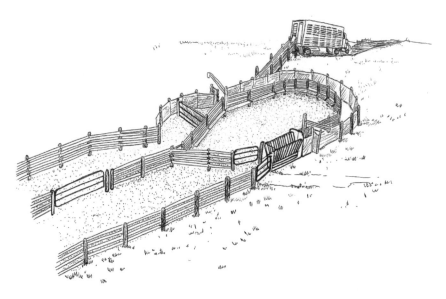

Figure 5.3   Basic cattle handling facilities.

- **Alleyways:** Well-designed alleyways and chutes are curved, solid-sided, constructed of the same material (including color and texture) throughout.
  - **Alleyway Use (Working Chute, Race):** Many procedures, such as vaccinations, spraying for external parasites, and applying pour-on insecticides, can be performed on cattle without restraining their head in a head catch (stanchion or headgate). They can be pressed together in an alleyway by using blocking gates or butt bars. Working front to back helps keep them tight together.
  - **Construction of Working Alleyways:**

- o **Walls:** A working alleyway should have walls 5 ft high. If Brahman cattle will be handled, the height should be 66 to 72 inches. Flaring the walls outward from the floor forces the feet of cattle to not spread out and helps prevent attempted turnarounds and associated balking. Vertical gaps in alleyways (*man-passes*) allow safety escapes or movement from one side of an alleyway to another.
- o **Width:** The center width should be 18 inches for small calves and up to 28 inches wide for adult cows. Large bulls may need up to 32 inches. The bottom should be 15–18 inches wide.
- o **Curved Alleyways:** Alleyways should be curved with a radius of 12 to 20 ft that permits cattle to see only two cattle lengths ahead. No corner in an alleyway should be more than 30 degrees. The minimum length should be 30 ft, but much longer alleyways may allow cattle to stand in one place too long and some will lay down.
- o **Ventilated Walls:** If solid sides could create ventilation problems, a 1–2 ft wide rail at cow eye height may be a useful compromise to a solid sided alleyway. The solid sides may also be flaps of canvas or rubber which allow the handler to reach into the alleyway to help move the cattle, if needed.
- o **Emergency Release Side Panels:** Emergency release panels allow cattle that go down to get out and regain their feet.
- o **End Gate:** The gate at the end of the alleyway should be made of bars to allow vision of the outside and encourage forward movement to the end.
- o **Overhead Restrainers:** Overhead restrainers 5 ft above the alleyway can stop rearing, turning around, and falling over backwards.
- o **Flooring:** Drains and grates should be located outside alleyways to avoid being a cause for cattle balking in an alleyway. Concrete in alleyways and crowding pens should be grooved in 8-inch squares or diamonds for better footing. Deep groves should not be used in milking parlors or other daily traffic areas due to excessive wear on hooves.
- **Catwalks:** Catwalks keep the handler above the sight of cattle helping forward movement. Handlers should step up on catwalks away from the cattle to prevent from startling them with a sudden appearance. Continually speaking in a normal tone also helps cattle be aware of handler presence and avoid startle responses.
- **Anti-Backup Gates and Butt Bars:** Alleyways should have drop down anti-backup gates rather than metal pipes (butt bars, slip rails) that are preferably worked with a control rope. If butt bars are used, they should block 6 to 8 inches below the average-sized cow's tail head.
- **Pens:** Types of pens can include holding pens, collecting pens, funneling pens, hospital pens, and quarantine pens.
  - **Size and Number:** Pens should be numerous, small, and with good gates. Pen fences should be 5 to 6 ft high.
  - **Handler Emergency Exit:** For pens in which handlers may be in with cattle, there should be a 16-inch clearance at the bottom of gates that can provide room for a handler to roll under in an emergency.
  - **Funneling (Redirection) Pens:** Funneling of small groups of cattle into single cattle-wide alleyways can be done with crowding pens (tubs) or with small pens with precisely located gates called Bud boxes.
    - o **Crowding Pens:** Crowding pens work cattle with handlers on catwalks outside the pen and are safer for inexperienced handlers or when working with aggressive cattle.
    - o **Bud Boxes:** Bud boxes require handlers with experience to be in the pen with cattle that enter a pen as a group through a large gate as they are redirected toward a small gate and into a single file alleyway.
    - o **Crowding Pen:** See Table 5.9 and Figure 5.4.
    - o **Bud's Box:** See Table 5.10 and Figures 5.5, 5.6, and 5.7.

Table 5.9 Use of a Crowding Pen

• When using a crowding pen ("forcing" or "sweep" pen), a handler should not fill the pen/tub with too many cattle at a time as this prevents movement needed to turn and to go the correct direction into an alleyway (Figure 5.4)
• Most crowding pens for cattle have a 12 ft radius designed for five to ten head, but inexperienced handlers tend to overfill them
• When moving cattle into the alleyway, the large swing gate should follow them and not shove the cattle
• Working fewer cattle at a time enables the entire job to take less time
• Crowding pens for domestic cattle should be filled to half to three-fourths full capacity
• Entrances to alleyways from crowding pens for cattle must gradually funnel them into the single file alleyway and not have a sharp angle between the crowding pen and alleyway
• Crowding pen walls and gates should be solid to block cows' vision from outside distractions
• The alleyway gate should be self-closing or have a self-closing latch.

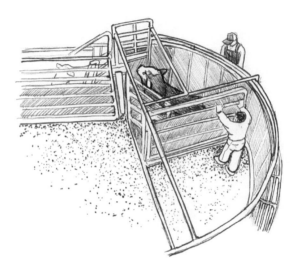

Figure 5.4 Crowding pen.

Table 5.10 Use of a Bud's Box

• A Bud's box is a pen constructed of pipe rails or thick board planks with a large group gate and a small individual cow gate (Figures 5.5–5.7)
• The working principle is to bring cattle into a small pen via a large gate, close the large gate, and herd the cattle around the perimeter of the pen and through a small gate in a corner adjacent to the large gate
• The small gate leads to a single file alleyway
• The pen is typically 12 ft wide and 20 ft deep
• If handlers move the cattle on horseback the width can be 14–16 ft
• The depth can be up to 30 feet if used to fill transport trailers
• The portion of the pen opposite the gates can be rounded or have blocked corners to turn cattle more easily and should permit visibility beyond the end of the pen so that cattle move into a pen without hesitation
• Four to 20 cattle can be funneled at a time depending on their size and length of the exit alleyway.

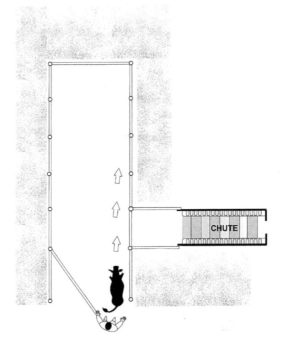

Figure 5.5 Entering Bud's box.

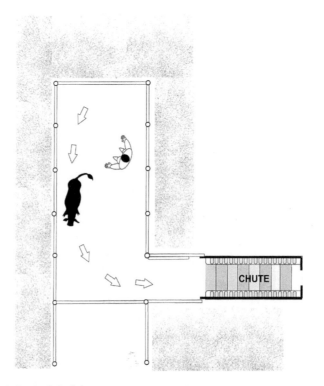

Figure 5.6 Redirecting in Bud's box.

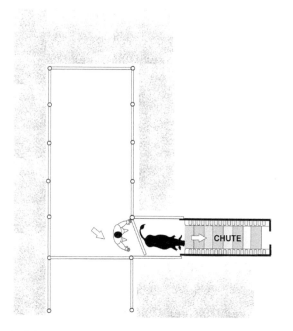

Figure 5.7   Exiting Bud's box.

- **Squeeze Chute:** Squeeze chutes are metal boxes with a headgate to entrap individual cattle. Headgates are head catches that close on the cow's neck preventing it from escaping forward or back but can also open as a front gate. Squeeze chutes are integrated with a headgate.
    - **Uses:** Procedures that are best performed in a squeeze chute and headgate are vaccinating, giving injectable medications, drenching, bolusing, castrating, dehorning, treating eye conditions, giving fertility exams, implanting, ear tagging, branding, bolus administering, stomach tubing, and collecting blood from the jugular vein.
    - **Accessibility in Squeeze Chutes:** A squeeze chute can press on the sides of the cow's body to prevent side-to-side movement. The upper section of the sides has drop down bars and the lower section has removable panels to provide access to different areas of the cow's body (Figure 5.8).

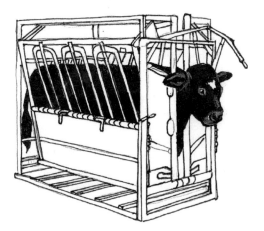

Figure 5.8   Cattle squeeze chute with scissors headgate.

- **Stability:** All squeeze chutes, including portable ones, should be securely fixed to the ground to prevent tipping or sliding.
- **Strength of Construction and Padding:** A squeeze chute and headgate should be 1-inch steel rods welded flush with the floor in scales and squeeze chutes. Equipment should be padded where steel hits steel. The headgate should move smoothly, quietly, and quickly.
- **Proper Placement Outdoors:** Outdoor squeeze chutes should be oriented north-south to prevent cattle facing the sun when approaching the chute. Single file alleyways leading to restraint chutes should be curved.
- **Chute Sides:** Squeeze chutes are V-shaped with the lower portion about half to two-thirds the width of the shoulder space which encourages the cattle to slow down when entering the chute.
- **Floor Width:** The lower aspect of the V-shape is about 16 inches wide and twice as wide at the top. The width of the floor in the squeeze chute should be set to 6 inches for 400–600 lb. calves, 8 inches for 600–800 lb., and 12–16 inches for adult cattle. The squeeze should work from both sides to prevent unbalancing the cow.
- **Texture of Flooring:** The flooring should be non-slip. Cattle will move into a chute if the flooring is the same color and texture as the alleyway floor. If that is dirt, dirt should be thrown onto the chute floor.
- **Squeeze Cattle Slowly:** Application of squeezing the sides should be slow and steady to reduce agitation.
- **Side Access Panels:** Squeeze chutes typically have removable 2 ft high side panels for access to the lower aspects of the cow with individually removable vertical bars for access to different areas of the cow's upper body. The entire side of the chute should open to rescue a cow that is down in the chute to regain her feet.
- **Potential for Arm, Hand, and Head Injuries:** Handlers should always open and close swinging gates in livestock enclosures, including headgates, with outstretched arms to reduce the risk of being knocked down by a bumped gate. A cow restrained in a headgate will typically put her head down and then jump forward bumping her shoulders against the gate while raising her head.
- **Manual or Hydraulic Operation:** Squeeze chutes and headgates can have either manual or hydraulic action. Most hydraulic chutes operate at 500 psi and have pressure release valves. The pressure setting should not squeeze excessively which can frighten or injure cattle, and squeezing should be slow and steady to limit movement without unneeded pressure.
- **Headgates:** The headgate in a squeeze chute entraps the cow's head just behind its ears. Cattle are driven into the chute and caught by vertical bars as soon as the ears go through and before the shoulders get into the headgate. As soon as the head is caught, a bar is placed behind the cow to prevent it from pulling back on its jaw and ears (Figure 5.8).
  - **Chute Assisted Restraint:** Depending on the restraint needed, the sides of the chute may be squeezed against the cow to limit movement.
  - **Neck Bars:** Headgates can have straight or curved bars to catch the neck. Curved bars limit the vertical movement of the head more than straight stanchions which reduces the risk of being butted by an upward head movement, but curved bars can cause choking if the cow goes down.
  - **Head Bars and Nose Bars:** Headgates may have adjunct swinging bars. A head bar is a straight bar that goes over the back of the neck preventing the head from being thrown upward. A nose bar has a bend in the middle that fits over the bridge of the nose preventing the head from thrusting forward.
  - **Stanchions:** A stanchion is a simple head catch without a chute.
  - **Types of Headgates:** There are four types of headgates: scissors, fully opening, positive control, and self-catching. The most common type is scissors.

- ○ **Scissors:** A scissors stanchion has halves that pivot from the bottom and squeeze the sides of a cow's neck. It opens from the front, and the bars may be straight or have a curve at the points of contact with the neck. This headgate may have accessory head table or nose bar attachments to limit vertical head movement.
- ○ **Fully Opening:** The fully opening headgate has headgate halves that work like sliding doors. It permits an easier exit for large cows and bulls.
- ○ **Positive Control:** The positive control (guillotine) headgates close from above and below which can cause choking. Positive control headgates were more common when horned cattle were popular. Release is relatively slow, requiring the cow to back up releasing its head and then opening the front like a swinging gate or releasing from the side of the chute.
- ○ **Self-Catching:** The self-catching headgate works by a cow's shoulders hitting the stanchion bars and moving them forward to close. This can malfunction and allow escape if not properly adjusted for the size of each animal.
- ● **Headgate Bars:** Straight bars allow the head to easily move vertically. Curved bars may put pressure on the carotid arteries and cause the cow to faint. Prolonged procedures, like many veterinary medical procedures, should be performed in straight bar headgates.
- ● **Tying Lead Ropes to Cleats:** When tying a lead rope to a cleat on the side of the headgate, the handler must pull and hold the line while making wraps and ending with half hitches on the cleat. The wraps should be done with the heel of the hand to protect fingers from getting trapped if the cow suddenly tugs on the lead rope.
- ● **Manual Levers:**
  - ○ **Types:** Manual levers can be ratchet-latch or friction-latch. Ratchets are noisier. Friction latches can become insecure with wear.
  - ○ **Protruding Levers:** Protruding levers on manual chutes are dangerous and can cause operator head and hand injuries and even death. Protruding levers are eliminated with hydraulic chutes.
- ● **Training for Squeeze Chutes and Headgates:** Although it is an uncommon procedure in the U.S., cattle should be trained for restraint in squeeze chutes and headgates (Procedural Steps 5.2).

Procedural Steps 5.2   Initial Training Cattle for Squeeze Chutes and Headgates
First Step: The first step is to allow the cattle to walk through the chute several times as quietly as possible.
Second Step: The next step is to stop cattle in the chute without squeezing them and then release.
Final Step: Cattle are stopped in the chute and the sides squeezed gently and released without any other procedures being done on them.
NOTE: After each training step, the cattle should be fed a small amount of grain or choice hay.

- ● **Maintenance Training for Squeeze Chutes and Headgates:**
  - ● **Time for When Not Struggling:** When procedures (ear tagging, vaccinations, castration, etc.) are performed on them in the future, release from the chute should be timed for when they are not struggling. Otherwise, they are likely to run out and have a perception that they have escaped. Unstressed cattle come out of a squeeze chute and headgate at a walk or slow trot.
  - ● **Calm Time with Food and Other Cattle:** Cattle that are normally released from a squeeze chute with a headgate should be penned with other cattle and provided with water, salt, molasses blocks, or choice hay to calm down before release into a pasture.

- **Backup Prevention Bars and Gates:** Bars or gates that slide across the alleyway or gates that drop down should be used to prevent backups, but a bar or gate should never be placed behind a handler who is in an alleyway moving cattle.
  - **Butt Bars:**
    - ○ **Uses:** Butt bars prevent backing up when released through the front of a chute. Butt bars are also placed behind the first cow in an alleyway and the last cow.
    - ○ **Caution:** If using a butt bar, the handler should always keep their body at the end of the bar in case the other end is suddenly hit by a cow and the handler's end is swung forward or backward. Butt bars in squeeze chutes can break the arm of someone doing a rectal palpation if the cow suddenly goes down.
  - **Drop Down Gates:** Drop down gates to block backing up are safer than butt bars if counterbalanced to prevent injury to cows' backs.
- **Collection Pens:** A collection pen should be located in front of the headgate and the side opening of the squeeze chute. This will enclose cattle that get too far through the headgate to catch them in front of the shoulders as desired and are caught by the hips and then must be released through the front of the chute. It will also contain cows that go down in the chute and are rescued by a side opening gate.
- **Stanchions without Squeeze Chutes:** Stanchions without squeeze chutes are common in dairies. Self-catching stanchions (headlocks) trap the most dominant cows first at feed bunks allowing others to then find a place to get to food. Stanchions are also incorporated in most veterinary clinic bovine stalls for cattle restraint during exam and treatment.
- **Loading and Unloading Chutes:** A loading chute is a loading platform or ramp that is used when cattle are moved between a trailer or truck and a working facility.
  - **Location:** Cattle will best move onto loading chute directly from a crowding pen or a Bud's box. Long single file alleyways to a loading chute should be avoided, and they should face north-south to prevent cattle facing the sun when loading.
  - **Construction:**
    - ○ **Single File with Foot Traction:** Cattle should be loaded single file in a chute that is a minimum of 12 ft long and 26–30 inches wide. Traction should be provided with cleats every 8 inches.
    - ○ **Catwalks:** Catwalks alongside the chute are helpful in encouraging smooth loading.
    - ○ **Incline and Gaps:** Fixed chutes should not exceed 20 degrees of incline. If concrete ramps are used, the ramp should be stair-stepped 12 inches deep with 4-inch rises. Gaps between loading chutes and transport vehicles should be blocked with self-aligning bumpers and telescoping sides.
- **Optional Restraint Facilities:** Optional additions include a weighing scale, palpation cage, tilt table, calf tilt table, shed over the working area, concrete flooring, or man-gates and man-passes.
  - **Weighing Scales:** Cattle scales are inserted at floor level and enclosed as a small pen or stall positioned just before a squeeze chute or after the squeeze chute. They should be off the main alleyway and entered only when being weighed. Some scales are built into the floor of squeeze chutes, but these can cause balking of the cattle at the chute and more often go out of adjustment.
  - **Palpation Cage:**
    - ○ **Purposes:** Palpation cages are used for pregnancy exams of cows, artificial insemination, fertility testing of bulls, and castration of calves.
    - ○ **Handler Gates:** Palpation cages have handler gates in the alleyway immediately behind a catch or squeeze chute. The gate swings into the alleyway

and away from the chute and can be latched to block other cattle in the alleyway from going forward until their turn in the chute. This allows a handler to inspect or treat a cow from behind by entering behind the caught cow in the chute and not be injured by other cattle in the alleyway.

- **Artificial Insemination (AI) Dark Box:** Artificial insemination should be performed in restraint chutes that are not used for painful procedures such as vaccination, ear tagging, or medical treatments. AI dark boxes are preferable. The chute for AI does not need to squeeze or have a head catch.
  - **Description:** AI dark boxes are 28 inches wide with solid sides, front, and top. A cloth hangs on the back of the box and drapes over the cow's rump.
  - **Wild Cattle Modification:** If wild cattle are handled, the dark box should be the length of two cows, so that a calm cow can be run in first and aid in pacifying the back cow to be inseminated.
- **Tilt Tables:** Tilt tables in vertical position allow attachment of a cow to the table which is then moved to a horizontal position with the cow restrained in lateral recumbency.
  - **Purposes:** Tilt tables facilitate working on the flank, udder, feet, or legs of cattle.
  - **Restraint of the Cow:** The cow is led or herded next to a vertical tabletop. The halter rope is tied to restrain the head first. One belly strap goes under the front part of the chest and a second strap goes under the abdomen, and the legs are strapped down.
  - **Tilting the Table:** The vertical position of the tabletop is then tilted to the horizontal plane. This type of tilt table may be on a hydraulic pedestal and able to go up, down, or flush with the floor. Smaller tilt tables may be transportable for field work.
- **Calf Tilt Table:** Calf tilt tables are reduced size versions of the tilt tables used for adult cattle (Figure 5.9). They work best for calves less than 500 lb.

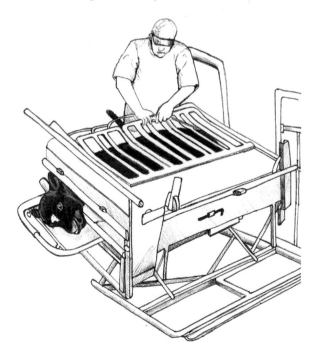

Figure 5.9   Calf tilt table.

- ○ **Advantages:** Calf tables are much safer than inexperienced handlers trying to rope calves. Calf tables also permit handling of calves with fewer people involved.
- ○ **Disadvantages:** Use of tilt tables for working calves is slower than the rope and drag method. A tilt table also results in greater separation from herd members.
- **Tables Compared to Rope and Drag:** The "rope and drag" method of working calves is still practiced by some western U.S. ranches. The reason is not because of tradition, but because some handlers believe that the 30 seconds it takes for six efficient calf handlers to vaccinate, ear tag, brand, castrate, and dehorn a calf is less stressful to calves and safer than being sorted, run up alleys, having their neck caught, and being squeezed in a chute. In addition, the procedures to perform on the calves take more time due to the obstructions to access created by the restraint equipment.
- **Rotary Chute:** A rotary chute is a squeeze chute with a headgate on a circular track which turns a cow on either side. After the cow is caught in the squeeze chute, the chute can be rotated 90 degrees until the cow is laying on its side and the side of the chute is like a horizontal tabletop (Figure 5.10).

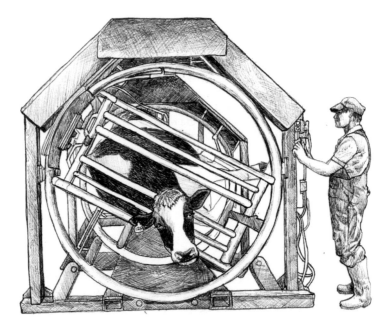

Figure 5.10   Rotary cattle chute.

- ○ **Advantage and Disadvantage:** Rotary chutes are safer for both cattle and handlers, but they limit access to the cow's side more than a tilt table.
- ○ **Risks:** Cattle should not be held on their sides for more than 30 minutes due to the risk of rumen gas accumulation.
- **Sheds:** Sheds are helpful over working alleys and squeeze chutes, especially if equipped with lights, outlets, and a water source for cleaning.
- **Concrete Flooring:** Concrete floors under the working alleys, squeeze chute, and crowding tub can improve footing and drainage.
- **Man-Passes and Man-Gates:** *Man-passes* are fence gaps 12 to 18 inches wide for handler safety escapes. *Man-gates* are 2 to 4 feet wide at convenient locations for handler movement and safety.

- **Dip Tank:** Dipping of cattle for ticks has been replaced in most areas by acaricidal sprays, pour-ons, dusts, and ear tags.
  - **Entrance:** Dip tanks should have a funneled entrance that permits only one cow to enter the dip tank at a time. Otherwise, incoming cattle may jump onto a cow that is already in the tank.
  - **Ramps:** The in ramp and out ramp should be cleated for traction and not exceed 20 degrees of inclination above water. The decline in the lower aspect of the in ramp that is under water can be a steeper drop off.

MOVING CATTLE

Other than transporting cattle, there are three methods of moving cattle: leading, driving, or herding.

- **Basic Considerations:**
  - **Avoid Stress:** Moving of cattle should be done quietly and without pain.
  - **Time of Day:** Moving cattle is preferably done in early morning or evening when it is cool. Cows with calves are best moved in the evening. When the herd is stopped, calves will lay down and the herd will stay with the calves.
  - **Detrimental Memories:** Cattle will file memories of places, people, weather, odors, and other environmental stimuli and react favorably or adversely on second exposure based on memory. Bad handling experiences are remembered by cattle for at least three years.
- **Calling and Leading:** Leading is the least stressful means of moving cattle.
  - **Motivate with Food:** Cattle can be trained to come or follow in anticipation of being fed. If a call or noise is used prior to and during feeding, cattle will learn to respond to the call. Sweet feed (grain with molasses) can be used to train cattle to be led.
  - **Call to Pasture or Range Feeding:** If training cattle to come to be fed in a pasture or range, they should be trained to associate food with a sound, not the sight of a truck or wagon to prevent crowding the truck or wagon prior to distributing the feed.
  - **Calm Leader Cattle:** Having a quiet leader steer or cow can be extremely helpful in moving cattle. In the great Texas cattle drives of the 1800s, nervous leader cattle were killed. Old Blue was a famous longhorn steer that wore a leather collar with a bell and calmly led more than 10,000 head of cattle over eight years to railheads.
  - **Training to Be Led:**
    - **Initial Steps:** Teaching new cattle where to go can be begun with leaving small piles of grain in a trail to the destination planned for them. If a cow gets too close to the handler, the handler should reaffirm dominant social status by spreading the arms and waving a herding stick in the air. If that does not result in moving the cow away, the handler should tap her on the nose with the herding stick.
    - **Training with a Visual Lure:** When walking among cattle for them to adjust to a handler's presence, the handler can feed them treats from a feeding bucket such as carrots, apples, or sweet feed (molasses and grain). This will teach them to follow if the handler carries the same bucket.
    - **Management of Reluctant Cows:** Cows that do not follow can be sorted and kept alone in a pen until the others are moved. The penned cow will seek out the others after she is released.
    - **Food Frenzy Caution:** A barrier or platform such as a truck bed should be used when training cattle with food. They respond better when hungry but could become dangerous if the handler is on foot.

- o **Do Not Lead Nursing Cows:** Cows with nursing calves should not be called to be led. The anticipation of food rewards may train the cow to leave her calf.
- o **Consistency Is Critical:** Over time, cattle can be taught to follow a quiet, leading handler. Frequent presence among the herd and the appropriate use of rewards, such as access to different food and fresh water, is required.
- o **Handlers Who Lead Cattle Cannot Herd the Same Cattle:** If training cattle to lead or leading trained cattle, a handler cannot switch to herding the herd and back to leading. If a herd must be herded, other handlers should do it. Once a herd is taught to lead, some herd members should be retained as tutors for new herd members if the remainder of the herd is to be sold.

- **Driving:**
  - **Driving Compared to Herding:** Driving and herding are often used as synonyms, but they are not. Driving cattle is less organized and involves the use of some degree of fear. Moving cattle by cracking whips, yelling, and waving objects is driving cattle.
  - **Driving Is Stressful:** Driving cattle uses the method that group hunting predators use to move animals for a kill. It is the oldest and most animal-stressful means of moving them.
    - o **Frightening toward a Goal:** At its core, driving involves positioning the cattle between the site to move them to and the handlers. Handlers then invade the flight zone, frightening the cattle to move in the direction desired. Driven cattle often move at a pace faster than a walk.
    - o **Multiple Handlers Required:** Driving cattle effectively toward a desired destination requires multiple handlers to try to guide the frightened cattle.
- **Herding—Flight Zones and Balance Points:**
  - **Herding:** Herding cattle mimics the means that a dominant herd member would use to move other herd members. It is a less animal-stressful method than driving, but experienced handlers are needed to accomplish herding.
    - o **Tempered Invasion of Flight Zones:** Herding cattle is accomplished by a rhythmic push on the periphery of the cattle's flight zone, followed by a slight retreat, slight push, slight retreat, etc.
    - o **Desired Pace:** The pace of herding is at a walk. Cattle should never be chased. If they are successful in escaping to another side of a pasture or somewhere else they can find rest, they will always attempt to run and escape if their flight zone is approached.
  - **Zones:** There are three psychological response zones around prey animals encountered when herding. Controlling the flight zone is critical in herding cattle (Table 5.11).

Table 5.11	Three Psychological Response Zones of Prey Animals
•	**Recognition**—The largest zone, alert response initiated
•	**Flight**—The middle-sized zone, movement initiated
•	**Fight**—The smallest zone, aggressive body language initiated.

- o **Flight Zones Are Variable:** If the flight zone is aggressively invaded, the fight zone will be reached. Factors that affect the flight zone are the time of day and season of the year, the weather, previous experiences, presence or absence of herdmates and their proximity, the terrain, the presence of obstacles between the animal and the herder, genetic tendency to be nervous or calm, and the herder's size, angle of approach, speed of approach, and demeanor as well as the number of herders and dogs.

- ○ **Average Flight Zone Size:** A typical flight zone for domestic cattle is an oval with a diameter of about 5 to 300 ft. Most dairy cattle have a flight zone of 5–10 ft.
- ○ **Northern versus Southern Beef Cattle:** Beef cattle that are around handlers on a regular basis have flight zones of about 15–25 ft. Beef cattle raised in southern states in the U.S. have a larger flight zone than the same breed raised in northern states because of regular, close exposure to humans that occur in winter feedings in northern states.
- ○ **Changing Flight Zones:** Flight zones are dynamic, changing depending on current conditions and past experiences. The easiest method for a handler to reduce a flight zone is to wait, be quiet, and let the animals settle and adjust to the handler's appearance and behavior. Squatting or turning sideways reduces a handler's silhouette and pressure on the animals' flight zone.
- **Balance Points:** Cattle, like all herd animals, have a side balance point at their shoulder for other animals or handlers to signal movement forward or backward.
  - ○ **Forward or Backward:** If the handler is located to the side and in front of the cow's shoulder, she will back up. If the handler is behind and to the side of the cow's shoulder, she will move forward (Figure 5.11).

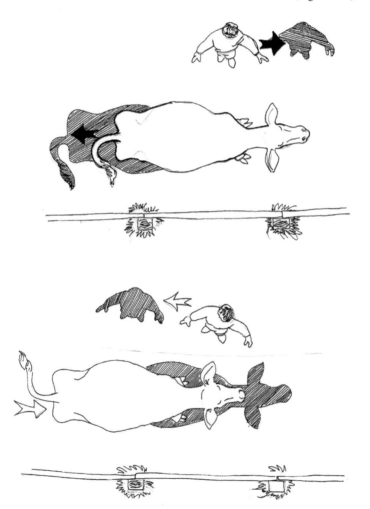

Figure 5.11 Moving a cow forward using its side balance point.

○ **Turning Right or Left:** The middle of the nose and middle of the tail are front and back balance points, respectively. When the handler is directly in front or behind a cow and moves to the left, a cow will move to the right. When the handler is directly in front or behind a cow and moves to the right, a cow will move to the left (Figure 5.12).

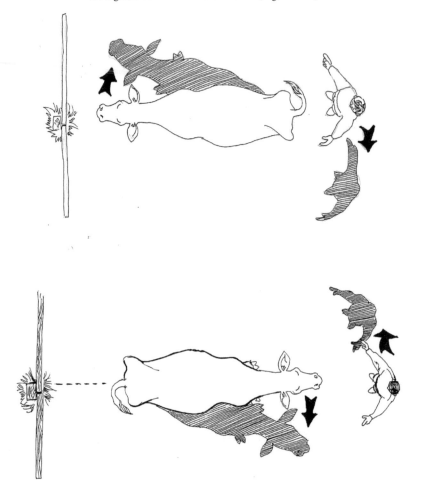

Figure 5.12   Moving a cow using its front and back balance points.

● **Initiating and Maintaining Movement:**
○ **Starting:** Methods for a handler to cause movement are to stare directly at the animals, facing the animals while increasing the profile (raise arms, spread legs), and directly approaching the animals.
○ **Stopping:** Stopping is achieved by removing the pressures to move, such as the handler lowering the arms to the side and standing at a 90-degree angle to the cattle.
○ **Feeding Effects:** It is best to herd cows without calves in the morning after cattle eat. Hunger decreases tolerance to stress.
○ **Concentrate on Leaders:** When starting cattle to move from a rest, handlers must concentrate on getting leaders moving in any direction and after they begin to move, direct their movement.

○ **Walking near Alleyways with Cattle:** If cattle are in an alleyway and cannot back up, a handler walking in the opposite direction to the cattle and close to them will encourage the cattle to move forward as the handler passes their side balance points. This can be repeated by the handler making a wide circle away from the cattle to again pass closely to them going in the direction opposite of the cattle direction (Figure 5.13).

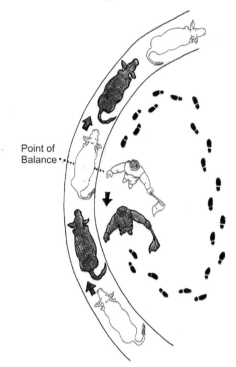

Point of Balance

Figure 5.13 Passing balance points to move cattle forward in an alleyway.

○ **Avoid Blind Spot:** Cattle cannot determine if a handler has invaded their flight zone if the handler is directly behind them. Herding must be performed from an angle (ideally, 45 to 60 degrees behind their shoulder) that allows the handler to see an eye of the cow to be moved to ensure they can see the handler. The handler should zig-zag while behind the herd to get out of the blind spot and be seen alternately with both eyes of the cattle.

○ **Competing Factors to Movement:** Factors that adversely affect the direction of movement are a desire to avoid icy, muddy, or rocky surfaces. Cattle will avoid new objects unless they have time to settle and develop curiosity. The location of others of their own species and especially their own herd has drawing power that can be advantageous to handlers.

○ **Handlers' Positions:** Although one handler can herd a large group of cattle, two handlers are more effective. The forward handler pushes on the herd leaders' flight zone. The rear handler pushes on the flight zone of straggling submissives.

○ **Move in Straight Lines:** Handlers should move in straight lines with confidence and change directions with angles, not curves. Circling movements mimic predator behavior and should be avoided.

○ **Focus on Dominants:** Flight zone pressure on a dominant herd member will result in it moving toward the center of the herd. Handlers who herd cattle must apply pressure from the side and behind the balance point of dominants, not directly from behind the group. Pressure on a low-ranking herd member may cause it to circle the herd, and if sufficiently frightened, take off on its own.

- ○ **Avoid Pressure on Submissives:** Submissive herd members, including young calves, follow in the back of the herd. Trying to move a herd from behind will push the submissives into the dominants, an action that is socially intolerable and leads to the submissives being driven away by the dominants.
- ○ **Reduction of Pressure on Flight Zone:** Reducing stress on herded cattle includes being moved by a familiar handler, looking away from the animals, pausing in pressing on the flight zone, occasionally taking a well-timed step backward, reducing the handler's profile by presenting a side profile, slouching, kneeling, or turning away. Fight or flight is decreased by dim light and rhythmic sounds and music, such as a low monotonous tone of singing, humming, or whistling. Fight or flight can also be reduced by leaving the agitated cattle alone for 20–30 minutes.
- **Herding with Horses, ATVs, and Dogs:**
  - ○ **Horses:** Although cattle are less frightened by a handler on horseback than a handler on foot, they will more readily move if a horse and rider invade their flight zone. Being on horseback increases the perceived size of the herder.
  - ○ **All Terrain Vehicles:** The noise of All Terrain Vehicles (ATVs) stimulates driving the cattle, not herding. ATVs cannot change directions abruptly and sharply enough to be very effective. In addition, ATVs require too much of the rider's attention as they are traversing the terrain, which detracts from appropriate attention needed for herding cattle.
  - ○ **Herding Dogs in Open Range versus Pens:** Well trained herding dogs can be helpful in finding and moving stray cattle on open ranges or in large pastures out of brush, but once the cattle enter a collecting pen, few dogs are useful. Herding dogs should generally not be used to move cattle in pens.
  - ○ **Dogs for Long Distance Herding:** When moving cattle a long distance, cattle naturally string out in a single file. They are easier to move in a long line than if they are forced to bunch up. Maintaining long lines is different than the herding tactics most dogs use when moving cattle.
  - ○ **Exclude Dogs:** Dogs' presence around collecting pens can be distracting and disturbing to the cattle causing danger to handlers by stirring the cattle in close quarters. Dogs should never be used to herd cows with nursing calves. The only result is putting the mother cow in fighting mode.
- **Moving Large Herds:**
  - ○ **Handlers:** Large herds should be herded with eight handlers (four pairs). These are (from front to back) the point, swing, flank, and drag pairs.
  - ○ **Train Herd:** Prior training of cattle is very helpful. Select, older cows that herd calmly should be kept as role models for younger ones.
  - ○ **Rate Speed of Movement:** To control the rate of movement, handlers go up sides of moving cattle to slow the herd. To speed the herd up, handlers move down the sides of the herd.
  - ○ **Moving through Gates:** Point riders open the gate in advance of the herd arrival. They then ease in behind about 20 cows and the others will follow. After the herd gets through the gate, they are allowed to mingle for about 30 minutes for calves to rejoin their mothers before the herd begins to move again.
- **Moving Bulls:** Moving adult bulls requires extra precautions.
  - ○ **Work in Pairs:** Handlers should work in pairs when handling bulls and neither handler should ever take eyes off the bull until it is contained separately from the handler.

- ○ **Dogs:** Trained dogs can be helpful in moving bulls by being a distraction to the bull if the bull gets aggressive toward the handler.
- ○ **Using a Truck or Tractor:** Riding in a truck or on a tractor to move bulls is safer for moving bulls on foot or horseback.

COLLECTING CATTLE

Introducing cattle to a collecting facility prior to handling them for routine or medical procedures will reduce their stress when the time comes for them to be collected for purposes other than training.

- **Location:** Collecting pens are best located between pastures, so that when changing pastures, the cattle have to walk through the collecting pens with a reward of fresh pasture on the other side. Gates should be located at the top of a rise, not the bottom. Entry to yards should be wide and along a fence line on level ground or uphill.
- **Pen Construction:** A collection pen must be strong enough to hold cattle in close confinement and not be constructed of wire fencing.
- **Handling in a Collection Pen:**
  - **Allow Initial Calming Period:** After moving cattle into a collection pen, they should be allowed to settle for 20–30 minutes.
  - **Move Cattle Quietly:** Cattle in close confinement will bruise or injure each other during sorting, especially if not done quietly and efficiently. Cattle movement in the pen should be directed with flags. Handlers should not yell at or hit the cattle.
  - **Move into Alleyways Slowly, One at a Time:** When most of a group in a crowding pen are facing the alleyway, a handler should slowly swing the crowding gate to have them enter the alleyway one at a time. A drop down gate should be at the entrance of the squeeze chute which is raised to let one cow at a time into the chute.
  - **Avoid Distractions to Cattle Movement:** People should not be visible to the front or side of the squeeze chute.
  - **Tail Twist Hold:** Careful use of a tail twist hold (released immediately with the slightest forward movement) can be used to train cattle to move forward when touched on the rump (Figure 5.14).

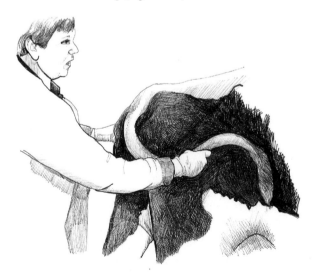

Figure 5.14   Tail twist to encourage forward movement.

- **Electric Prods:**
  - ○ **American Veterinary Medical Association's Policy on Livestock Handling Tools:**

    Electrical devices (e.g., stock prods) should be used judiciously and only in extreme circumstances when all other techniques have failed. Electrical devices should never be applied to sensitive parts of the animal such as the face, genitalia, or mucous membranes. See Figure 5.15.

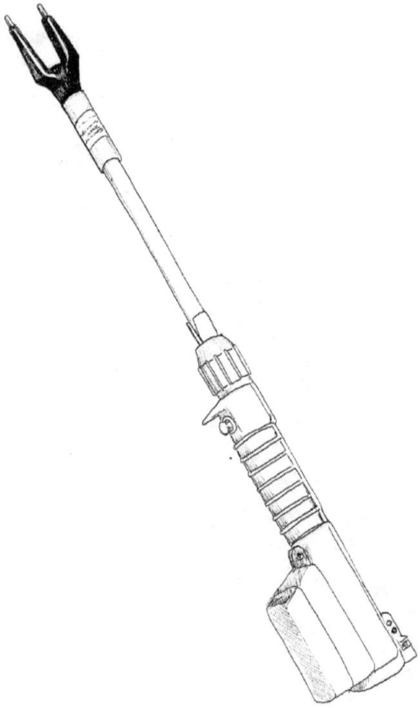

Figure 5.15   Electric cattle prod.

  - ○ **Justified Uses:** In some situations, if the cow does not get up or move, her life may be in danger, for example if she does not move to shelter before storms. Electric prods may be necessary to get a cow to move to save a handler's life if the handler is knocked down in a pen or chute and is in danger of being stomped or crushed.
  - ○ **Proper Application:** Electric prods deliver 2,200 to 9,000 volts. Before using it, an electric prod should be discharged on something metal near the cow since the sound of the buzz may be enough to cause movement, especially if they have been shocked before. After using it, the end should be touched to a metal surface to discharge any residual electricity.

SORTING CATTLE

Sorting may be for separating cattle by age, sex, state of health, and other reasons.

- **Separate in Pairs:** Separating cattle from a larger group should be done in pairs. Sorting a cow into a pen by itself can cause it to panic. In addition, a cow that is removed and isolated from a herd for 24 hours or more will be harassed when it rejoins the herd.
- **Return to Herd as Soon as Possible:** Separated cattle should be returned as soon as possible. If separation is more than 24 hours, the member should be returned when the herd is actively engaged in something else that distracts it, such as grazing in a new pasture or being fed grain. Returned cattle usually assume the same rank in the herd as they had previously.
- **Methods:**
  - **Sorting Alleyway:**
    - **Alleyway into Pens:** One method of sorting is to move cattle from collecting or holding pens into a sorting pen alleyway which is 12 to 14 ft wide and then they are separated into sorting pens. Slick flooring of sorting alleyways should be treated with sand or crushed limestone.
    - **Cattle First down Alleyway:** The handler should plan for the largest cattle to move down the alleyway to last sorting pen. Sorting can be done more quietly with poles and small flags.
    - **Least Excitable Separated First:** It is best to sort out the least excitable first. For example, separate cows from bulls, cows from calves, and older from younger cows. Alleyway sorting requires at least two handlers.
  - **Sorting at Pen Gate:**
    - **Turn Desired Cows Back:** Sorting can also be done while moving cattle quietly out of a pen by stepping in front of a cow's side balance point when wanting to turn one back into the pen. Movements should be slow, deliberate, and measured.
    - **Calm the Group:** The group to be sorted should be calmed for about 20 minutes. The handler should be visible, quiet, and present a small profile (turn to side, squat, sit) during the calming period, but should never turn their back to animals near an exit.
    - **Inducing Desire to Exit:** If an exit from a pen is provided but cattle are reluctant to leave, a shirt or jacket can be tied to a rope and dragged slowly through the pen and out the gate. Often, the leaders of the group will follow it.
    - **Slowing the Exit:** If cattle rush through a gate, a handler can stand nearby inside the pen and move slightly toward the gate in front of the leader's side balance point, and as soon as the cattle slow down, the handler should step back. This back and forth movement may need to be repeated to regulate the speed of additional cattle movement through the gate.
  - **Round Pen or Modified Bud's Box:** A handler in a round pen or a modified Bud's box with side pens can encourage movement of the cattle along the inside edge of the pen, while a handler opens the appropriate sorting gate at the optimum time. The side pens should have gates that swing either into or out of the sorting pens to aid in sorting regardless of the direction they are moving around the round pen or Bud's box. It is best to work small groups of cattle in a sorting pen so they can move more freely.
  - **Cutting Horse:** Sorting can also be performed horseback using trained cutting horses and experienced riders. Sorting with horses requires fewer facilities than sorting using special pens and handlers on foot. The maintenance time and expense for training and maintaining the needed horse and rider skills is high.

HANDLING FOR COMMON MEDICAL PROCEDURES

Most handling and restraint of cattle can be and should be done without tranquilization, sedation, hypnosis, or anesthesia. However, some handling and restraint procedures should be restricted to veterinary medical professionals due to the potential danger to the animal or handler. These require special skills, equipment, or facilities, and possibly adjunct chemical restraint or complete immobilization by chemical restraint.

RESTRAINT OF INDIVIDUAL CATTLE AND PORTIONS OF THEIR BODIES

Restraint of the head of cattle eliminates most of their struggling when restrained. Any other restraint that does not restrain the head well will result in continued struggling. Methods of head restraint include the use of halters, nose leads, nose rings, and stanchions.

- **Head Restraint:**
  - **Rope Halters:**
    - ○ **Advantage:** Use of a halter is the safest method to restrain a cow's head because a cow or bull may go down and be injured if it is tied only by a nose lead, nose ring, or neck rope. However, putting a halter on a cow, especially when it is in a stanchion, can be hazardous for handlers.
    - ○ **Rope Halters:** The most commonly used halter is a rope halter that extends into a lead (Figure 5.16). Rope halters for ruminants are made with twisted rope and created with splicing techniques. Rope halters are used to lead halter-broke cows, calves, and steers.

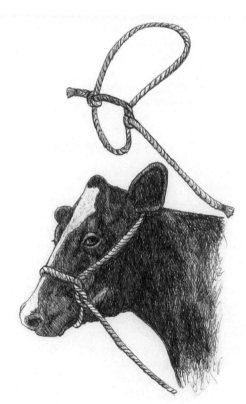

Figure 5.16   Rope halter for cattle.

○ **Application:** To put a halter on a cow on properly, a handler should remember: "the part that draws goes under the jaws." Care must be taken not to place the nosepiece portion of the halter lower than the bony part of the nose or the nostrils may be pinched shut causing the animal to panic. Rope halters may be applied while a cow or calf is in a stall, a stanchion, or when restrained by a neck rope and snubbing post (Procedural Steps 5.3).

Procedural Steps 5.3	One-Hand Application of Rope Halter on the Left Side
1.	The adjustable portion and lead rope portion should be on the left side of the cow's head.
2.	With practice the halter can be held at the crownpiece with the right hand and placed on the cow's head with a backhand movement of the right hand while standing to the left of the cow.
3.	The left hand holds the lead portion of the halter.
4.	The crownpiece goes over the right ear and then the left.
5.	The muzzle part should be open enough to fall under the cow's jaw.
6.	The halter is then tightened and adjusted into place.
7.	This method does not require a handler to be pressed against the cow to place a halter or risk injury to the handler's hip.

○ **Two-Hand Application of a Rope Halter:** Some handlers prefer to use two hands and catch the muzzle first and then place the top part over of the ears. If the handler's hip is not pressed against the cow, a swing of the cow's head may fracture the handler's hip. Furthermore, two-handed haltering can result in bending close enough to a cow's head that a butting injury to the handler's head is possible.

○ **Reversible:** A cattle rope halter extends into its own lead rope and exits the halter on either the right or left side of the animal's cheek (i.e., it is reversible). When leading a cow, the lead rope should be on the cow's left side. If a cow is caught in a stanchion, it should be on the same side of the face that will be tied to the chute's cleats.

● **Nose Leads:** A nose lead is a blunted, scissors-like clamp with two arms called *tongs*. The tongs are best placed in nostrils with a sweeping motion from the side while the cow is in a stanchion and the handler faces it at a safe distance.

○ **Description:** Functional nose leads should have smooth blunted ends on the tongs, a 1/8-inch gap between closed tongs, and a smooth rope lead (Figure 5.17). Chains on nose leads are undesirable since they can kink, pinch, and pull open.

○ **Application Requires Neck Restraint:** Nose leads should only be used if the neck is restrained in some form of stanchion or headgate.

○ **Limit Use:** Use of nose leads to restrain the head is more likely to make the animal more resistant to future handling than will the use of rope halters. Therefore, nose leads should not be used for procedures that have to be frequently repeated.

○ **Advantages:** Nose leads allow the cow's head to be pulled to either side without being removed and reversed (flipped) as necessary with a halter. A nose lead also allows the cow's head to be pulled further to the sides or upward, which can facilitate jugular venipuncture in some cows.

○ **Disadvantages:** Nose leads risk injuring the nasal septum in cattle, but this is very rare if the balls of the leads do not touch when the leads are closed and the lead rope is always kept tight so the cow does not sling its

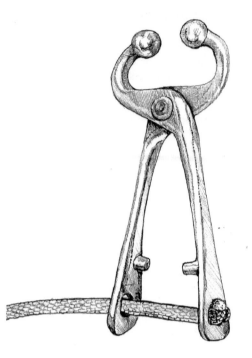

Figure 5.17 Nose lead with rope attachment.

head. Cattle restrained by a nose lead should not be tied firmly to a chute cleat in case they go down and could hang by their nose and possibly tear their nasal septum. The nose lead rope should instead be wrapped around the chute cleat and held by an assistant.

○ **Application of Nose Leads:** See Procedural Steps 5.4.

	Procedural Steps 5.4 Application of Nose Leads
1.	When applying nose leads to a cow, the handler must take care not to lean over the cow's head or be within forward striking distance of the cow's head if it should lunge forward in the headgate.
2.	The handler should not approach the cow from a straight-on direction with the nose lead as this will intensify its efforts to dodge placement of the lead.
3.	Nose leads are applied by holding the lead with one hand with the palm up.
4.	The handler stands in front of the cow's head while the cow's head is retrained in a head catch or stanchion.
5.	The tongs are separated and held open using the ring and little finger.
6.	A sweeping movement is used from the handler's right to left if the tongs are held with the right hand.
7.	As the right tong goes in the cow's left nostril, the left tong immediately follows into the right nostril, and tongs are quickly closed by a tug on the lead rope.
8.	Tension must be kept on the lead rope until the tongs are removed.
9.	Nose leads should not be applied for more than 20 minutes.

○ **Alternative Application Method:** A less safe method is for the handler to press a hip against the cow's head, putting a hand on the other side of the jaw, and putting the tongs in while trying to partially immobilize its head.

○ **Brief Hand Restraint of the Nose:** For brief restraint, a handler can grasp a cow's nasal septum with a thumb and middle finger and use the fingers in the same manner as metal nose tongs.

● **Nose Rings:**

○ **Purpose:** For the handler's safety, nose rings are used in all adult dairy bulls and some beef bulls (Figure 5.18). Most have a nose ring placed between 1 to 2 years of age, before they become territorially aggressive.

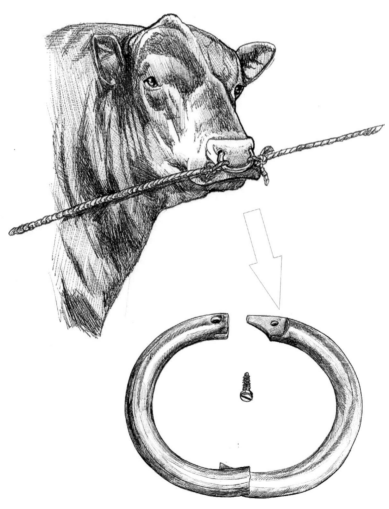

Figure 5.18   Bull nose ring.

- ○ **Use of Nose Rings:** The safest means of moving a bull with a nose ring is with two handlers, one on each side with a bull staff. A bull staff is a pole that has a hook or snap on one end that attaches to the nose ring. A bull staff is usually used in combination with a halter to lead a bull.
- ○ **Placement of Nose Rings:** Placement of nose rings should be done by a veterinarian since the use of local anesthesia and post-surgical pain relievers are needed. A chute with a headgate and nose bar should be used for nose ring placement.
- ○ **Risks of Handling a Bull Calf:** People should never play with a bull calf since this can eliminate the natural respect most have for human personal space. A bull calf should be culled if it shows signs of dominance aggression, such as head shaking, staring at people within the bull's enclosure, pawing the ground while facing a person, or deliberately showing its side to a person.
- • **Whole Body Restraint:**
  - • **Stanchions and Tying Posts:** Stanchions or tying posts can be used to restrain halter trained cattle. Either stanchions or posts should be strong enough to hold adult cattle that might resist the restraint with all their strength. Tie rings on tying posts should be at a cow's natural head height or slightly higher.
  - • **Improvised Chutes and Hay Bale Barriers:** A gate that swings against a wall can be used as an improvised treatment squeeze chute when other facilities are not present. Square bales of hay or straw can be used behind restrained cattle to reduce the risk of the handler being kicked if work is needed round their rump, such as rectal palpation.
  - • **Rope and Snubbing Post:**
    - ○ **Technique:** If adept with a lariat, a handler can toss a lariat loop around a cow's neck and pull it to a stout stationary post. The restraint should be brief or a halter should be placed on the cow's head and the lariat removed.
    - ○ **Temporary Halter:** Alternatively, a bight can be run underneath the neck loop at the throat and then placed over the cow's nose to make a temporary halter. This will relieve some of the pressure around the cow's neck.
    - ○ **Indications:** A rope and snubbing post should be used when less stressful means are not available and the need for the restraint is more important than the stress that might result.
  - • **Chest Twitch:** A chest twitch is a rope looped around the chest and pulled tight. This may calm a tied, agitated cow.
  - • **Casting:** Casting methods are means to lay a cow down and immobilize it when restraint chutes or tilt tables are not available or appropriate for the procedure to be done. Any time a cow is laid on its side there can be risk of displaced abomasum or bloat if handled roughly or forced to remain recumbent for too long. Cows within 2 months of calving should not be cast due to the risk of induced abortion.
    - ○ **Appropriate Surface to Lay a Cow Down:** An appropriate ground surface should first be selected. The ground selected for casting should be clear, smooth, and somewhat soft.
    - ○ **Techniques:** Cattle will lay down if a rope squeezes their chest and their abdomen (half-hitch method) or puts pressure beneath their front legs and over their back (Flying W method). With either method, the lead rope should be held by an assistant or tied low, near the ground, to a sturdy object. Both methods require 40 ft of rope.
    - ○ **Half-Hitch Method:** This is also referred to as *Reuff's method*. See Procedural Steps 5.5 and Figure 5.19.

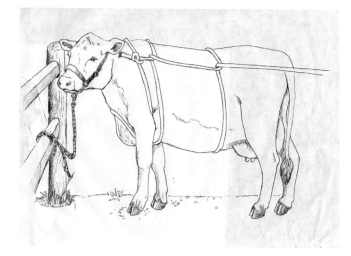

Figure 5.19   Half-hitch method of casting.

Procedural Steps 5.5	Application of the Half-Hitch Method of Casting
1.	A loop is placed around the cow's neck and tied with a bowline knot.
2.	A half hitch is placed around the chest just behind the cow's elbows.
3.	The rope is thrown under the cow or a pole with a hook that can be used to retrieve the rope on the other side.
4.	Another half hitch is placed around the abdomen, avoiding the udder or prepuce.
5.	The remaining line is pulled back steadily in line with the cow's spine and the cow is gradually laid down on its side.
6.	Cattle should be laid either on their back (ventrodorsal) and propped with hay bales with their front legs stretched forward and their back legs stretched back with cotton ropes, or on their right side so that the left side can be uppermost and observed for gas accumulation.
7.	If laying on its right side, the front legs are tied with 6 ft cotton ropes after flexing the leg so that the hoof is near the elbow and restrained with a clove hitch around a pastern, leaving about 8 inches extra.
8.	The long end is wrapped around the radius and the pastern 3 to 4 times and then the rope is tied with a slip knot (sheet bend with a bight for quick release) to the 8 inches left over from the clove hitch.
9.	Similar ties can be used on flexed hind legs with a clove hitch on a fetlock, figure 8 wraps incorporating the fetlocks and tibia just above the hock, and slip knot tie.
10.	Since recumbent ruminants rise with their front legs first, tying the hind legs securely is of more importance than the front legs.

○ **Flying W Method:** This is also called the *Criss-Cross method* or *Burley method*. The Flying W method is preferred by dairymen since the ropes are not placed in front of the udder and the cow goes down on its sternum and must be pushed over on its side. There is no pressure on the chest or udder and no knot to tie around horns, neck, or front leg. Although its application and release are quicker and there is control of which side the cow rolls onto, it is harder to pull two ropes with enough strength to cast a cow than one rope with the half-hitch method (Figure 5.20).

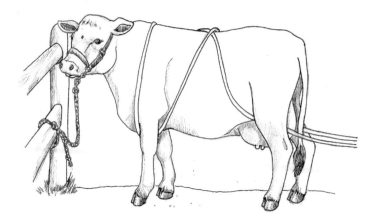

Figure 5.20   Burley method of casting.

- **Restraint of the Tail:** The tail of a cow can inflict serious injury to a handler since the coccygeal (tail) vertebrae nearly extend to the end of the tail.
  - **Quick Release Sheet Bend:** A quick release sheet bend can be used as a simple, effective hitch using the long hair (switch) at the end of the tail. The long hair of the end of the tail is bent around the tie rope to begin making the hitch.
  - **Anchor Only to Cow's Body:** A tied tail should only be secured to the cow's body in case the cow goes down during the restraint. The other end is tied around the cow's neck using a bowline knot to prevent the rope from tightening around the neck (Figure 5.21). Alternative ties to further reduce or to eliminate the risk of pressure on the windpipe are to put the rope around the neck and behind a front leg on the opposite side to the side that the tail is bent toward, or around the horns instead of the neck on horned cattle.

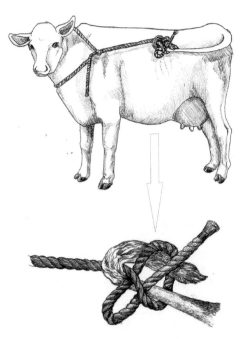

Figure 5.21   Tail tie.

- **Lifting Feet:**
  - **Be Brief:** Lifting a cow's foot should only be done for brief periods. Standing on three legs will quickly exhaust a cow and it may go down.
  - **Use Ropes:** Cow legs should not be lifted by hand as done with horses. Dairy cattle can be resentful or sullen and fall on the handler. Beef cattle that are not halter trained will not tolerate an attempt to pick up a front leg.
  - **Front Leg Method:** To lift a front leg on a dairy cow, a rope with a quick release honda is placed around the pasterns below the dewclaws, and the standing end looped over an adjacent bar or the cow's back and held by an assistant.
  - **Hind Leg Method:**
    - **Requires Restraint Chute:** Lifting a hind leg is usually done in a chute. A rope with a quick release honda is placed around the cow's cannon bone and looped over a bar above and behind the leg. Another wrap is made with the standing end around the leg just above the hock, the leg is hoisted, and the rope is held by an assistant (Figure 5.22).

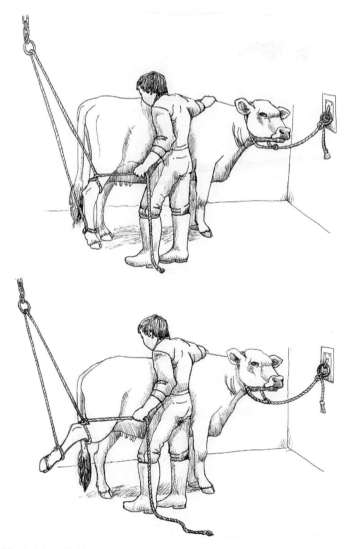

Figure 5.22   Hoisting a hind leg.

- o **Leg Must Be Stretched Backward as Well as Upward:** If the bar used to lift the leg is not sufficiently behind the cow, the hind leg will not be stretched back, and the leg will have too much freedom to kick back and forth for safe restraint.
- **Anti-kicking Methods:** Calves may kick with both hind legs, but adult cattle usually kick with one. However, they are more flexible in their ability to kick than horses. Cattle can reach forward to their shoulder and sweep outward when they kick.
  - **Tail Jacking:**
    - o **Basis:** Cattle are reluctant to kick if the tail is bent backward toward their spine.
    - o **Method:** The handler stands to the cow's side and grasps the tail about one-third down from the base of the tail. The tail is raised as the handler steps close behind the cow, holding the tail straight up and bent slightly toward the spine (Figure 5.23).

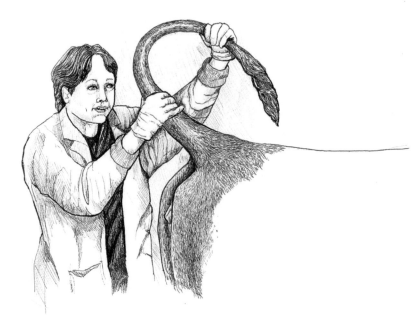

Figure 5.23 Tail jacking to inhibit kicking.

- o **Avoid Excessive Force:** Only moderate pressure should be used to prevent injury to the tail.
- o **Uses:** Tail jack restraint hold is used for venipuncture of the ventral vein of the tail; to examine, clean, or treat the mammary glands; and for castration.
- **Frank Pressure:**
  - o **Grasping a Flank Fold:** Grasping a flank fold and lifting the skin can inhibit kicking, but the handler's position to apply the hold is dangerous from the risk of being kicked first, or in spite of the hold.
  - o **Rope around the Flank:** A rope loop with a honda pulled tight around the flank will inhibit vigorous kicking, but it will not prevent subdued attempts to kick.
  - o **Metal Flank Clamp:** Large metal flank clamps that close with a screw mechanism or telescoping rods with button-pin spring locks are available to exert pressure in the flank to inhibit kicking (Figure 5.24).

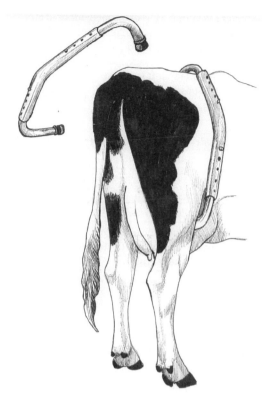

Figure 5.24   Anti-kick flank clamp.

- **Hind Leg Hobbles:**
  - **Metal Clamps and Hobbles:** Tendon clamps or metal U-shaped hobbles placed above a hock on the Achilles (gastrocnemius) tendon prevent cows from kicking in milking parlors. Hobbles are connected by a chain which must be long enough to permit the cow to keep its hind legs sufficiently apart to keep its balance. While standing next to the cow's side, hock hobbles are applied to the far side's Achilles tendon first and then to the near side tendon.
  - **Rope Hobble:** A 4 ft cotton rope may also be used to hobble the hind legs. A bight in the middle of the rope is placed above the hock on one leg. The two standing ends are twisted several times to provide sufficient length between the legs for the cow to stand normally and then the ends are wrapped around the other leg above the hock and tied with a sheet bend knot.

WORKING WITH DOWNED CATTLE

Downed (downer) cattle are those that have lost their desire or ability to stand and move. Common causes include milk fever, leg injuries, or calving (obturator nerve) paralysis. Downed cattle may recover but need shelter and nursing during the recovery period. Downed cattle cannot be sent to commercial slaughter for human consumption.

- **Inherent Danger for Handlers and/or Cattle:** Working with downed cattle can be especially dangerous for handlers due to the risk of falls. However, cattle that are down and cannot escape inclement weather may die if not moved to shelter and a more favorable treatment environment.

- **Feasible Management Methods:** Most of the methods used for rescuing downed horses can be applied to cattle. However, financial constraints preclude the extraordinary efforts that are more commonly used on downed horses. A local veterinarian should always be called to provide any needed medical care, sedation, or guidance in a rescue effort.
- **Getting a Downed Cow to Stand:** It is always best to try to have downed cattle stand with their own strength, if possible.
    - **Basic Method:** See Procedural Steps 5.6.

Procedural Steps 5.6	Encouraging a Downed Cow to Stand
1.	Determine if the cow is physically able to stand.
2.	Make sure that there is sufficient room for the cow to stand and that the surface is non-slip.
3.	All of its legs need to be underneath the cow's body.
4.	Provide incentive and sufficient time for the cow to stand by clapping, shouting, and slapping the cow's neck or chest, preferably with a used grain sack or other means of making a noise without bruising.
5.	If the cow stands, she should be permitted several minutes to adapt to standing before encouraging any walking.

- **Alternative Methods:** Another method that is often effective is for a handler to rock the cow's body with the knees. In extreme situations, an electric prod should be used sparingly. Twisting or lifting with the tail should not be done due to risk of causing a fracture or paralysis.
- **Lifting a Downed Cow:** Attempts to lift a downed cow should be done over a non-slip surface to provide traction if efforts are made by the animal to support its own weight. Straps or ropes under the chest and abdomen can be tried on smaller cattle. Placing a large air bag underneath the torso and inflating it can be effective.
    - **Web Strap Harness Sling:** A web strap harness sling may be used underneath the torso so the cow can be lifted with a pulley system or power lift.
    - **Hip Hoist:** A hip hoist is a clamp placed over the pin bones of the hip to lift the rear of a dairy cow (Figure 5.25). The pelvic bones of beef cattle are usually not prominent enough to use a hip lift.

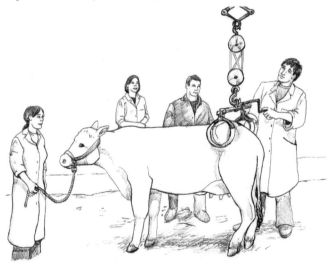

Figure 5.25 Hip hoist.

- ○ **Advantages:** Hip hoists avoid any pressure on the abdomen or mammary glands when lifting.
- ○ **Disadvantages:** The cow must have enough strength in her front legs to support her weight for the hip lift to be effective. The lift does not support the cow's body. It only assists their own efforts to stand.
- ○ **Short Term Use Only:** Slings and hip clamps are for brief periods of lifting and should not be used for extended periods (i.e., more than 1 hour).
- **Aquatic Rehabilitation Tubs:** Rehabilitation tubs for aquatic therapy are available for cattle in some veterinary hospitals. These support much of the weight of a cow by the buoyancy of their body. The water should be maintained at 100°F and the cow's head supported with a halter and lead rope.
- **Moving a Downed Cow:**
  - **Glides:** Downed animals should never be dragged because of friction injuries to their skin. Downed cattle can be pulled onto a flatbed trailer or livestock trailer using a glide (heavy canvas may be an adequate substitute), a ramp, and a block and tackle.
  - **Travois:** To move short distances, downed cattle can be pulled or rolled onto a skid, such as a detached farm gate that acts as a travois and then pulled by a tractor.
  - **After Moving:** After removing the cow from the glide or travois, it should be assisted to lie on its sternum, propping it with hay bales if needed. If the cow cannot stand without assistance within a day, it should be assisted with a hip clamp or sling, if available.

INJECTIONS AND VENIPUNCTURE

- **Access to Veins:**
  - **Jugular Vein:** The most common site for collecting blood samples or administering intravenous medications in cattle is the jugular vein. The restraint most commonly used is a squeeze chute with a headgate and a halter. Downed cattle in sternal position can be restrained for jugular venipuncture by using a halter and lead rope, pulling the cow's head to the side of the most accessible hind leg, and tying the lead above its hock.
  - **Coccygeal Vein:** The coccygeal vein on the lower aspect of the tail can provide access to the bloodstream. The restraint used is the tail jack hold.
  - **Subcutaneous Abdominal Vein:** The subcutaneous abdominal ("milk") vein is very prominent but should not be used for venipuncture. There is risk to the handler of being kicked and of large hematomas developing on the cow.
- **Injections:**
  - **Subcutaneous:** Subcutaneous injections in cattle are usually administered on the side of the neck.
  - **Intramuscular:**
    - ○ **Anterior Neck Area:** Intramuscular injection sites for cattle are restricted to the anterior neck area only, in accordance with Beef Quality Assurance guidelines. The injections are given about 4 inches below the top of the neck and 4 inches in front of the shoulder (Figure 5.26).
    - ○ **Inject While Cattle Movement Is Minimized:** The back of the hand with the syringe should be laid on the cow's neck and held there until the cow quits moving. The hand and syringe are then rotated and the injection is performed. Injections should not be given to cows in alleyways or chutes by reaching through narrow spaces between bars or planks.

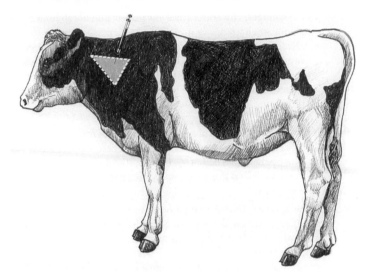

Figure 5.26 Intramuscular injection site in cattle.

ADMINISTRATION OF ORAL MEDICATIONS

Giving tablets (*bolusing*) or liquids (*drenching*) to cattle is achieved with head restraint and a balling gun or drenching syringe, respectively. Sufficient restraint usually requires a restraint chute for adult cattle. Calves may be crowded into an alleyway and treated individually.

- **Oral Administration Instruments**
  - **Balling Guns:** Balling guns are metal syringes for solid medication called boluses (i.e., large tablets) (Figure 5.27). Prior to using a balling gun, the handler should check it for rough or sharp protrusions or edges and file them smooth.

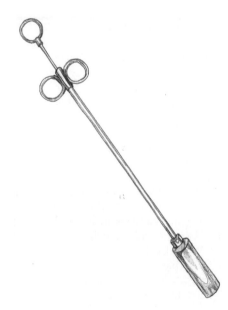

Figure 5.27 Balling gun.

- **Mouth Speculum:** Mouth speculums (*Frick speculums*) are placed in the mouth in a similar manner to oral syringes. These are cylindrical tubes that are protective conduits for passing soft stomach tubes. As the stomach tube is presented to the back of the cow's mouth, the cow's nose needs to be lower than its poll to reduce the possibility that the stomach tube can enter the trachea.
- **Method with Chute Restraint:** See Procedural Steps 5.7 and Figure 5.28.

Procedural Steps 5.7	Oral Administration of Medication Using Chute Restraint
1.	Remove the halter if the cow is wearing one.
2.	A handler places the left hip next to the cow's head while bringing the left thigh underneath the right side of its jaw.
3.	The handler places the left arm over its head, behind and under its ear, and runs a hand down underneath the cow's left mandible (Figure 5.28).
4.	Care must be taken to keep the handler's head as far from the cow's head as is practical.
5.	An oral syringe, a gag, or speculum is put into the right corner of the cow's mouth with the handler's right hand.
6.	If necessary, the left hand is used to open the mouth by sticking the hand in the corner of the mouth and pushing up on the palate.

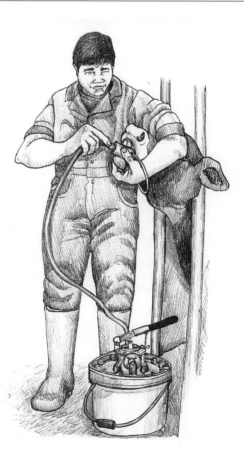

Figure 5.28   Restraint for oral administration.

- **Packed Calves Method:** See Procedural Steps 5.8.

Procedural Steps 5.8	Oral Administration to Packed Calves in an Alleyway
1.	The calves should be crowded together and the handler wades backward while catching calves and drenching them using their packed bodies to provide the restraint.
2.	Chalk markers are used to identify ones previously treated.
3.	While standing beside a calf or straddling it, the handler puts a thumb into a corner of the calf's mouth at the interdental space and presses the tongue with the thumb while squeezing the lower jaw to open the calf's mouth.
4.	The handler must avoid putting fingers into the back of the mouth where they could be bitten by the calf's upper and lower premolar teeth.
5.	The other hand places the balling gun or oral dose syringe into the mouth and over the hump of the tongue.
6.	The plunger on an oral dose syringe must be pushed slowly to prevent the liquid from being sprayed into the trachea.

TRIMMING HOOFS AND TREATING FEET

How often hoofs need to be trimmed depends on the surfaces cattle have to walk on. Foot problems and lameness is common in dairy cattle, particularly in their hind feet. Examination, trimming, and treatment are often needed.

- **Variable Means of Restraint:** There are several methods of trimming possible and different means of restraint, including lifting one leg at a time with a rope, casting with ropes, tilt tables, or rotary chutes.
- **Preferred Restraint:** Tilt tables and rotary chutes are the most effective and safest for both the cow and the handler.

MAMMARY EXAMINATION AND TREATMENTS

Mammary examination and treatments in dairy cows require restraint in stanchions. Resistant cows must be restrained in squeeze chutes with a headgate. The tail jack hold or hock hobbles may be needed to control kicking.

TRANSPORTING CATTLE

Because of its relative novelty to the cattle, loading well-handled cattle into a truck or trailer is more difficult than into an alleyway and squeeze chute. As with other aspects of cattle handling, allowing extra time to accomplish the loading with minimal stress is desirable.

DETRIMENTAL EFFECTS OF TRANSPORT STRESS

- **Decreased Meat Value:** Transport stress causes muscle to become dark and tough. If the cattle are going to be marked "dark cutters," they are less valuable.
- **Weight Loss:** Cattle that are stressed defecate more often, drink less, and lose weight, which also makes them less valuable at their destination.
- **Impaired Immunity:** Stress lowers their immune responses to infectious organisms and puts them at higher risk for infectious diseases.

PROVISION OF APPROPRIATE TRANSPORTATION

- **Cattle Trailers:** Cattle trailers should be adaptable to ensure sufficient ventilation, wind protection, and cover for protection from excessive sunlight or inclement weather.
  - **Ramp Construction:** Loading ramps should have solid sides, be one cow wide, and not exceed a 20-degree incline. Steps with 4-inch rises are preferred to cleats. If cleats are used, the distance between cleats should be about 8 inches.
  - **Position Vehicle Flush with Ramp:** No gaps should be left between the transport vehicle and the ramp sides before loading.
  - **Avoid Glare:** The loading ramp should be positioned so that cattle do not face glaring sunlight when loading.
- **Feed and Water before Transport:** Cattle should never be transported if they have not been watered and fed recently. Access to water should be provided up until 2 hours prior to loading and to grass hay until the time to load. Legume hay or grain rations should be avoided because of the risk of causing scours (diarrhea) and in turn, slick footing.
- **Transportation Compartment:**
  - **Flooring:** The transport compartment should be clean and have bedding that reduces the risk of slippage.
  - **Appropriate Packing of Cattle:** The cattle should be packed for transport close enough to reduce the chance to fight or fall but not so closely as to cause overheating. Partitions should be used to eliminate excess space.
  - **Avoid Mixing Cattle of Different Origins, Sizes, or Genders:** Cattle from different herds or pens should not be mixed during transport to minimize fighting. Different-sized cattle should be sorted and loaded into trailer compartments by similar weight. Adult bulls should be transported in separate individual compartments.
  - **Avoid Mixing Species:** Cattle should not be transported with other species.
- **Condition of Cattle:**
  - **Freshened Cows:** Freshened cows must be milked out prior to being transported. If dairy cattle are in transport for 12 or more hours, they should be unloaded, milked, fed, and watered.
  - **Calves:** Calves that have a dry navel and are able to walk may be transported, if they can remain dry and the temperature is not less than 60°F.
  - **Pregnant Cows:** Cows in late pregnancy should not be transported. If transport is unavoidable because of natural disasters or need for veterinary care, they should be in individual compartments with enough room to lie down.
  - **Lameness:** Cattle that are lame at a walk should not be transported. Those with fever should not be transported for anything other than veterinary care.
- **Weather Concerns:** If transporting cattle in cold weather, they should be checked for signs of cold stress, such as eating bedding material, frozen nasal secretions, or shivering. If signs of cold stress occur, further travel should be delayed if adjustments to the transport vehicle cannot be done to improve protection from inclement weather.
- **Excessive Transportation Times:** U.S. Code 49, Chapter 805, Section 80502 requires that animals cannot be transported more than 28 hours without stopping for food, water, and rest for at least 5 consecutive hours.

BIBLIOGRAPHY

1. American Veterinary Medical Association. Welfare implications of tail docking in cattle. https://www.avma.org/resources-tools/literature-reviews/welfare-implications-tail-docking-cattle. Accessed 08/29/2014, 2014.

2. Cote S. Stockmanship: A Powerful Tool for Grazing Lands Management. USDA Natural Resources Conservation Service, Boise, ID, 2004.
3. Grandin T. Livestock Handling and Transport. 4th edition. CABI Publishing, New York, 2014.
4. Grandin T, Deesing M. Humane Livestock Handling. Storey Publishing, North Adams, MA, 2008.
5. Hansen AL. Beef Cattle. BowTie Press, Irvine, CA, 2006.
6. Kilgour RJ, Uetake K, Ishiwata T, et al. The behavior of beef cattle at pasture. Appl Anim Behav Sci 2012;138:12–17.
7. Lindahl C, Pinzke S, Keeling LJ. Human-animal interactions and safety during dairy cattle handling—comparing moving cows to milking and hoof trimming. J Dairy Sci 2016;99:2131–2141.
8. Stafford KJ. Cattle Handling Skills. AAC WorkSafe. Massey University, New Zealand, 2005.
9. Thomas HS. Storey's Guide to Raising Beef Cattle. 3rd edition. Storey Publishing, North Adams, MA, 2009.
10. Tone I, Irwin A. Watch out for the bull! Farmer risk perception and decision-making in livestock handling scenarios. J Agromed 2022;27:259–271.
11. Toxel TR. Cattle Working Facilities MP239. University of Arkansas, Division of Agriculture, https://www.uaex.uada.edu/farm-ranch/animals-forages/beef-cattle/beef-cattle-handling-facilities.aspx, 2022.
12. WorkSafe. Safe Cattle Handling Guide. WorkSafe New Zealand. https://www.worksafe.govt.nz/topic-and-industry/agriculture/working-with-animals/working-with-cattle/safe-cattle-handling-guide/, 2017.

6

SMALL RUMINANTS

DOI: 10.1201/9781003110910-6

Domesticated small ruminants in North America are listed in Table 6.1. Sheep and goats became the first domesticated livestock about 10,000 years ago by nomads in the Middle East. Domestic goats originated in Iran. Llamas and alpacas were domesticated 4,500 years ago in Peru to be used for meat, wool, and transportation. They are now also used as property guardians.

Table 6.1 Domesticated Small Ruminants
• Domestic Sheep
• Domestic goats
• Llamas
• Alpacas.

SPECIES CHARACTERISTICS

SHEEP AND GOATS
- **Appearance:** Some sheep and goats have a similar appearance.
  - **Tails:** Goats carry their tail up unless they are sick or frightened. Sheep carry their tails down. Sheep tails are often docked to reduce the risk of infections caused by feces smeared on and around the tail.
  - **Upper Lip:** Sheep have a philtrum (groove) in their upper lip; goats do not.
  - **Horns:** Most goats have horns, and most sheep do not. Sheep horns curl more than goat horns do.
- **Breed Variations:** There are more than 200 breeds each of domestic sheep and goats.

SOUTH AMERICAN CAMELIDS
- **Unique Features of Camelids:**
  - **Long Neck:** Camelids have long necks that they tend to put through holes in fences, among other places, and get caught or injured.
  - **Pacing Gait:** Camelids have a pacing gait like that of Standardbred horses. The front and rear legs on the same side move forward and backward at the same time.
  - **Footpads:** South American camelids do not have hooves. They have two toes with large nails and a large soft footpad. Their sternal area is heavily callused for long periods of rest in sternal position.
  - **Fighting Teeth:** Males and some female camelids have vestigial incisors, canine teeth, and large premolars which become six fighting teeth that begin to erupt at 2 years of age and are completely erupted by 4 years of age. There are two pairs on the upper arcade, just behind the dental pad, and one pair below on the mandible. Fighting teeth are sharp and angled backward (Figure 6.1).
- **Appearance:** Llamas and alpacas appear similar.
  - **Adult Size:** Adult llamas are larger, taller, and stronger than alpacas. Alpacas are about 1 to 2 ft shorter at the shoulder than llamas.
  - **Ear Shape:** Llamas have banana-shaped ears while alpaca ears are more like a Teddy bear's.
  - **Tails:** Alpacas have lower-set, stubbier tails and a more sloping rump.
- **Breed Variations:** Two breeds of alpacas exist, but there is only one breed of llama.

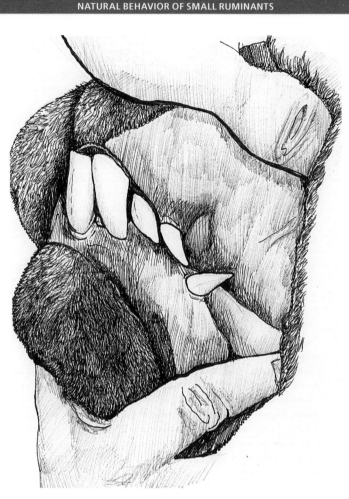

Figure 6.1 Fighting teeth in a llama.

NATURAL BEHAVIOR OF SMALL RUMINANTS

BEHAVIORS COMMON TO ALL SMALL RUMINANTS
- **Fears:** The fears of small ruminants are identical to those of cattle. For example, moving into dark areas, loud noises, high-pitched noises, flapping materials, shiny objects, unfamiliar people, and dogs can cause fear in small ruminants.
- **Social Structures:** Their social structures, like cattle, include leaders, dominants, and submissives.
- **Group for Defense:** Small ruminants usually move in groups and are distressed when removed from a herd. They will bunch up in 90-degree corners of holding pens. They will not readily intermingle with other breeds and tend to stay near family units within a herd.
- **Use of Special Senses:** Their vision, hearing, smell, taste, and touch senses are similar to cattle.

SHEEP

- **Social Bonding:**
  - **Strongest Social Bonding of All Domestic Animals:** Sheep have the strongest social ties of any domestic animal. They hate to be alone but will act distant or aloof to animals other than sheep.
  - **Group Defense:** The main defense of sheep is to run as a flock, sacrificing the young, weak, and slow on the periphery of the flock to predators to ensure the survival of the flock in general.
  - **Natural Groupings of Ewes:**
    - **Old Ewe Leaders:** In the wild, ewes form flocks of approximately 20 who are led by the oldest ewe. The oldest ewe with the greatest number of offspring is usually the flock leader. Within a flock, subgroups form, particularly among ewes and their direct descendants.
    - **Group Location of Leader:** The most dominant ewes will position themselves furthest from possible threats.
  - **Natural Groupings of Rams:** Rams form separate smaller flocks. Horn size is a significant factor in horned breed flock hierarchy.
- **Low Sleep Requirements:** Sheep are awake 16 hours a day and sleep 4 to 5 hours a day, which is much less than cattle.
- **Grazing Habits:**
  - **Dawn and Dusk:** Sheep spend half of their daylight hours grazing short, young grass and clover. Dawn and sunset are favored grazing times.
  - **Close Grazers of Grass and Short Weeds:** Sheep apprehend grass with their dental pad and lower incisor teeth and graze closer to the ground than cattle. Cattle cannot graze where sheep have recently grazed.
  - **Prefer Higher Ground:** Sheep prefer to graze on higher ground facing into the wind to better monitor for the smell of predators.
- **Communications:** Sheep communications include body language, visual, olfactory (smell), and vocal signals.
  - **Vision:** Sheep vision is similar to cattle vision, except in those with long wool around their face. These "closed face" breeds have a portion of their range of peripheral vision blocked, called "wool blindness." Sheep have good depth perception which allows them to move among rocks with sure-footedness.
  - **Body Language:** Lowering of the neck and head is a visual submissive posture. Stamping with a front foot is a threat for aggressiveness. Lowering and twisting the head is a horn threat suggesting aggression.
  - **Vocal:** Vocal communications include bleating to locate others or relate distress. Ewes "rumble" to lambs, and the "snort" of rams indicates irritation and possible aggressiveness.
  - **Odor:** Odor is important among sheep for identification. They have three pairs of scent glands: suborbital face glands beneath their eyes, groin glands on each side of the udder, and interdigital glands between the toes on each foot.

GOATS

- **Social Bonding:**
  - **More Independent Than Sheep:** Goats are herd animals, but unlike sheep, goats can be independent and will scatter if endangered. They are also more inquisitive, quicker, and more agile than sheep.
  - **Easily Discernible Leaders:** Social status is more evident in goat herds than in sheep flocks. Each herd is led by a dominant female, the *queen*. The head buck is usually the oldest and largest.

- **Natural Groupings:** Wild goats form variable-sized groups, but groups of three to five does are most common. Bucks group separately, except at breeding seasons. Horns, size, and age determine social dominance among able-bodied goats.
- **Grazing Habits:** Goats are browsers, eating weeds, leaves, vines, and shrubs while grazing for about half their daylight hours. They are more selective about what they eat than sheep.
- **Seek Shelter from Adverse Weather:** Goats try to avoid being caught in rain and will seek shelter from inclement weather more often than sheep.
- **Communications:**
  - **Body Language:**
    - **Nibbling and Butting:** Goats will nibble to investigate and communicate. They will butt to play or to re-establish their dominance.
    - **Buck Aggressiveness:** Bucks will stamp and sneeze when acting aggressive. They will flick their tongue just before rearing to begin a charge to butt an opponent.
  - **Odor:** Males have scent glands in their skin behind the horns, above their hocks on the inner surface of their legs, and under their tail which produce strong odors during rutting (mating) season. In addition, bucks will urinate on their face, beard, chest, and front legs. All these odors are rubbed on territorial markers and possessions, especially during mating seasons.
  - **Vocal:** When kids are handled and become frightened, they may shriek with childlike sounds to distract a handler and call for adult goat help.

SOUTH AMERICAN CAMELIDS

- **Social Bonding:** The herd social structure of llamas and alpacas are more similar to sheep than goats.
- **Protective of Territory:** Male camelids are very protective of their territory, especially male llamas. This instinct prevents overpopulation in areas with sparse vegetation and assures genetic diversity in the wild.
- **Communications:**
  - **Body Language:** Although social animals, individuals act aloof and do not like touching. Pinning the ears back can be a signal of possible aggression.
  - **Vocalizations:** Camelids, particularly alpacas, produce various vocalizations, but humming is the most common. Llamas may snort or make clicking sounds, if agitated. When frightened, camelids may scream.
- **Defense:**
  - **Sexually Intact Males:** Adult males fight by pushing with their shoulders, battering by swinging their necks, and biting. Kicking may also be used in defense, more so with alpacas than llamas.
  - **Females:** Overt defense tactics include kicking (they usually do not strike), spitting, and sometimes biting. Spitting is a spraying of rumen contents that is preceded by a gurgling sound. The spray may be effective for up to 6 ft and is usually a prelude to an attempted escape or an impending attack.
  - **Distrust of Dogs:** Camelids have an innate fear of dogs.
- **Averse to Temperature Extremes:**
  - Camelids have poor tolerance to heat.
  - They are adapted to cold but not frigid temperatures (less than 10°F).
- **Kushing:** Kushing is laying down on their sternum. It can be a means of adjusting to overheating by cooling their abdomen on cool ground, but it also is a passive means of defense (Figure 6.2).

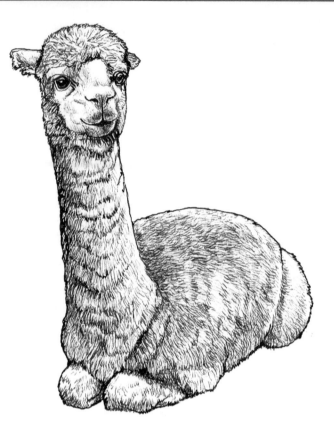

Figure 6.2 Kush position for a camelid.

SAFETY FIRST

HANDLER SAFETY
- **Sheep:**
  - **Deceptively Dangerous:**
    - **Panicked Group Danger:** If pressured or startled, adult sheep can bolt en masse and knock handlers down, trampling them. Even a single sheep is capable of knocking a handler down, often in an attempt to rejoin a flock.
    - **Danger to Children:** Children that are 5 years old, or less, should not be allowed in pens with sheep.
  - **Rams:**
    - **Potentially Lethal Attacks:** Rams are heavier and stronger than the average human and may butt with enough force to kill a handler. Bending over in a pen with a ram can be perceived as a challenge and can result in being charged. Handlers of sheep should never take their eyes off of a ram.
    - **Handling of Ram Lambs:** Ram lambs being raised for breeding should be minimally handled. Otherwise, the ram lamb may lose its inherent respect for humans and become dangerous as an adult. It should not be played with by patting it on its head, or otherwise encouraged to butt.

- ○ **Indications of an Intention to Butt:** Rams will back up in preparation to charge with their head tucked low. Also, stotting or pronking is a stiff-legged jump that is used by small ruminants to signal alarm to a perceived threat.
- ○ **Preventing Aggressive Acts:** See Table 6.2.

Table 6.2	Management of Aggressive Rams
•	Moving a ram with one hand under its jaw aids in controlling its attempts to be aggressive
•	A side hobble (a strap from front to hind leg on the same side) can also be used to discourage ramming
•	Attaching a clog (wood block) to a foreleg with a one leg hobble can discourage ramming (and jumping fences)
•	A dangerous ram can be hooded with a leather "ram shield" to see only down and to the rear.

- ○ **Response to an Attack:** Stepping 90 degrees to the side, at the optimum time, when charged by a ram is an effective defense tactic when needed. Throwing water on a ram during a charge may discourage some from further attempts to ram a handler.
- ○ **Ram Rivalry:** Rams that are not familiar with each other will butt one another with risk of serious injury. To allow a few days of acclimation, they should be put together in a small pen to eliminate the ability to run at each other.
- **Goats:**
  - **Intolerant of Rough Handling:** Goats can be very gentle, but they do not tolerate rough treatment and will butt when provoked.
  - **Potential Danger with Postpubertal Bucks:** Bucks are particularly dangerous after they reach puberty at 5 to 10 months of age. Signs of puberty include urinating thin streams of urine on their legs, mouth, beard, bellies, and lower aspect of their chest. Scent glands near their horns become active and secrete a strong odor that they will try to smear on animals and people to mark them as their possessions.
  - **Rutting Season Aggression:**
    - ○ **Seasonal Aggression:** Intermate rivalry or aggression becomes intense during the rutting season. Rutting season is fall to midwinter for some breeds, particularly dairy goats, but it can be year-round for other breeds, primarily meat goats. Aggression can also be directed at humans, especially men.
    - ○ **Buck Rivalry:** Adult bucks are especially aggressive to each other during mating season and should be housed individually with aisles separating their pens.
    - ○ **Signs of Aggression:** Signs of aggression can be staring, ducking the chin to present horns forward, pressing horns or forehead against an opponent, and rearing with or without a following charge. No one should be allowed to play with or tease a buck. Scratching or pushing on its head must always be avoided.
    - ○ **Avoid Aggravating an Attack:** A goat handler should never ignore a buck goat during rutting season. If threatened by a buck, a handler should not stomp feet or stare at the buck's eyes because both of these actions are indications of a challenge to bucks. Bucks do not back up in preparation to charge as do rams.
    - ○ **Plan an Emergency Exit:** Handlers should never allow a rutting buck to get between the handler and a route of exit.
  - **Aborting an Attack by a Buck:**
    - ○ **Body Language and Manual Restraint:** A handler may get the buck to delay or abort a charge by spreading the arms out and standing in an erect

position to look as large as possible. If close to the buck, the handler can grasp its beard and hold on to it while walking backwards to an exit.
- **Tennis Balls on Horns:** If working with horned goats, a small X-shaped incision can be cut into old tennis balls so that they can be jammed on the end of the horns until the handling procedure is finished.
- **Cull or Nose Ring:** Dangerous buck goats should be culled or a ring placed in their nasal septum, as with dairy bulls, for safer handling.
- **Danger to Children:** Children should be forbidden to be around bucks.
- **South American Camelids:**
  - **Aloof and Non-Aggressive, Except for Adult Males:** Camelids generally have an aloof, nonaggressive attitude and are easy to handle.
    - **Male Aggression:** Males are more likely to bite, strike with their heads and necks, and bump with their shoulders.
    - **Kicking:** Alpacas tend to kick in defense.
    - **Spitting:** Camelids, especially female alpacas, will spit a fine mist of regurgitated rumen contents, if made angry. They usually warn a potential spit victim with gurgling sounds first. A hand towel can be stuffed under the nose piece of a halter to protect a handler against spit if handling a gurgling camelid.
  - **Territorial Guardians:** Llamas are highly territorial. As a result, young, gelded llamas, 18–24 months old, that have been socialized with other llamas can be removed and socialized with other species to become guardians for those species, such as sheep. Sexually intact males cannot be housed together and should not be used as guardians.
  - **Beware Head Down Posture:** Camelids, particularly alpacas, may attempt to avoid a handler by holding its head down. The handler must be prepared when near the camelid for the possibility that its head may suddenly be raised. Otherwise, the camelid could hit an ill-prepared handler in the face.
  - **Bezerk Male Syndrome:**
    - **Overhandling of Young Males:** Camelids are believed to be easier to handle if "imprinted" (handled within the first few hours of life). However, overhandling a young sexually intact male that is raised in isolation to other camelids can result in a failure to respect human handlers, a condition called "bezerk male syndrome." Excessive handling of young male camelids should be avoided and orphaned male llamas that have had repeated human handling should be castrated before weaning.
    - **Manifestations:** Aggressive male camelids will put their ears back and their face dangerously near the handler's face. They may stick their head forward and horizontal with the ground and charge to bump the handler with its shoulders and try to knock the handler to the ground. If successful in pinning the victim, it will bite at the victim's face, neck, knees, and groin.
  - **The Handling Approach:** See Table 6.3.

Table 6.3	Handling Approach for Camelids Is Similar to Handling Horses
•	Avoid feeding treats by hand to discourage crowding and invasion of a handler's personal space
•	Allow crias to learn by watching well-behaved adult camelids being handled
•	Teach to be led with a halter and lead rope by gentle pressure and well-timed release
•	Teach patience and respect by being tied by a halter and lead rope for increasing periods of time.

SMALL RUMINANT SAFETY
- **Care of Small Ruminants:**
  - **Avoid a Rush:** All small ruminants should be handled slowly and quietly. They all have relatively fragile bones that can break much easier than horse or cattle bones.

- **Avoid Overheating:** With the exception of some goats, small ruminants have thick wool or long hair that makes them susceptible to overheating and should not be exerted or crowded during warm or humid weather.
- **Birth in Pens:** Newborn lambs may be abandoned by ewes in a flock that is grazing large areas. Penning them together for the first few days after birth allows the lambs to become stronger and the ewe to bond better with her lamb.
- **If Packing, Do Not Overload:** When goats or camelids are used for carrying packs, the packs should be balanced, properly mounted, and not exceed 20% of the ruminant's body weight.

- **Danger of Predators:**
  - **Many Predators Exist:** Small ruminants are prey to a larger range of carnivores than horses and cattle. One-third of all sheep and goat losses are from predators. All small ruminants have an innate fear of carnivores, but they can become socialized early in life to the presence of dogs.
  - **Protection from Canids:**
    - **Coyotes:** The leading predator of small ruminants in western states is the coyote, but in the eastern U.S., it is the roaming dog.
    - **Dogs:** All small ruminants need protection from roaming carnivores, such as dog-proof ruminant enclosures or herd guardian dogs or donkeys. Roaming dogs are usually not true predators. They are serial killers that chase sheep for fun rather than food and may maim them without a killing bite or kill them and not eat them.
  - **Other Predators:** In addition to coyotes and dogs, other predators of small ruminants include bears, cougars, bobcats, foxes, feral hogs, birds of prey (hawks, eagles), and carrion birds (vultures, ravens). Predators primarily kill weak, injured, or low-ranking sheep. Large flocks of sheep, sheep on open range, and those in areas with abundant predators should have two or more guardian dogs or other guardian animals.

- **Guardian Dogs and Other Guardian Animals:**
  - **Value of Guardian Animals for Sheep and Goats:** Guardian animals are highly recommended for the safety of sheep and goats that are in open pastures. The animal most adapted to guarding sheep is the guardian dog. Most guardian dog breeds for protecting sheep appear somewhat like sheep which enables them to visually blend in with flocks.
  - **Mission:** Guardian animals are intended to protect flocks from predators and serial killer canines. Care must be taken in approaching flocks when a guardian animal is present since a strange handler may be perceived as a predator.
  - **Guardian Dogs:** Guardian dogs are the most efficient guardians, but more than one is needed. Two should be available to chase a predator in increased confidence and safety while a third or more remains to protect the sheep from other predators. Guardian breeds are Akbash, Anatolian shepherd dog, Briards, Great Pyrenees, Komondor, Kuvasz, Maremma, Shar Planinetz, Spitz, and Tibetan Mastiff.
  - **Guardian Donkeys or Llamas:**
    - **Castrated Males:** Single castrated (gelded) male donkeys or llamas can also be acceptable guardians if properly selected, prepared for guarding, and maintained as a member of a sheep or goat herd. Sexually intact male donkeys or llamas are too aggressive toward sheep and goats, and sometimes people. A female llama may be an effective guardian if it cannot be used for breeding.
    - **Limit to One:** More than one castrated male donkey or llama will bond with their own species rather than sheep and goats, if given the chance.

- ○ **Limitations:** One gelded donkey or llama can be effective against coyotes, which do not hunt in packs or against single dogs. However, they are not effective against packs of dogs or wolves. Donkeys are not selective with threats and will bray at or strike at an innocent dog while llamas tend to be less aggressive to innocent dogs, foxes, and other non-threatening pasture invaders.
  - ○ **Adequate Size:** Standard-sized donkeys should be used as herd guardians because miniature donkeys are too small to protect a herd, or themselves, from dogs and coyotes.
- **Training Required:** All guardian animals have to be trained to protect sheep.
  - ○ **Dogs:** See Table 6.4.

Table 6.4	Training Required for Guardian Dogs to Protect Sheep
•	Guardian dogs should be socialized with sheep at an early age (just after weaning) by being kept in separate, adjoining enclosures with sheep
•	Socialized guardian dogs between 4 months and 9 months of age can then be allowed in pastures with sheep
•	Guardian dogs should be socialized to human handling and routinely handled but reside with the flock at all times
•	A guardian dog's focus should remain on the flock, while herding dogs bond and focus on the handler
•	Herding dogs should live with the owner; working guardian dogs should not.

- ○ **Llamas:** Gelded male llamas should be socialized with other llamas until the age of 18 months to 2 years and then socialized for guarding sheep or goats. In that time, it will have attained the physical size and strength needed and had exposure to the territorial behavior of its elders.
  - ○ **Donkeys:** Donkeys less than a year old should be introduced to small ruminants in adjacent pasture or paddock until they bond with the sheep or goats. Guardian donkeys should be kept away from dogs, including herding dogs.
- **Llamas Compared to Donkeys as Herd Guardians:**
  - ○ **Social Behavior:** Donkeys are often gregarious and seek human attention. Llamas tend to be aloof.
  - ○ **Dietary Requirements:** Llamas eat the same vegetation and require the same vaccinations as sheep and goats. Donkeys have different feed, vaccination, and hoof care requirements.
  - ○ **Heat Tolerance:** Donkeys tolerate hot weather much better than llamas.
- **Avoid Pampering Guardians:** Care must be taken not to overfeed or over handle guardian animals or they will become complacent and lethargic.
- **Other Protections from Predators:** Other methods for reducing predators include putting bells on some ewes so that there is an auditory alert to a flock being chased, mesh fencing, and gathering sheep in well-lit pens near a handler's residence.

KEY ZOONOSES

(NOTE: Apparently ill animals should be handled by veterinary professionals or under their supervision. Precautionary measures against zoonoses from sick animals are more involved than those required when handling apparently healthy animals and vary widely. The discussion here is directed primarily at handling apparently healthy animals.)

Apparently healthy domestic small ruminants pose little risk of transmitting disease to healthy adult handlers who practice conventional personal hygiene. The risks of physical injury are greater than the risks of acquiring an infectious disease (Table 6.5).

Table 6.5 Diseases Transmitted from Healthy-Appearing Small Ruminants to Healthy Adult Humans

Disease	Agent	Means of Transmission	Signs and Symptoms in Humans	Frequency in Animals	Risk Group*
Butting and Trampling (Sheep and Goats), Kicking and Biting (Llamas)	—	Direct injury	Crushing, butting, or bite injuries which can be permanently disabling or lethal	All small ruminants can inflict serious injuries. Injuries from adult males can be fatal.	3
Cryptosporidiosis	*Cryptosporidium* spp.	Direct, fecal-oral. Indirect from contaminated water	Diarrhea	Common, particularly in young small ruminants	2
Brucellosis	*Brucella melitensis*	Direct—secretions, especially placental fluid	Undulant fever, muscle aches, and lethargy	Very low, due to U.S. federal eradication program	3
Orf	Parapoxvirus	Direct contact with mouth or oral secretions	Blisters and lumps on the hands and face	Common	2
Q Fever	*Coxiella burnetii*	Direct with body secretions, particularly milk or placental fluids. Indirect from inhalation of contaminated dust.	Flu-like signs and atypical pneumonia	Moderate in cow-calf operations	2
Leptospirosis	*Leptospira* spp.	Direct from exposure to urine. Indirect from urine-contaminated water.	Kidney infection	Common in some locations and varies with vaccination	3

*Risk Groups (National Institutes of Health and World Health Organization criteria. Centers for Disease Control and Prevention, Biosafety in Microbiological and Biomedical Laboratories, 5th edition, 2009.)
1. Agent not associated with disease in healthy adult humans.
2. Agent rarely causes serious disease and preventions or therapy possible.
3. Agent can cause serious or lethal disease and preventions or therapy possible.
4. Agent can cause serious or lethal disease and preventions or therapy are not usually available.

SANITARY PRACTICES
- **Wear Appropriate Attire:** A handler of small ruminants should wear appropriate dress to protect against skin contamination with hair and skin scales or saliva, urine, and other body secretions. Gloves should always be worn when handling the mouth or nose of sheep and goats due to the risk of *contagious ecthyma* (*soremouth, orf*).
- **Control Ectoparasites and Rodents:** Ticks should be controlled. Contact with wildlife should also be controlled, especially rodents.
- **Maintain Basic Personal Sanitation:** Basic sanitary practices should be practiced, such as keeping hands away from eyes, nose, and mouth when handling small ruminants, in addition to washing hands after handling them.
- **Contain and Isolate Sick Small Ruminants:** Special precautions are needed if sick small ruminants are handled, and sick small ruminants should be isolated from apparently normal small ruminants. New herd members should be quarantined for at least 2 weeks to reduce the risk of transmitting a disease that new animals could be incubating before introducing them to the rest of the herd.

SHEEP

Common sheep breeds and terms for sheep age and genders are provided in Tables 6.6 and 6.7.

Table 6.6 Common Sheep Breeds and Their Use
• **Meat**—Suffolk, Hampshire, Southdown, and Cheviot
• **Fine Wool**—Rambouillet and Merino
• **Long Wool**—Lincoln, Romney, and Border Leicester
• **Dual Purpose**—Columbia, Corriedale, and Targhee
• **Hair**—Dorper and Katahdin
• **Minor Breeds**—Clun Forest, Jacob, and Shetland.

Table 6.7 Age and Gender Terminology for Sheep
• **Ram**—Adult sexually intact male sheep
• **Wether**—Castrated male sheep
• **Ewe**—Adult female sheep
• **Lamb**—A young sheep, less than 1 year old.

APPROACHING AND CATCHING
- **Initially Contain the Group:** To catch an individual sheep, it is necessary to herd the desired individual with the flock into a small catch pen with ten to 15 other sheep. Temporary corrals can be created using welded wire at least 40 inches high and steel T posts, or similar fencing. Herding flocks into the pen can be facilitated with a properly trained, herding-breed dog.
- **Approach the Individual to Be Caught:** Once the flock is packed in the pen, the handler should quietly approach the desired sheep straight from behind with the intent to stay in their blind spot.
  - **Basic Restraint Holds:** The capture is done by placing one arm under the sheep's neck and the other arm behind the rump (Figure 6.3). If needed, the sheep may be briefly immobilized by grasping a thigh just above the stifle. This may give enough time to get the other hand under its neck.

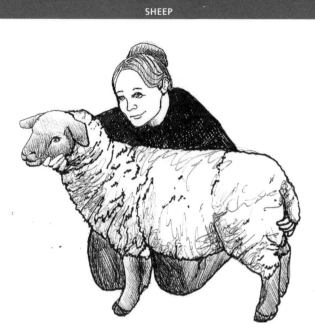

Figure 6.3   Loose restraint of a sheep that does not pull its wool.

- **Do Not Grasp the Wool:** Handlers should never grab or pull the wool to restrain sheep.
- **Cornering a Sheep:**   If 90-degree corners are present in the pen, the handler can move the desired sheep toward a corner. Cornered sheep will face the handler, who should grasp its head and neck with both hands and move the sheep's front end to the side. The sheep will try to move forward and the handler grasps the loose skin of both flanks to slow or stop it before grasping the neck and rump.
- **Shepherd Crooks:** Shepherd crooks are either for the neck (about four fingers wide at the bend) or for the hock (less than 2 inches wide at the bend) (Figure 6.4). Neck crooks are safer for sheep, but leg crooks may be more useful for horned sheep. Leg crooks have the potential to injure legs if used roughly or if the sheep strongly resists.

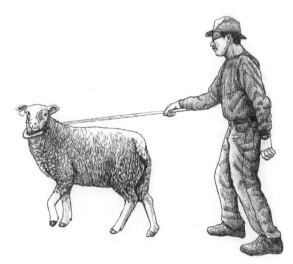

Figure 6.4   Capturing a sheep with a neck crook.

HANDLING FOR ROUTINE CARE AND MANAGEMENT

- **Basic Equipment and Facilities:**
  - **Commercial Handling Equipment:** Sheep handling equipment is commercially available, which is the reduced size versions of the equipment used on cattle.
    - ○ **Basic Equipment:** Basic handling equipment for sheep includes a collecting pen, crowding pen, alleyway, and sorting pens. Gates should be drop down style.
    - ○ **Optional Equipment:** Optional equipment includes a sheep tilt table, squeeze chute with headgate, elevated platform, scales, foot troughs, dipping tanks, and a loading ramp (Figure 6.5).
  - **Collecting Pen:** The collecting pen should provide 5 to 6 sq ft/sheep. The crowding pen should have an 8 ft radius.
  - **Alleyways:**
    - ○ **Purpose:** Alleyways are used for individual treatment and sorting.
    - ○ **Dimensions:** An alleyway should be up to 28 inches wide, at least 8 ft long, and 3 ft high with sloping sides that adjust to different size sheep. Higher alleyway sides may be needed for taller breeds.
    - ○ **Solid Sides:** Alleyways should have solid sides but with a 4-inch gap at the bottom to allow air circulation to the floor.

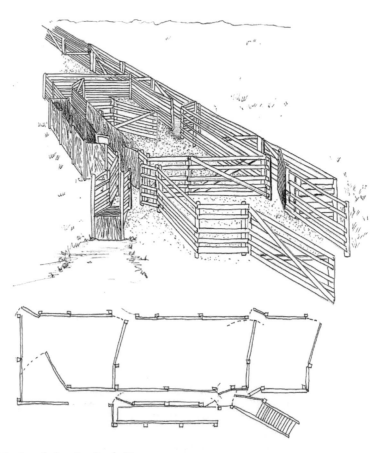

Figure 6.5   Example sheep handling facility.

- **Squeeze Chute:** A squeeze chute tilt table is helpful in trimming hooves, checking fertility of rams, and performing multiple procedures on one sheep.
- **Dip Tank:**
  - **Need:** Because of their thick wool, sheep are better treated for external parasites using dip tanks than with sprays or pour-ons.
  - **Construction:** Dip tanks should be 6 ft deep, 12 ft long, and 6 ft long at the level bottom. The other 6 ft are cleated slopes. It should be 2 ft wide at the top and 1 ft wide at the bottom.
  - **Shearing:** Dipping is best done 1 week after shearing in the spring. Just two sheep are driven in at a time. Young lambs do not need to be sheared first, and lambs under a month of age should not be dipped.
- **Packing Alleyway:**
  - **Use of Handler Legs for Packing:** A 3 ft alleyway can be used to pack groups of sheep facing the same direction. One handler packs the group with their legs and vaccinates, drenches, or ear tags one sheep at a time and then pushes finished ones behind, gradually working through the whole group (Figure 6.6).
  - **Exclude Adult Rams:** Adult rams cannot be included since they become aggressive after being turned back behind the handler.
  - **Backing with a Trained Herding Dog:** The group can be cleared out of a packed alleyway by a herding dog trained to "back" sheep. To back sheep the dog jumps on the sheep's backs and moves toward the front of the group, jumps down and turns the front sheep, and herds them out of the alleyway.
- **Moving Groups:**
  - **Leading:**
    - **Food Lures:** Sheep can be moved a short distance by enticing them to follow the handler who provides an opportunity for the sheep to eat a small amount of grain along the way.
    - **Lamb Lure:** A ewe with a newborn lamb can be moved by a handler carrying the lamb near the ground (no more than a foot high) and the ewe will follow.
    - **Lead Ewe Lure:** Capturing the lead ewe in a flock and moving or leading her will result in the rest of the flock following.
    - **Bellwether Sheep and Judas Goats:** A bellwether (leading sheep with a bell on a collar) or a "Judas" goat can be trained to follow a handler while leading sheep.
  - **Herding:**
    - **Flight Zones and Balance Points:** Herding sheep is achieved using flight zones and balance points as with herding cattle.
    - **Balking in Order to Fight Does Not Occur:** Unlike cattle, sheep do not stop and turn nor attempt to fight.
    - **The Flock Draws Potential Wanderers Back:** If a sheep briefly strays from the flock, keeping the flock together will result in the stray sheep returning.
    - **Teach to Be Herded:** Teaching sessions in a small pen with at least six sheep consist of moving them around the pen at a walk and occasionally stopping them in a corner to rest. Practice sessions should be about 20 minutes for at least three consecutive days. Repeat herding exercises should be done once per month.
  - **Herding Dogs:**
    - **Size Compared to Guardian Dogs:** Herding dogs are usually moderate-sized (30–50 lb.) intense, workaholic athletes. Guardian dogs are large breeds often exceeding 100 lb.
    - **Behavior Compared to Guardian Dogs:** Guardians like to rest near flocks and watch sheep during the day, although they are protective and

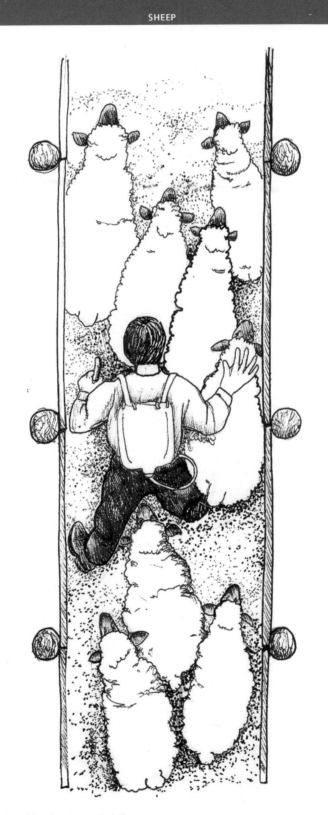

Figure 6.6 Drenching sheep in a packed alleyway

should become aggressive with possible predators. Guardian dogs are effective for goat herds, but goats do not flock together in danger like sheep and cannot be herded by dogs as effectively as sheep.

- ○ **Herding Dogs—The Gathering Types:** The gathering breeds are border collies, kelpies, Australian shepherds, collies, and bearded collies. Border collies and kelpies dominate in sheep gathering competitions. Herding dog trials use four to six sheep because a group of three sheep will scatter if over-pressured by handlers or herding dogs, but a group of four or more will usually not separate when herded.
- ○ **Herding Dogs—The Tending Types:** The tending breeds are Belgian Malinois, Belgian sheepdogs, Belgian tervurens, Bouvier des Flandres, Briards, German shepherd dogs, Beauceron Pyrenean shepherds, and Pulis. These were originally bred with the intent to have them patrol the perimeters of a flock and keep the sheep in a particular grazing area.
- ○ **Herding Dogs—The Driving Types:** The driving breeds are Rottweilers, Welsh corgis, Old English sheepdogs, and Australian cattle dogs. They were originally used on sheep to drive them to market and assist in moving sheep in stockyards.
- **Sorting Panels:** Sheep can be moved and sorted by herding into a small pen and using 4 ft portable sorting panels (hurdles). Groups of three to four sheep should be sorted at a time. Sorting individual sheep will cause a sheep to panic.
- **Restraint of Individual Sheep and Portions of Their Body:**
  - **Halters:** Appropriately sized halters can assist in restraining sheep. Most of the bridge of the nose is cartilage and can be compressed by a poor fitting halter. The nose strap should go over the bony part of the bridge of the nose and close to their eyes.
  - **Pressing against a Wall:** Sheep can be restrained against a wall by a handler backing the sheep into a corner with a solid wall. It is pressed against the wall with one of the handler's legs between its neck and shoulder and the other leg against its chest (Figure 6.7). Additional restraint can be accomplished with a hand under the sheep's neck, near its head.

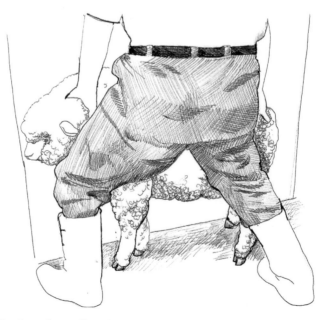

Figure 6.7   Pressing against a wall restraint.

- **Straddling:**
  - **Purposes:** Straddling is restraint for using a bolus gun or drenching syringe on a sheep, taking rectal temperatures, and performing eye or mouth examinations.
  - **Method for Restraint:** The handler backs a sheep into a corner, straddles its neck facing the same direction as the sheep, and holds it still with the knees on both sides of its neck. Straddling the sheep's chest and using one hand under the neck to block forward escape provides more control, but only one hand is free to perform examinations and treatment (Figure 6.8).
  - **Method for Moving:** If the handler is tall enough, straddling can also be used to move a sheep a short distance. The handler places a hand under the jaw, straddles the sheep's body facing the sheep's head, and places one hand on its rump or tail. The handler can then shuffle forward while holding the sheep's jaw and rump.

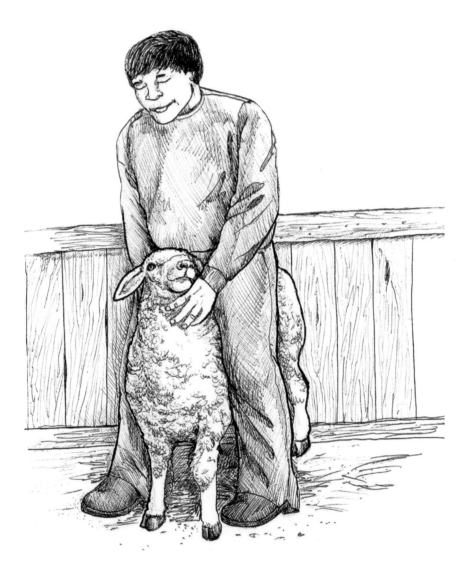

Figure 6.8 Straddle restraint.

- **Tipping ("Set Up," "Rumped"):**
  - ○ **Sitting Position Restraint:** Sheep have a rump padded by wool and fat, and downward positioned tails. This allows them to tolerate being placed on their rumps while leaning backward against a handler's legs. However, this will be resented if the tail has not had sufficient time to heal from being docked.
  - ○ **Purposes:** Sheep are tipped for shearing, crutching (clipping wool from around the rump), and hoof trimming.
  - ○ **Method:** See Procedural Steps 6.1 and Figures 6.9, 6.10, and 6.11.

Procedural Steps 6.1	Tipping Sheep
1.	The sheep does not have to be lifted to accomplish being tipped.
2.	The handler stands alongside the sheep's body, the sheep's head is turned away from the handler, and its rump is pushed down (Figure 6.9).
3.	After it sits with the legs away from the handler, its front legs are lifted and body turned slightly so that its back is leaned against the handler's legs (Figure 6.10).
4.	The sheep is tilted slightly onto one hip which makes it more comfortable and facilitates the handler freeing both hands to be able to shear.
5.	The sheep's head is tucked under an elbow as needed for better visibility and access to the lower chest and neck (Figure 6.11).

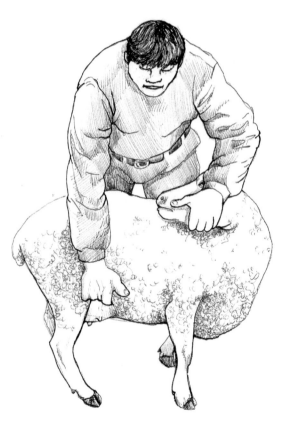

Figure 6.9   Initiating tipping a sheep.

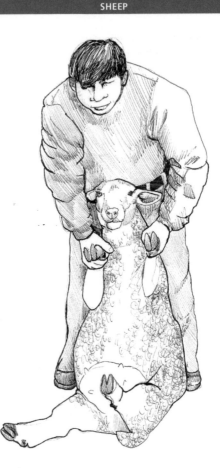

Figure 6.10   Sheep in tipped position.

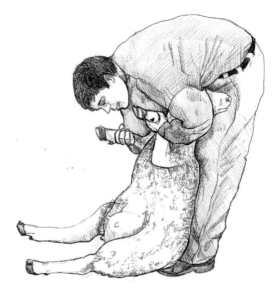

Figure 6.11   Restraint of head in tipped position.

○ **Sheep Chair:** Sheep chairs are restraint slings to hold a sheep in tipped position without the need to lean on the handler's legs (Figure 6.12).

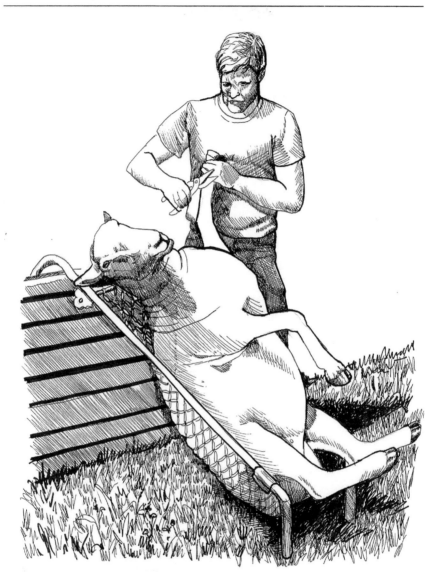

Figure 6.12   Sheep chair.

● **Backward Walk:** Moving a sheep a short distance is sometimes performed most easily by assisting it to walk backwards. The handler straddles the sheep facing the same direction as the sheep, picks up the sheep's front legs and has the sheep stand up on its hind legs. Continuing to hold its front legs, the handler walks backward to his destination while the sheep backpedals (Figure 6.13).

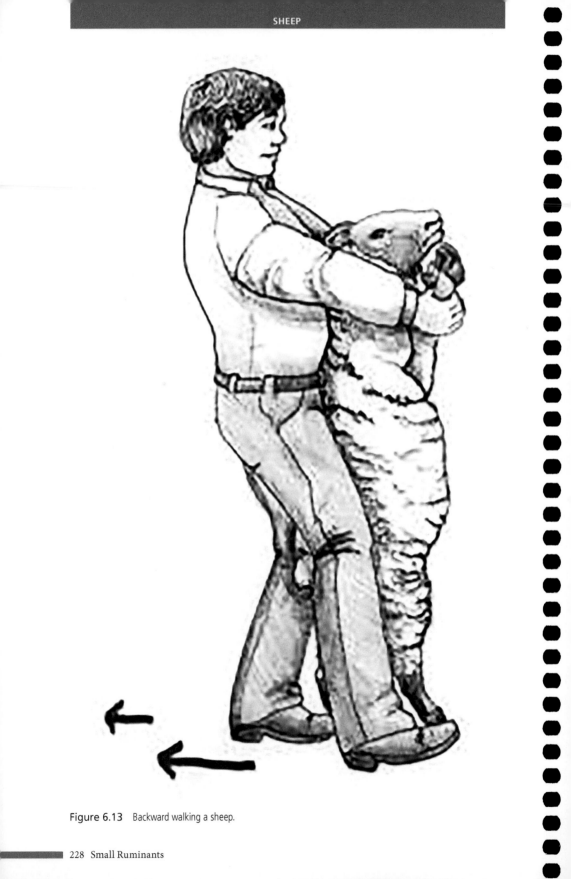

Figure 6.13   Backward walking a sheep.

- **Tying Up:** As with calves, sheep can be restrained by tying their legs with a rope that loops over the back of their necks. Using a fixed loop of rope, a half hitch is placed around each hind leg above the hocks and the rest of the loop between front legs and over the back of the neck. With the sheep on its side, the head is positioned level with the body or pointed up an incline to aid in eructating rumen gas and preventing bloat.
- **Gambrel:** A plastic W-shaped gambrel can be placed on the top of the neck and both front legs placed in the crooks on each side. Sheep cannot lift their legs out of the gambrel while their head is pressed down by the gambrel (Figure 6.14). Gambrels are used for short-term restraint during transit or treatment.

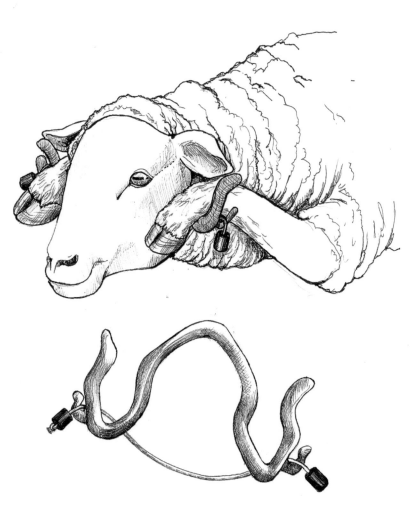

Figure 6.14   Gambrel for restraining sheep in sternal recumbency.

- **Trimming Hooves:**
  - **Purpose:** Small ruminant hooves that do not get worn down by rocky surfaces may need to be trimmed as often as every 8 weeks. Hoof trims every 6 months is about average.

- - **Assessing Need:** Front hooves carry more weight and will wear down faster. To check whether trimming is needed, the rear hooves should be checked.
  - **Trimming Instruments:** Hoof trimmers for small ruminants look like garden pruners, but true hoof trimmers are sharper and easier to handle than pruners.
  - **Method:** See Procedural Steps 6.2.

Procedural Steps 6.2	Trimming Sheep Hooves
1.	To trim hooves, the sheep is restrained to a stationary object and a foot picked up and the leg bent so that the bottom of the hoof is visible without causing discomfort to the animal.
2.	Other options are to place the sheep in tipped position against the handler's legs, in a sheep chair, or on a small tilt table.
3.	The bottom of the hoof is cleaned with a stiff hoof brush.
4.	The edge of the hoof should be trimmed until it is even with the sole.
5.	Any softened areas between the hoof wall and the sole need to be scooped out, and any excess growth between the heels should be trimmed.
6.	Uneven areas of the sole should be pared, but not enough that pink color appears.
7.	A light brush with a fine-toothed rasp can aid in leveling the bottom surface of the hoof.
8.	The dewclaws should be checked and carefully trimmed in small amounts, if needed.

- **Restraint of Lambs:**
  - **Carry Hold Restraint:** Lambs are captured as if picking up a small dog with a hand under its torso. Small lambs can be carried with one hand by a wrist and forearm under their chest and abdomen and the hand grasping the lamb's front leg nearest the handler's body.
  - **Castration and Tail Docking Restraint:** In the first 2 weeks of life, lambs are castrated and their tails are docked to prevent fecal accumulation and flystrike. Both these procedures can be done with the lamb held head up with its back toward the handler. The handler restrains the lamb's right front and rear legs with his right hand and the left front and rear legs with his left hand, or the same hold can be used while the handler sits to hold the lamb on its back (ventrodorsal position) on the handler's lap.
  - **Larger Lamb Restraint:** Larger lambs can be restrained by straddling the lamb, holding the body by pressing the lamb just behind the shoulders with the handler's calves while the handler blocks forward movement with a hand on the lower aspect of its neck behind the lamb's jaws. Another method is to straddle the lamb, grasp each front leg and raise the lamb onto its hind legs and hold its chest between the handler's thighs.

HANDLING FOR COMMON MEDICAL PROCEDURES

- **Injections and Venipuncture:**
  - **Assess to Veins:** Sheep can be tipped on their rump for jugular or cephalic vein venipuncture. The femoral vein may be accessed with a sheep in lateral recumbency.
  - **Injections:**
    - **Subcutaneous:** Subcutaneous injections are generally given under the skin behind an elbow, in the inguinal area, or fold of the flank.

- ○ **Intramuscular:** Intramuscular injections (IM) should only be administered in the side of the neck, except for nursing lambs (Figure 6.15). Nursing lambs should receive IM injections in the semitendinosus and semimembranosus in the back aspect of the thigh.

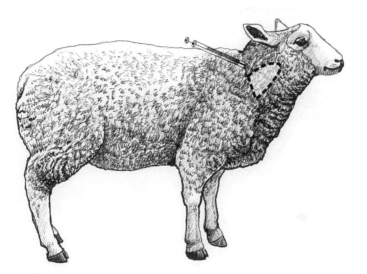

Figure 6.15   Site for IM injections in sheep.

- **Administration of Oral Medications:**
  - **Drenching (Administering Liquids):**
    - ○ **Method:** To drench a sheep, a handler straddles its back, places a hand under its lower jaw, and raises its head slightly. The nozzle of the drench syringe is inserted between the cheek and the back teeth. The plunger is pushed in slowly allowing the sheep to swallow the liquid medication.
    - ○ **Personal Protective Equipment:** Handlers should wear gloves and not put their fingers in the sheep's mouth.
  - **Bolusing (Administering Solid Medications):**
    - ○ **Balling Guns:** Balling guns are plunging instruments used to administer solid medications. The balling gun is inserted in the mouth and the plunger pushes the bolus onto the back upper surface of the tongue.
    - ○ **Method:** Sheep are caught individually, backed into a wall, and straddled. The sheep's head is lifted under the jaw but its nose should not be lifted higher than the poll. Otherwise, its ability to swallow will be impeded.
  - **Oral Speculums:** An oral speculum to protect the insertion of a flexible stomach tube is placed in the same way as a balling gun.

GOATS

Methods of handling goats vary and depend on if they are dairy goats, meat-producing goats, wool-producing goats, brush clearers, or companion pets (Table 6.8).

Table 6.8 Common Goat Breeds and Their Use

•	**Dairy**—Alpine, La Mancha, Toggenburg, Nubian, Oberhasli, and Saanen
•	**Meat-Producing**—Boer
•	**Wool-Producing**—Angora and Cashmere (Kashmir)
•	**Brush Cleaners**—Alpines, Boer, and Pygmy
•	**Companion Pet**—Pygmy.

Terms for age and gender of goats are provided in Table 6.9.

Table 6.9 Age and Gender Terminology for Goats

•	**Buck (Billy)**—Adult sexually intact male goat
•	**Wether**—Castrated male goat
•	**Doe (Nanny)**—Adult female goat
•	**Kid**—A young goat, less than 1 year old.

APPROACHING AND CATCHING

Approach and capture should be done gently or the goat will become aggressive and try to butt.

- **Signs of Aggressiveness:** Signs of aggression in bucks are curled tail over back, raised hair on the back, sneezing and snorting, stamping the forefeet, and rearing up on its hind legs. Goats do not bite or kick.
- **Use Their Curiosity:** Domestic goats are curious and will come to a handler doing another task in their pen. After the goat approaches the handler and the handler pets the goat, most will allow gentle restraint by holding at the base of the skull with both hands or grasping its collar if it has one.
- **Neck Crooks for Evasive Goats:** A shepherd's neck crook can be used if the goat is evasive. Leg crooks should not be used due to the risk of leg injury.
- **Catch Pens:** A catch pen is advisable, particularly for meat goats that are not frequently handled.
  - **Training for Catch Pens:** The pen should be used to feed and water to desensitize goats to the catch pen for future captures and handling. To accustom them to a catch pen and handler presence, the handler should feed grain in a small pile for each goat and kneel down near them and talk to them. Practice captures of short duration should be performed at a regular time when the goats are in the catch pen.
  - **Beware Bucks:** If a buck is in the group, the handler must be watchful of their own actions.
- **Neck Chains or Collars and Halters:** Dairy goats often have neck chains or collars for handling and identification.
  - **Plastic Chains or Flat Web Collars:**
    - **Purpose:** Colored plastic neck chains or flat web collars can be used to identify groups of goats by age, family, productivity, or other criteria. Goats can be led by their collar, or a separate leading collar with a leash can be used for leading and tying them for restraint.
    - **Cooler and Drier:** Nylon web or plastic chain collars permit better air circulation and drying of the skin than leather collars. Leather collars will trap moisture and will lead to bacterial or fungal infections. Other goats will often chew off a herdmate's leather collar.

- Breakaway: Plastic neck chains for routine use should break under moderate strain to prevent entrapment on a fence, by another goat's horns, or on other objects.
        - Aggressive Buck Neck Chains: Aggressive bucks should wear a neck chain. This allows them to be captured with a bullstaff. A halter with a lead rope can then be placed on their head and control exerted by the dual use of the staff and lead rope.
    - Dog Collars: Dog collars are hazardous because of the metal buckles which can become caught and cause strangulation.

HANDLING FOR ROUTINE CARE AND MANAGEMENT

- Basic Equipment and Facilities: Meat or milk goat handling equipment is commercially available that are reduced size versions of the equipment used on cattle.
    - Basic Equipment: Basic handling equipment for meat goats includes a collecting pen, crowding pen, alleyway, and sorting pens. Gates should be drop down style. Since goats are more independent and good jumpers, the sides of alleyways and pens must be higher (up to 6 ft) than those used for working with sheep.
    - Optional Equipment: Optional equipment includes a goat tilt table, squeeze chute with headgate, elevated platform, scales, foot troughs, and loading ramp.
- Moving and Separating:
    - Train to Follow: Milk and companion goats should be trained to follow rather than attempting to herd them.
        - Goats Are Capricious: Goats are more independent thinking than sheep. The Latin word caprine, referring to goats, is related to root for "capricious," meaning doing things on a whim.
        - Queen Goats: Rather than herding goats, it is more effective to identify the lead goat, usually an alpha doe (herd queen), and capture and lead her so the others will follow to a smaller pen for sorting or capture.
        - Luring with Food: By routinely feeding goats, they will follow the handler as they do the herd queen, but if the handler tries to drive them, then they are likely to scatter. If it is during breeding season, the handler may be challenged by bucks.
    - Psychological Barriers to Herding: Goats do not like to move from light into dark. They like to move to more open spaces, uphill rather than down, into the wind rather than downwind. They do not like to cross water or go through narrow openings, and they hate getting wet.
    - Leading Individuals: Goats can be trained to be led by a halter, but most are led by a collar around their neck. Bucks may need a halter and a bull staff clipped to their collar to control their movement, preventing the handler from being butted or stuck by a horn.
    - Odor Effects on Bucks: Bucks have strong odors that come from scent glands that are especially active during breeding season and the urine that they spray on their beards and front legs. Handlers should take care not to stand in front of bucks or within urination range of bucks during breeding season. Because of their odor and aggressiveness at breeding season, bucks are not handled as frequently nor can they be handled as gently as doe goats.
    - Do Not Herd Goats with Dogs: Dogs are generally ineffective in herding goats. Goats will climb, scatter, and fight, all of which are incompatible with effective herding with dogs.
- Restraint of Individual Goats and Portions of Their Bodies:
    - Pressing against a Wall: A goat can be restrained by backing the goat into a corner with a solid wall. The handler then presses it against a wall with one leg between its neck and shoulder and the other leg against its chest.

- **Jaw and Neck Hold:** Small and medium-sized goats can be restrained by a hand under their jaw and the other hand on the upper part of the back of their neck.
- **Straddling:** Some goats can be straddled for restraint. The goat is backed into a corner and the handler straddles its neck facing the same direction as the goat holding the goat still with the knees on both sides of the goat's neck. Straddling can be hazardous if attempted on horned goats or adult meat goats.
- **Flanking:** See Procedural Steps 6.3.

Procedural Steps 6.3	Flanking a Goat
1.	A handler can flank a goat by standing next to it and reaching over the neck to grasp the foreleg nearest the handler's body while his other hand grasps the flank.
2.	While lifting the goat, it should slide down the front of the handler's leg onto its side.
3.	The hand on the flank is moved to the bottom hind leg and the handler's elbow presses on the goat's neck while the hand on the front leg continues to restrain that leg.

- **Platform and Stanchion:**
  - **Milking:** Milking of goats is typically done with the doe standing on an elevated stand. Some include stanchions similar to cattle chutes with headgates. The goat may voluntarily walk up onto a platform if trained with grain as a reward, or led by its collar up to the platform.
  - **Foot Trims and Grooming:** Stanchions also aid in performing foot trimming and grooming.
- **Side Sticks and Neck Cradles:** Sticks from a halter to a chest strap (surcingle) or neck cradles can be used to prevent chewing on the legs or to prevent a dairy goat that has learned how to nurse itself.
- **Spanish Halter:** Spanish halters are similar to a tiedown used for horses. A strap or cord from a halter is run between the front legs and attached to a surcingle. The Spanish halter allows most normal grazing but prohibits the goat from eating from lower tree branches.
- **Tattooing:** Most goat breed registries require an identification tattoo on the ear flap or, in breeds with small ears, the tail web. The method of restraint used is manual restraint of the head or placing the head in a stanchion.
- **Trimming Hooves:**
  - **Frequency:** Hooves need to be trimmed about every 8 weeks depending on how abrasive the ground is in their enclosure.
  - **Method:** Goats are usually trimmed while they stand in the same manner as horses. An assistant handler may be needed to manually restrain the head and is preferred rather than tying the goat by a halter lead. Elevated platforms or small tilt tables may also be used for hoof trimming restraint.
- **Restraint for Kids:**
  - **Carry Hold Restraint:** Kid goats are captured as if picking up a small dog. Small kids can be carried with an arm under their chest and abdomen while the hand of the same arm grasps the kid's front leg nearest the handler's body. Kids should never be restrained by an ear, horn, the neck, or a leg.
  - **Castration Restraint:** Kids up to 20 lb. can be held with their heads up and back to the handler and the handler restraining the kid's right front and rear legs with the right hand and the left front and rear legs with the left hand. The same hold can be used while the handler sits and holds the kid on its back on the handler's lap.

- o **Larger Kid Restraint:** Larger kids can be restrained by straddling the kid facing the same direction as the kid, holding the body by pressing the kid just behind the shoulders with the handler's legs while the handler blocks forward movement with a hand behind the kid's jaws. Another method is to straddle the kid facing the same direction as the kid, grasp each front leg, and raise the kid onto its hindfeet and hold its chest between the handler's thighs.
- o **Disbudding Restraint:** Goats should be disbudded to prevent horn growth. Horns present a hazard to other goats and to handlers. In addition, the goat may entrap its head more easily with horns than without (Procedural Steps 6.4).

Procedural Steps 6.4	Disbudding Kids
1.	Kids should be disbudded within four days of birth.
2.	Properly performed disbudding will also remove the adjacent skin containing the scent glands.
3.	Restraint for disbudding a small kid is to hold the kid on the handler's lap in sternal recumbency while restraining the head movement with both hands on the neck and thumbs just behind its ears.
4.	Alternatively, a goat holding box may be used which is similar to a suitcase but with a hole for the goat's head to stick out.

HANDLING FOR COMMON MEDICAL PROCEDURES

- **Avoid Tipped Restraint:** Most handling and restraint of goats are similar to the methods used in sheep, except goats should not be restrained in the tipped position unless they are obese or very muscular. Since goat tails are held in an elevated position rather than against their anus like sheep, tipping goats may also injure their tail.
- **Avoid Restraint by Their Horns:** A goat should not be restrained by its horns or pulling on an ear which will be resented and cause struggling. Grasping the base of a horn of an adult may be done with little risk of it breaking off, but grasping the end of a horn or anywhere on a young goat horns may result in the horn breaking off and bleeding profusely.
- **Catatonic and Myotonic Responses:**
  - **Catatonic Response:** Some goats become catatonic with fear. The proper handler response is to back off and resume moving or handling in a less intimidating way.
  - **Myotonic Response:** Catatonic response is different from fainting goats which have a genetic disorder called myotonia. Fainting goats do not really faint. Their muscles will go into involuntary extreme contraction causing them to stiffen and fall on their sides.
- **Segregate Large, Horned, and Buck Goats:** Groups in small pens can become aggressive against small or timid members. Large goats should not be penned with small ones. Horned goats should not be penned with goats without horns, and bucks should not be penned together.
- **Injections and Venipuncture:**
  - **Assess to Veins:** Goats are haltered and tied or placed in a stanchion for jugular or cephalic vein venipuncture. The femoral vein may be accessed with a goat in lateral recumbency.
  - **Injections:**
    - o **Subcutaneous:** Subcutaneous injections are generally given under the skin behind an elbow or fold of the flank.

    ○   **Intramuscular:** Intramuscular injections should only be administered in the side of the neck, except for nursing kids (Figure 6.16). Nursing kids should receive IM injections in the semitendinosus and semimembranosus in the back aspect of the thigh.

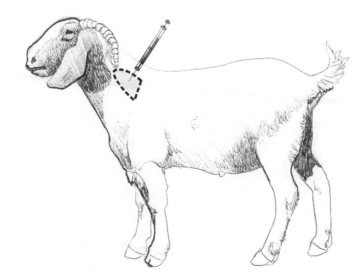

Figure 6.16   Site for IM injections in goats.

- **Administration of Oral Medications:**
  - **Drenching:** For up to 8 to 10 ounces, drenching is more practical than using a stomach tube (Procedural Steps 6.5).

Procedural Steps 6.5 Drenching a Goat	
1.	To drench a goat, a handler straddles its back, places a hand under its lower jaw, and raises its head slightly.
2.	The nozzle of the drench syringe is inserted between the cheek and the back teeth.
3.	The plunger is pushed in slowly allowing the goat to swallow the liquid medication.
4.	Handlers should wear gloves and not put their fingers in the goat's mouth.
5.	A speculum for insertion of a stomach tube is placed in the same way.

  - **Balling Gun:** Balling guns are used to administer solid medications (Procedural Steps 6.6).

Procedural Steps 6.6 Using a Balling Gun	
1.	Goats are caught individually and backed into a wall and straddled facing the same direction as the goat.
2.	The goat's head is lifted under the jaw but its nose should not be lifted higher than the poll as this would risk its ability to swallow.
3.	The balling gun is inserted in the mouth and the plunger pushes the bolus onto the back upper surface of the tongue.
4.	The balling gun should not be inserted too far, which could impair swallowing and allow the bolus to go into the larynx or trachea.

SOUTH AMERICAN CAMELIDS (LLAMAS AND ALPACAS)

The llama is a beast of burden that can carry 25–30% of its weight when conditioned. It is also bred for their meat, hide, and sinew. The smaller alpaca is bred for its fine wool. There is one breed of llama and two breeds of alpacas (Table 6.10).

Table 6.10 Common Breeds of South American Camelids
• **Llama**—Llama
• **Alpaca**—Huacaya and Suri.

Terms for age and gender of camelids are provided in Table 6.11.

Table 6.11 Age and Gender Terminology for South American Camelids
• **Machos**—Adult breeding males
• **Geldings**—Castrated males
• **Hembras**—Adult females
• **Crias**—Young camelids.

APPROACHING AND CATCHING
- **Herd Group into a Small Enclosure:**
  - **Catch Pen or Alleyway:** Even docile, well-handled camelids are often resentful of being caught. They can be difficult to impossible to catch in a large pasture. To catch them, they can be herded into a small catch pen or funneled into an alleyway.
  - **Mobile Rope Enclosure:** Herding may be more effective by *sweeping*, which is done by two handlers holding a 30 ft rope about 3 ft off the ground and moving camelids toward a fence. One handler can tie one end to the fence while the other maintains the trapped camelids. The free handler can then catch and halter the desired camelid.
- **Training to Be Caught:**
  - **Food as a Lure and Reward:** Typically, camelids must be trained to enter small catch pens that are 10 × 30 ft, or smaller, where they are often fed to desensitize them to the enclosure. They should be approached in a calm direct manner in the pen using an approach and retreat method similar to catching an evasive horse.
  - **Risk of Haste:** Rushing an approach can cause camelids to panic and injure themselves.
  - **Managing Fright:** Camelids that are frightened should be caught in a shelter or building with one or more calm companions to prevent attempts to jump over a fence.
- **Manual Restraint:**
  - **Neck Hug:** The basic restraint of a camelid is for the handler to wrap an arm around the camelid's neck near its head and pull it close to the handler's body. The handler's other hand pushes down on its shoulders or holds the camelid's shoulder and chest close to the handler's body.
  - **Alternative or Assisted Holds:** An alternative hold to holding its shoulder is to grasp the base of the tail. However, grasping their tail may cause

some to kush. Pinning them against a solid wall may also assist with restraint.

- **Avoid Touching Ears:** The ears should never be used for restraint. Causing pain or fear from handling their ears will teach them to dangerously swing their head and neck in efforts to escape.

- **Dogs Not Allowed:** Dogs should not be allowed within sight nor sound of camelid catch pens.

HANDLING FOR ROUTINE CARE AND MANAGEMENT

- **Basic Equipment and Facilities:**
  - **Catch Pens:** Catch pens for camelids are small pens, 10 × 30 ft or smaller and at least 5 ft high. At least two or more camelids should be herded into a catch pen for ease of sorting and reducing anxiety in camelids separated from the main group.
  - **Camelid Stocks:**
    - **Need:** A restraint chute similar to horse stocks is advisable for ease of restraint of llamas (Figure 6.17). Alpacas respond better to loose restraint with a halter and lead rope.

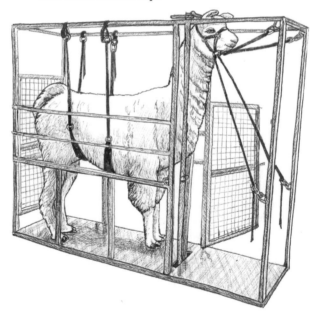

Figure 6.17 Camelid stocks.

- **Top-Heavy Construction:** Camelid stocks are tall and narrow. If they are not constructed of anchored posts, stocks should be bolted to the floor to prevent it from being tipped over on its side.
- **Dimensions:** The size should be 2 ft wide, 5.5 feet long, and 45 inches to the top rail.
- **Access:** There should be access to the camelid from all sides.
- **Cinches:** A front and rear cinch attached to side rails is required to keep camelids from kushing in the stocks. Cinches should be 8 to 10 inches apart for llamas and closer for alpacas. A third cinch may be needed for some camelids to go over the withers to prevent rearing or jumping.

- o **Cross-Tie Rings:** Cross-tie rings should be in forward positions to prevent the tied camelid from moving backward in the stocks. Quick release ties should be used, if lower cinches are not used to prevent kushing.
- **Moving and Separating:**
    - **Catch Pens:** Camelids are extremely herd-oriented and are best moved as groups. Separation of individuals from the herd is ideally completed by using a series of catch pens that gradually get smaller until an individual can be caught.
    - **Mobile Rope Corral Method:** Another method of separation involves two handlers holding a 30 to 40 ft rope about 3 feet off the ground to sort camelids.
    - **Avoid Blindfolds:** Blindfolds should not be used in an attempt to move camelids because they will kush.
- **Restraint of Individual Camelids or Portions of Their Body:**
    - **Halters and Lead Ropes:**
        - o **Training to Be Restrained by a Halter:** Camelids can be taught to be haltered and led. This is basic training for llamas to be used as pack animals.
        - o **Method:** Camelids are principally handled from the left side and led from their left side. Placing the halter is done with a bear hug approach as with haltering horses.
        - o **Appropriate Halter:** A camelid halter should be used. Pony halters should not be used because the noseband is too low for camelids.
        - o **Fitting a Halter:** The noseband should be at least 1 (inches above the end of the bony part of the nose. At least two fingers should be able to be placed under the lower aspect of the band and the jaw so that it can chew. The cheekpieces should be at least 1 inch below the eyes (Figure 6.18).

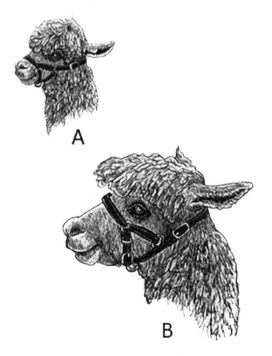

Figure 6.18   Positions of a camelid halter's nosepiece: A—incorrect, B—correct.

- Use Halters Only When Handling: Halters should be removed when not handling the animal because of the risk of it catching on brush, fences, and other objects if the camelid is on pasture.
- Handling Crias:
  - Small Crias: Small crias can be flanked and laid in lateral recumbency or pressed against a solid wall as with sheep or goats.
  - Medium-Sized Crias: Crias are handled similarly to foals by boxing in their forward and backward movements with the handler's arms without squeezing them.
  - Chukkering: If a cria kushes in resistance to being restrained, a handler should bend down on their knees and straddle its chest facing the same direction as the cria and hold the upper area of its neck. They can be kept in kush position by *chukkering*, which is the use of a folded loop of rope over the back in front of the pelvis with the ends of the loop around the fetlocks of the flexed hind legs. This prevents them from being able to rise and allows a handler to perform jugular venipuncture or administer oral medications.
  - Training: Cria should be handled for brief periods (less than 20 minutes) on a regular basis to gradually desensitize them to being haltered and led, loosely restrained, and having their legs and feet handled. This will prepare them for necessary toenail trimmings 3 to 4 times per year if their enclosures are not abrasive enough to wear the nails down.

HANDLING FOR COMMON MEDICAL PROCEDURES

- Injections and Venipuncture:
  - Access to Veins: Venipuncture is generally from the jugular vein or the ventral tail vein.
    - Jugular Vein: South American camelids have thick skin in the neck and large transverse processes of the cervical vertebrae that obscure the jugular vein. The most accessible points are high in the neck or low in the neck. The high location is preferred because of the proximity of the carotid artery to the lower region of the jugular vein.
    - Cephalic Vein: The cephalic vein may be accessed if the camelid is in kush position.
  - Injections:
    - Intramuscular: Intramuscular injections are generally given in the triceps muscle in the forelegs or the semitendinosus and semimembranosus muscles of the hind legs. Intramuscular injections should not be given in the neck of camelids regardless of age.
    - Subcutaneous: Subcutaneous injections are given under the loose skin low on the chest just behind the elbow.
- Administration of Oral Medications: Oral administration of liquids is the same as with sheep and goats, except straddle restraint is not possible. Restraint is similar to horse restraint and is achieved with a halter and lead rope or camelid stocks.

TRANSPORTING SMALL RUMINANTS

LOADING CHUTES

- Divide Loading Chutes with Partitions: Loading chutes for sheep and goats can be side by side and should be solid walled on the outside to prevent seeing handlers and high enough to prevent attempts to jump out. Partitions between chutes for sheep should be see-through so that they can see other sheep moving forward.

- **Narrow Chutes to Prevent Turn Around:** There should be narrow divisions in the loading chutes to prevent animals from being able to turn around in the chute. Cleats are needed in floors to eliminate or reduce slipping.

SHEEP OR GOATS

- **Transport Two or More:** Sheep or goats should not be transported alone. They should be transported with at least one favored herdmate.
- **Drive with Gentle Transitions in Speed and Direction:** As with transporting all live-stock, driving of the transport vehicle should be smooth. Accelerating or stopping suddenly should be avoided. Turning corners should be slow enough for the animals to shift their weight and stay on their feet.
- **Required Rest:** During travel, sheep or goats should be rested every 5 consecutive hours and off loaded, fed, and watered after 24 hours of travel, or more frequently. Title 49, U.S. Code, Chapter 805, Section 80502 prohibits 28 hours of continuous travel of livestock. However, sheep may be transported up to 36 hours if travel is completed at night.
- **Bedding:** Dust-free, mold-free bedding of sand or rubber mats should be used to provide foot traction and cushion, and to be able to clean soiling.
- **Sufficient Room:** Enough room between the animals should be allowed to permit moving without crashing into each other or the sides of the transport vehicle and to lie down, if desired. However, animals should be close enough to brace against each other when needed. If too much room is present, straw bales can be tied down to provide bumpers.
- **Horned or Aggressive Sheep or Goats:** Horned or aggressive sheep or goats should be partitioned from others or haltered and tied. The lead rope should be tied with just enough length to allow the animal to get up if they fall or lie down but not so long that it could easily get tangled.
- **Be Vigilant for Goat Escape Attempts:** Goats must be transported in completely enclosed containers to prevent escapes. Doubly latched dog crates can suffice, if they are large enough for the goat to stand up and lie down comfortably. Goat-sized livestock crates are available for the bed of pickup trucks.
- **Avoid Heat Stress:** Unshorn sheep, alpacas, and Angora and cashmere goats are especially susceptible to heat stress. They need to be provided extra space and ventilation. Travel should occur in the early morning, late in the day, or at night if transported in warm weather.

SOUTH AMERICAN CAMELIDS

South American camelids can be trained to travel in horse trailers or in the back of station wagons, minivans, or pickup trucks with stock sides. They kush during travel and because of this, they occupy relatively small space during travel. If they have enough room to stand as in a horse trailer and are tied, they should be tied with enough lead line to be able to kush.

BIBLIOGRAPHY

1. Birutta, G. Storey's Guide to Raising Llamas. Storey Publishing, North Adams, MA, 1997.
2. Hoffman C, Asmus I. Caring for Llamas and Alpacas: A Health & Management Guide, 2nd edition. Rocky Mountain Llama and Alpaca Association, Inc., South Fork, CO, 2005.
3. Mateo JM, Estep DQ, McCann JS. Effects of differential handling on the behaviour of domestic ewes (*Ovis aries*). Appl Anim Behav Sci 1991;32:45–54.

4. Sayer M. Storey's Guide to Raising Meat Goats. Storey Publishing, North Adams, MA, 1997.
5. Simmons P, Ekarius C. Storey's Guide to Raising Sheep. Storey Publishing, North Adams, MA, 2001.
6. WorkSafe. Safe Sheep Handling Guide. WorkSafe New Zealand. https://www.worksafe.govt.nz/topic-and-industry/agriculture/working-with-animals/working-with-sheep/safe-sheep-handling-gpg/, 2017.

7

SWINE

DOI: 10.1201/9781003110910-7

Domesticated swine are referred to as hogs or pigs depending on their size. Hogs are raised for their meat, hides, bones, and hair. Pork products are the most consumed meat product in the world. The U.S. has become the largest exporter of pork products in the world with 30% of its hog production being exported.

Age and size, plus gender terms are provided in Table 7.1 and 7.2.

Table 7.1 Age and Size Terminology for Swine	
•	**Piglets**—Young swine that are still nursing
•	**Pigs**—Swine from weaning to 120 lb. (also called shoats)
•	**Starter Pigs**—Pigs from 10 to 40 lb.
•	**Feeder Pigs**—Pigs from 40 to 80 lb.
•	**Hogs**—Pigs 120 lb., or more
•	**Finisher Hogs**—Hogs 150 to 220 lb.
•	**Butcher Hogs**—Hogs 220 lb., or more.

Table 7.2 Gender Terminology for Swine	
•	**Boar**—A sexually intact male hog
•	**Barrow**—A castrated male hog
•	**Gilt**—A female hog that has not had a litter of pigs
•	**Sow**—A female hog that has had a litter of pigs.

NATURAL BEHAVIOR OF SWINE

SOCIAL STRUCTURE
- **Prefer Small Groupings:** Swine in the wild live in groups, called "sounders" of two to six sows and their piglets. The sows will often pair up for foraging and sleeping.
- **Social Rank Based on Body Size:** Body size strongly affects social status in hogs and pigs. The superior social rank of heavier pigs is established in early play contests. Success in pushing other pigs away from food or other possessions reinforces social rank.

SPECIAL SENSES AND COMMUNICATIONS
- **Special Senses:** Swine have an extraordinary sense of smell, excellent hearing, and poor vision.
- **Vocalization:** Grunting vocalizations are auditory social contacts that are nearly constant if moving or nursing piglets. Squealing is a call to congregate.

DAILY ACTIVITIES
- **Group Interaction:** Hogs cannot reach most of their body with their mouth or their hind legs. In groups, they groom each other with their mouths. When deprived of this, they spend much of their time trying to scratch themselves on objects.
- **Foraging:** The natural behavior of swine is to forage for food (grubs, worms, roots, nuts) and investigate their surroundings by rooting with their snout for about 7 hours a day. Hogs have a disk-shaped snout cartilage that aids their ability to root. They root to find food and create wallowing areas to cool themselves.

- **Need for Mental Enrichment:** Hogs are highly intelligent and require much mental stimulation to prevent self-mutilation or aggression toward other hogs. Deprived of these mental challenges, food possession becomes more important and aggressiveness to other hogs increases.

HABITATS

- **Moderate Temperatures:**
  - **Preferred Temperature:** Hogs are adapted to temperate climates. They are most comfortable at temperatures between 55° and 85°F.
  - **Response to Hot Weather:** During hot weather, their activities in the wild are primarily nocturnal. In daytime, they wallow in mud and rest.
  - **Response to Cold Weather:** When cold weather occurs, their activities become more crepuscular and diurnal. When resting in cold weather, they huddle together to conserve body heat.
- **Natural Habitat:** Hogs are capable of living in a wide variety of habitats, but they prefer woodland marshes that provide escape from sunburn and heat, chances to wallow in mud to control flies and other external parasites, and their favorite foods, including acorns and earthworms.
- **Confinement on Concrete:** For economic benefits, 98% of swine in the U.S. are now raised in total indoor confinement on concrete. This prevents their primary natural behaviors, rooting and wallowing and has adverse effects (Table 7.3).

Table 7.3	Adverse Effects of Confinement on Concrete
•	**Lack of Rooting**—The natural 7 hours of mentally stimulating rooting are exchanged for 2 hours of eating from a pan or trough in a pen
•	**Lack of Wallowing**—Hogs normally wallow up to 3 hours per day to cool their body and for social activity; without a chance to wallow they have less mental stimulation and resort to vices
•	**Reduced Rest**—When hogs are prevented from rooting, they lie on their sternums more than their sides which is less restful and more stressful
•	**Tail Biting**—Tails are docked to prevent tail biting that results from the lack of the mental stimulus resulting from rooting and wallowing
•	**Iron Deficiency**—The inability for baby pigs to ingest dirt from the sow's teats while nursing and rooting will lead to iron deficiency anemia without administering iron supplements.

AGGRESSION AND DEFENSE

- **Aggression:**
  - **Crowding and Lack of Foraging:** Crowding and time limited access to food generates most aggression in hogs.
  - **Drug-Induced:** Hogs in large commercial operations may be given beta-adrenergic drugs to reduce fat in their muscle. Common side effects of beta-adrenergic drugs are nervousness and aggression.
  - **Breed Predisposition:** Breed affects social rank in mixed groups. Large Whites are more aggressive than Hampshires which are more aggressive than Durocs. Large Whites are the most common breed used in pork production in the United States.
  - **Gender Behavior:**
    - **Peak Aggressiveness:** Boars are most aggressive during breeding season and sows are especially aggressive when they have nursing piglets.
    - **Adult Boars Do Not Tolerate Young Males:** Once young boars are near the age of puberty, they are driven away by older, more dominant boars. They finish their development in bachelor groups until they are ready to challenge the dominant boars. The dominant boars tend to remain solitary except at breeding seasons.

- Marking Territory: Boars "champ" their teeth and produce some frothy saliva containing pheromones. They mark territory which they will aggressively protect with saliva and urine.
- **Defense Tactics:**
  - **Push and Bite:** Hogs defend themselves by pushing and biting.
  - **Bullet-shaped Body:** The bullet shape of their body is a passive means of defense that affords considerable protection from predators and adversaries. Their body shape facilitates quick escapes in thick bush and difficulty in being caught, especially if their body is wet and muddy from wallowing.
  - **Congregate in Danger:** They move in loose groups as a herd, but if alerted to threats by a herd member's squeal, other hogs will come to the member's defense.

SAFETY FIRST

HANDLER SAFETY

- **Squealing:**
  - **Exacerbates Aggression by Adult Hogs:** Restrained swine squeal very loudly. Handlers should not cause pigs to squeal in the presence of sows for procedures such as treating pigs' navels, clipping needle teeth, docking tails, notching ears, castration, or administering injections because the mother sow or other sows may become agitated enough to become aggressive and dangerous.
  - **Risk of Permanent Hearing Loss:** Feeding time in a swine building can have squealing intensity that reaches 95 to 130 decibels. Hearing loss can begin at 85 decibels. If a handler must raise their voice for someone to hear them speak that is standing an arm's length away, the decibels are above 80 decibels and ear protection should be worn.
- **Respiratory Dangers:** When working in hog total confinement buildings, respiratory problems are a risk to handlers.
  - **Causes:** Causes of respiratory difficulty in swine buildings can include dust (particularly particles of feed and fecal matter) and gases (especially ammonia from urine and hydrogen sulfide from feces).
  - **Respirator or Disposable Mask:** Wearing an appropriate respirator may be necessary. Disposable dust masks with two straps provide protection against inhaling larger particles, but do not provide protection against small particles of dust or gases.
- **Biting and Pushing:**
  - **Boars and Nursing Sows:**
    - **Handle Dominant Boar First:** The most dominant boar should be handled first so that the smell of subordinate boars will not stimulate aggression.
    - **Size Matters:** Breeding boars or nursing sows weigh more than 500 lb. They are often aggressive and dangerous, especially if they have been mishandled in the past, which includes not allowing them to socialize with other hogs when they were young.
    - **Gender Tactics:** Sows attempt to knock down intruders in their personal space and then bite them. Boars will attack intruders while they are still standing and can be extremely aggressive, if provoked.
    - **Maintain a Barrier to Leg Access:** Adult hogs, particularly boars, if aggressive may try to bite the inner aspect of the thigh and if successful can sever the femoral artery of a handler. This can quickly lead to life-threatening hemorrhage. Handlers should always keep a barrier (panel, fence, or other partition) between the themselves and a boar being handled.

- ○ **Wear Leg and Foot Protection:** It is advisable to wear knee boots and steel toed shoes when in hog or pig pens.
        - ○ **Handler's Last Defense:** If charged by a sow or boar, a slap on its snout with a shovel, cane, or long handled, heavy-duty flashlight may be enough distraction for a handler to quickly escape.
    - **Ensure Two Exits and Ability to Grasp a Stationary Object:** Handlers should always leave themselves two exits from a hog pen, always remain within reach of stationary objects to hold to prevent being knocked down, and never back a grown hog into a corner.
  - **Pen Gates Are for Hogs Only:** Gates in hog pens should only be used for moving hogs in and out. Handlers entering a pen should climb over the pen wall or fence since hogs can escape with speed and force if the gate is unlatched momentarily for a handler to enter.
  - **Separate Handlers for Breeding or Painful Procedures:** Handlers who routinely work with hogs should not be involved when breeding sows or boars or if painful procedures, such as vaccination or blood collection, are to be performed. Hogs are more likely to remain calm for daily activities if they do not associate pain or restraint with their routine handlers.

SWINE SAFETY

- **Risks of Intelligence, Independence, and Poor Eyesight:** Hogs and pigs are very intelligent and individualistic. They do not herd well in groups.
    - **Attempted Escapes:** Each one that becomes trapped in an enclosure will look for an opening and root around their enclosure in an attempt to find an escape. Pigs will pile on top of each other seeking escape. Attempts to escape can contribute to overheating and death from heat stroke if not handled quickly with as little stress as possible.
    - **Poor Vision:** They have poor vision and activate "fight or flight" responses quickly.
  - **Stimuli of Aggression:**
    - **Hunger:** Hogs are more aggressive to each other and to handlers, if hungry.
    - **Squealing of Other Pigs or Hogs:** Hogs will become agitated and sometimes aggressive to each other and to handlers by "mob action" if a member of the group seems in distress.
  - **Train to Reduce Stress of Handling:** Hogs and pigs should be desensitized to humans near their flight zones by handlers getting into their pen, getting the pigs up as quietly as possible, and having them move quietly around the pen, then leave when they are relatively calm.
  - **Provide Diversions When Handling:** To decrease fighting when mixing sows or pigs, groups should be established according to size; extra food should be provided during initial introduction; and hay, straw, and toys made available for mental stimulation and diversion. A new hog or pig being added to an established group is best introduced in a dark room.
  - **Clip Day-Old Piglets' Teeth:** The incisors and canine teeth are often clipped in 1-day-old piglets to reduce injuries to the sow's teats and to litter mates.

KEY ZOONOSES

(NOTE: Apparently ill animals should be handled by veterinary professionals or under their supervision. Precautionary measures against zoonoses from sick animals are more involved than those required when handling apparently healthy animals and vary widely. The discussion here is directed primarily at handling apparently healthy animals.)

Apparently healthy domestic hogs pose little risk of transmitting disease to healthy adult handlers who practice conventional personal hygiene. The risks of physical injury are greater than the risks of acquiring an infectious disease (Table 7.4).

Table 7.4 Diseases Transmitted from Healthy-Appearing Swine to Healthy Adult Humans

Disease	Agent	Means of Transmission	Signs and Symptoms in Humans	Frequency in Animals	Risk Group*
Bites	—	Direct injury	Bite wounds to hands and legs; death can occur from torn or severed arteries	All swine are capable of inflicting bites	3
Salmonellosis	*Salmonella* spp.	Direct, fecal-oral	Diarrhea, systemic disease and abscesses	Common	3
Swine Influenza	Influenza A, H1N1, and H3N2	Direct, airborne	Respiratory disease and possible death	Requires a rare mutation of common swine influenza virus	4
Leptospirosis	*Leptospira* spp.	Direct from contact with urine or indirect from urine contamination of water	Kidney infection and flu-like symptoms	Hogs recovering from leptospirosis can appear normal and shed the bacteria in the urine	3
Yersiniosis	*Yersinia enterocolitica*	Direct and indirect, fecal-oral	Diarrhea and occasionally reactive arthritis	Common and can transmit disease while appearing healthy	2

*Risk Groups (National Institutes of Health and World Health Organization criteria. Centers for Disease Control and Prevention, Biosafety in Microbiological and Biomedical Laboratories, 5th edition, 2009.)

1. Agent not associated with disease in healthy adult humans.
2. Agent rarely causes serious disease and preventions or therapy possible.
3. Agent can cause serious or lethal disease and preventions or therapy possible.
4. Agent can cause serious or lethal disease and preventions or therapy are not usually available.

SANITARY PRACTICES

- **Appropriate Personal Protection Equipment:** A handler of hogs should wear appropriate dress to protect against skin contamination with hair and skin scales or saliva, urine, and other body secretions.
- **Routine Basic Sanitary Practices:** Basic sanitary practices should be practiced, such as keeping hands away from eyes, nose, and mouth when handling hogs and washing hands after handling them.
- **Precautions if Hogs Appear Sick:** Special precautions are needed if sick hogs are handled, and they should be isolated from apparently normal hogs. New herd members should be quarantined for at least 2 weeks to reduce the risk of transmitting a disease that new animals could be incubating before introducing them to the rest of the herd.
- **Preventive Measures:**
  - **Influenza:**
    - **Vaccinations:** Influenza vaccinations should be maintained current in handlers and handlers sick with influenza should not handle hogs.
    - **Migrating Waterfowl:** Migrating waterfowl can transmit influenza to swine and should not be allowed contact with hogs.
  - **Leptospirosis:** Hogs should be vaccinated for leptospirosis, and wildlife, especially rodents, which are reservoirs for leptospirosis, should be controlled in swine-raising facilities.

APPROACHING AND CATCHING

AVOID STARTLING

- **Startling Hogs Can Cause Injuries:** In total confinement operations, hogs are restricted to crates or small pens in which catching is relatively easy. A startle reaction in hogs is to vocalize with a woof sound, jump to feet if recumbent, and then freeze in place. Regardless of whether hogs are in crates, small pens, large pens, or on pasture, care must be taken not to startle hogs, especially sows with pigs, by being too quiet or excessively noisy.
- **Alert at a Distance:** Hogs will become quickly agitated by the sight and sounds of a stranger. Normal level noise should be made at a distance so that hogs moderate their alert response before the handler gets near them.

PREVENT BITES AND BEING KNOCKED DOWN

Special precautions should be taken to prevent being bitten on the legs and knocked down in a hog pen.

- **Knee-High Boots and Objects to Grasp:** When entering a pen of hogs, a handler should wear knee high boots and stay near a fence or something else that is firmly stationary to grab to maintain balance if pushed on.
- **Sorting Panel and Poles:** A handler should carry a sorting panel or pole to keep curious hogs from crowding the handler.
- **Feed before Handling:** Hogs in total confinement are deprived of normal mental stimulation and become excited by the presence of a handler with whom they also associate with being fed. Smelling a handler's legs and inquisitive bites of boots is common. However, this can become dangerous if the hogs are large, have not been fed recently, or blood is present anywhere in the pen.

TRAIN TO COME WITH A CALL

Swine on pasture or in hog lots are usually taught to come for feeding by being called. Traditionally, the commands "suey" and "pig-pig-pig" have been used to call hogs.

RUB AND SCRATCH TO REDUCE STRESS

Hogs can be taught to appreciate being rubbed and scratched on the back, but this must be done firmly since light touches will be suspicious of danger. Minor procedures, such as vaccinations, can be done without stress on many hogs by restricting their movement, providing food, using a soothing voice, and scratching their shoulders and behind their ears during the procedure. The handler should never put hands within range of a hog's head where it could turn and bite.

SEPARATE BY SIZE

If collecting swine of different sizes, the largest hogs should be sorted out first. Sorting out by largest size to smallest should continue to reduce the risk of smaller pigs being trampled and crushed. Larger hogs or pigs are also easier to separate from smaller pigs than smaller pigs from larger pigs or hogs.

MANUAL CATCHING OF PIGS LESS THAN 50 LB.

- **While along a Wall, Grasp a Hind Leg:** Pigs less than 50 lb. can be caught as they run along a wall of a pen by the handler facing the same direction and sweeping an open hand back and under them to grasp the nearest hind leg, picking the pig up, and grasping the other hind leg. For example, a pig running to the left would be caught by its left hind leg by the handler's right hand.
- **Trap against a Wall with Sorting Panel:** Sorting panels or gates can be used as traps to catch pigs.

HANDLING FOR ROUTINE CARE AND MANAGEMENT

HIGH VOLUME FACILITIES

- **Components:** High-volume swine facilities may have collecting pens, crowding pens, alleyways, drop down gates, squeeze chutes, and scales.
  - **Crowding Pen:**
    - **Size:** Crowding pens for pigs should have a radius of 6 ft.
    - **Avoid Pile-ups:** Pigs will jam up and pile on top of each other if funneled from crowding pens into alleyways. The transition from a crowding pen to an alleyway should have an offset entrance to prevent jamming and piling (Figure 7.1).
  - **Bud's Box:** A Bud's box can be used rather than a crowding pen to funnel swine into an alleyway or into sorting pens.
  - **See-Through Middle Partitions:** Alleyways and ramps should be two pigs wide with a see-through middle partition.
- **Restraint Crates:** Most restraint on confinement hogs is done in their crates or single alleyways. This permits inexperienced handlers to handle and restrain hogs for various reasons relatively safely. Handling and restraint of pigs and hogs raised in hooped pens or on pasture requires more skill.

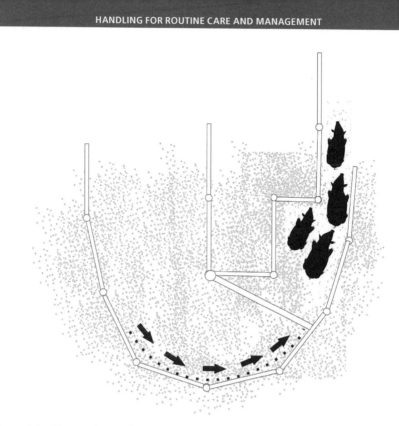

Figure 7.1 Offset entry into an alleyway prevents piling of pigs onto each other.

BASIC EQUIPMENT

- **Hog Snares, Sorting Panels, Snubbing Ropes, and Manual Restraint:** Specialized restraint facilities are not needed for routine handling and restraint of swine. Most procedures can be done by minor distractions (scratching the shoulders of a hog, gently holding a pig's thigh), hog snares, panels, snubbing ropes, leg holds, and holding small pigs in the same manner of small dogs.

    - **Restraining Piglets:**
        - **Need:** Within 1 day to 2 weeks of age, piglets have their needle teeth clipped, ears are notched, iron dextran injections are given, and males are castrated. In close confinement operations, the tails may be docked. Vaccinations may also be started before weaning.
        - **Method:** Nursing pigs (piglets) are less than 20 lb. and can be easily picked up and handled like a puppy. They should be removed from the sow's sight and hearing for all procedures to be done, but not for more than 1 hour.
    - **Leg Holds on Pigs:** Leg holds are performed on pigs up to about 50 lb. Handlers should wear ear plugs, coveralls, and high-topped boots.
        - **Inverted Standing Leg Hold:** An inverted standing leg hold ("head stand" hold) is accomplished by grasping each hind leg at the hocks, picking up the pig by its hind legs, and then placing the pig's back toward the handler. The pig's torso is caught between the handler's legs. The pig's chest and shoulders are held by the handler's legs (Figure 7.2). This hold is used for castration and subcutaneous injections.

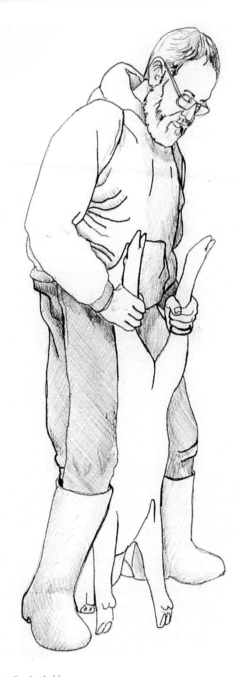

Figure 7.2 Inverted standing leg hold.

○ **Upright Standing Hold:** Oral medications and subcutaneous injections may be administered while pigs are held upright and standing. Holding the front legs allows the pig to bite the handler's hands, so gloves are recommended as well as squeezing the sides of the pig's neck with the handler's wrists while holding the pig's front legs. The hold is performed by straddling the pig, grasping the front legs, then the flanks are immobilized with the handler's legs (Figure 7.3).

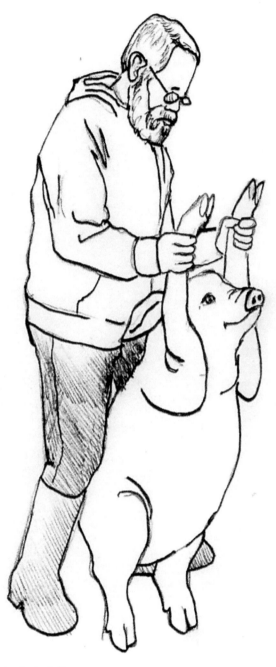

Figure 7.3   Upright standing leg hold.

- **Hog Snout Snare:**
  - **More Than 50 Lb. Pigs:** Pigs more than 50 lb. are usually captured with a snare, which is a hollow rigid tube with a wire that goes through the tube and forms a capture loop at the end (Figure 7.4).
  - **Over 100 Lb. Hogs:** See Procedural Steps 7.1.

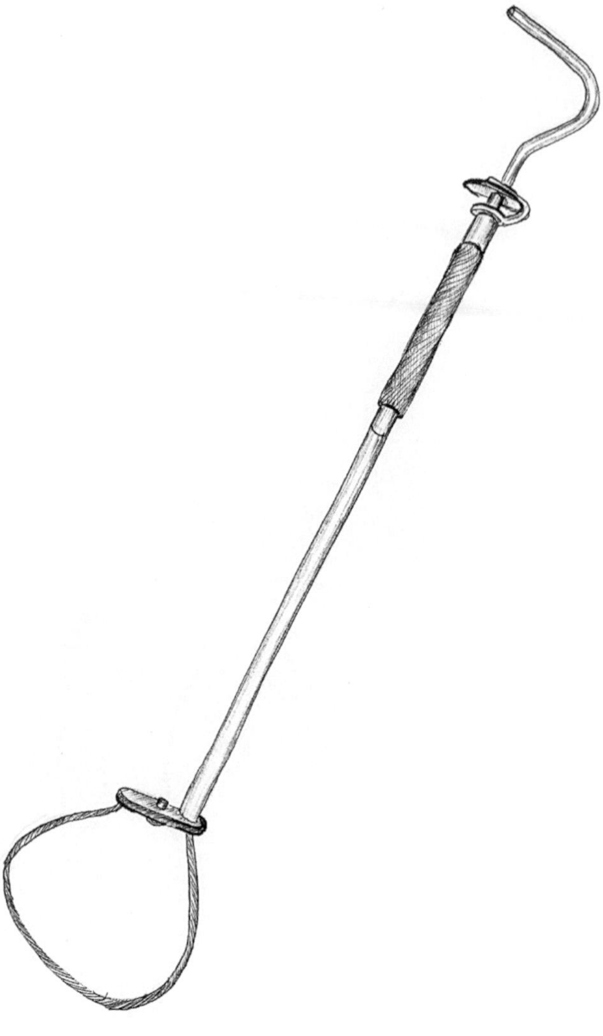

Figure 7.4   Hog snout snare.

Procedural Steps 7.1 Application and Use of Snout Snare	
1.	Large hogs should be positioned so that their attempt to back up while being snared is blocked.
2.	The loop is placed inside the hog's mouth and the loop is closed tightly around the upper jaw of the snout (i.e., the maxilla) (Figure 7.5).
3.	Care should be taken to get the snare loop far enough back in the mouth that when it is tightened it does not squeeze the soft tissue at the end of the nose where it would cause pain, shut the nostrils, and probably slip off.
4.	After tightening the snare, the handler moves in front of the hog as the hog will lean back and try to pull out of the loop (Figure 7.6).

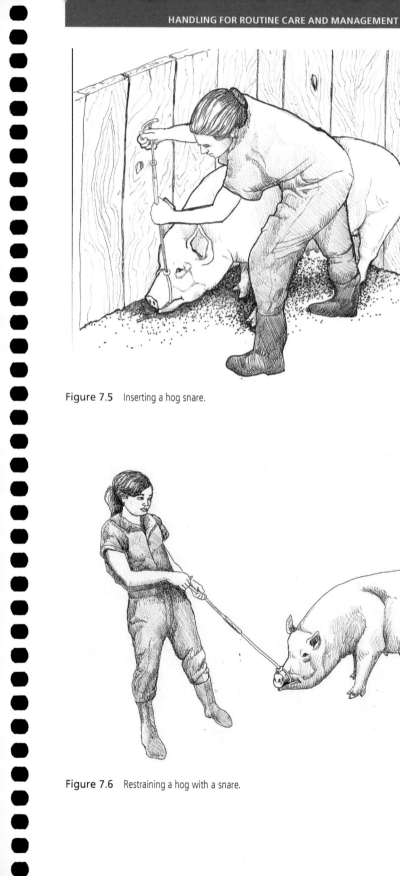

Figure 7.5   Inserting a hog snare.

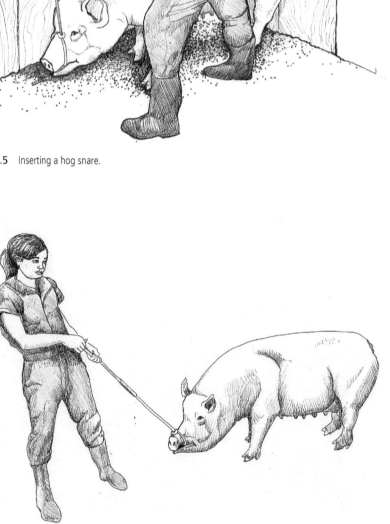

Figure 7.6   Restraining a hog with a snare.

- ○ **Limitations of Snout Snares:** Snares will lose their effectiveness with time and therefore should be employed for less than 10 minutes. The use of snares with hogs that have tusks can be dangerous when trying to remove the snare because the snare must be placed behind the tusks, complicating the snare's removal. Swine should never be pulled forward with a hog snare.
- **Snubbing Rope:**
  - ○ **Placement of the Loop:** Restraint of large hogs that are too strong for a handler to restrain with a snare pole may be achieved with a lariat and quick release honda if an assistant handler is available (Figure 7.7 and Procedural Steps 7.2).

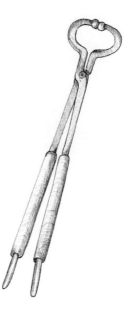

Figure 7.7 Long-handled bull nose tongs used to put pressure on a hog's neck.

Procedural Steps 7.2	Application and Use of a Snubbing Rope
1.	The handler stands to the side behind the hog's head and places the bottom of the lariat's loop in its mouth, around the upper jaw and pulls the loop down tight on its upper jaw (Figure 7.8).
2.	If the hog will not open its mouth, long-handled (3 ft) bull nose tongs can be used by the assistant to squeeze the neck behind the ears, which will briefly restrain the hog and make it open its mouth to insert the snubbing rope loop.
3.	The tongs on the neck can then be removed and the rope is run around a tie ring, or similar tie point, higher than the hog's head.
4.	If the snubbing rope will be briefly tied, the tie should be close (within a foot) of the snubbing post to reduce the risk of the hog being able to loosen the snare and spit it out.
5.	If an assistant plans to continue to hold the rope rather than tie it, it is helpful to tie the end to a short rod or pole to maintain a sturdy grip with both hands as the pig pulls backward.

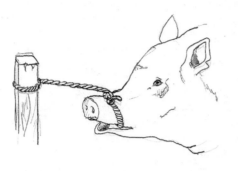

Figure 7.8   Snubbing rope restraint.

- ○ **Quick Release Metal Honda:** Use of a snubbing rope with a quick release honda permits easier and safer removal than a snare in a large hog with tusks, but it does not allow any pushing away option if the hog becomes aggressive and moves forward rather than pulling back. Two snubbing ropes that are cross-tied will reduce the risk of the handler being chased. A quick release metal honda should have a leather tether that will allow safer and quicker release of the latch.
- ○ **Forward and Backward Movement:** A hog should never be pulled forward with a snubbing rope. However, the hog may be allowed to move backward with a handler holding the rope while a second handler guides it by grasping its tail.
- • **Snout Rings:**
  - ○ **Purpose:** Hogs confined in dirt lots or pastures will root the ground with their snouts. If rooting is excessive, when the pigs are about 40 lb. they can be caught and metal snout rings clamped into the edge of the cartilage of the nose to discourage rooting.
  - ○ **Method:** Pigs less than 50 lb. can be caught by an assistant and held by their front legs. Leather gloves should be worn and the pig's front legs should be pulled back along the edge of the pig's face to block its ability to bite.
  - ○ **Boars Are Not Ringed:** Boars are not ringed since they use their nose to push on the female during breeding.
  - ○ **Interference with Self-Feeders:** If excessive rings are used or placed in poor positions, they can interfere with the pig opening lids of self-feeders.
  - ○ **Humane Snout Rings:** So-called "humane" snout rings are clamped into the nasal septum, leaving the rim of the snout free to open feeder lids without restriction.

MOVING PIGS AND HOGS

- • **Training Pigs for Moving:** Swine are not as whimsical as goats. They are much more independent and willing to try an individual escape than sheep and cattle.
  - • **Avoid Overheating:** In warm weather, swine should only be moved outdoors in early morning or late afternoon to reduce the risk of overheating.
  - • **Move in Small Groups:** Hogs move best if moved in small groups. Groups of three to six are recommended. Large groups tend to scatter or, if cornered, they may pile on top of each other.

- **Alleyway Dimensions:** Alleyways for moving hogs should be 18–20 inches wide.
- **Guiding with a Cane:** Adult hogs can be trained to be moved by the handler walking next to the hog, just behind its shoulder, and guiding it with a cane by taps on the shoulders and neck.
- **Need for Training to Be Handled and Moved:** In total indoor confinement operations, piglets are not allowed to learn to follow their mother. At weaning, they are separated from older swine. Handlers of indoor confined pigs should begin to train them for being herded just after weaning (Procedural Steps 7.3).

Procedural Steps 7.3	Training Weanling Pigs to Be Handled and Moved
1.	Training should involve being rubbed and scratched for short periods after being fed.
2.	Small reward treats should be offered.
3.	Later training periods should include being gently pushed in different directions and being briefly picked up and gently put down.
4.	Eventually, moving them in groups of five or six in a small pen (10 × 10 ft) and up ramps without generating any excitement should be practiced.

- **Distractions to Eliminate:** Like cattle, swine are reluctant to walk on strange flooring, move toward darkness, or past dangling or wiggly objects on fences. They should be moved toward better lit areas (but not blinding light), over familiar flooring without sharp contrasts in color or texture (cover with bedding if needed), and in alleyways without clutter for herding. Side-by-side alleyways with a see-through septation panel in the middle allows two pigs to move abreast and facilitates forward movement.
- **Canes, Poles, and Paddles:**
  - **Canes and Poles:** After brief introduction training, gently tapping the sides of the pig's or hog's face, neck, and shoulders with a cane or pole can redirect a hog without generating excitement. If canes or poles are used abusively, the hog may become frantic or aggressive.
  - **Rattle Paddles:** Rattle paddles can be more effective for hogs that are not trained to accept canes and poles.
- **Sorting Panels:** Portable solid sorting panels can block distractions and aid in directing the movement of swine.
  - **Construction:** Sorting panels (also called "hurdles") are flat panels of wood, plastic, or metal that are helpful in sorting, loading, and restraining pigs and hogs. They should be at least as tall as the hog and at least two-thirds as long (Figure 7.9). Panels have small holes along the top edge or one side for the handler's hands, but they should not have holes that allow the hog to see through which will encourage them to push through or under the panel.
  - **Method:** The smoothest side of the panel should be presented to the hog. The top should be tilted toward the handler and the bottom pressed on the floor and braced with the handler's foot to prevent a hog from rooting under the bottom.
- **Backing Bucket:** If a hog's head is covered with a bucket, it will move backward quickly. The speed and direction of retreat can be guided by a second handler holding its tail to move the hog a short distance. If they are in an alleyway and cannot turn, a scoop shovel in front of their face may aid in backing them toward a desired destination.

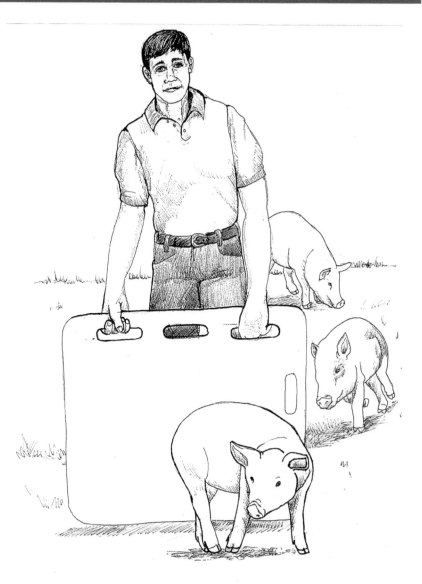

Figure 7.9   Sorting panel.

- **Rope Harness:** A rope harness for a pig can be created by putting a non-constricting loop tied with a bowline knot over its neck and a half hitch around its thorax. The harness can be effective for controlling the movement of pigs up to about 100 lb.
- **Plastic Trash Can on Wheels:** Weanling pigs and small pigs can be moved short-distances with less stress to the pigs by using a plastic trash can on wheels or a wheelbarrow with high sides.
- **Carrying or Lifting Pigs:**
  - **Small-Sized Pigs:** Small pigs (less than 10 lb.) can be scooped up with a hand under the body or caught by a hind leg and then grasped under their torso for their comfort and a feeling of security. They should never be captured or restrained by their ears.

- **Medium-Sized Pigs:** Pigs weighing 10–50 lb. can be caught by a hind leg, held by both hind legs proximal to their hocks, and carried short distances.
- **Large-Sized Pigs:** Pigs more than 50 lb. should be lifted by two people, each holding one hind leg.

HANDLING FOR COMMON MEDICAL PROCEDURES

Most handling and restraint of hogs can be and should be done without tranquilization, sedation, hypnosis, or anesthesia. However, some handling and restraint procedures should be restricted to veterinary medical professionals due to the potential danger to the animal or handler. These require special skills, equipment, or facilities, and possibly adjunct chemical restraint or complete immobilization by chemical restraint.

RESTRAINT OF INDIVIDUAL HOGS AND PIGS AND PORTIONS OF THEIR BODY

- **Whole Body Restraint:**
    - **V-Troughs:** V-shaped troughs can be used to restrain pigs less than 50 lb. on their backs for blood samples from the cranial vena cava. V-troughs can be tilted head down or head up depending on the needs of the procedure being performed.
    - **Canvas Slings:** Canvas slings with holes for each leg and an access hole to the neck can be used for collecting blood from the cranial vena cava in hogs less than 50 lb. This is less stressful, more comfortable for the hog and provides better restraint than V-troughs. However, it is not as flexible in holding a variety of sizes of pigs as the V-trough.
    - **Lateral Restraint and Casting Methods:**
        - **Small Pigs, Less Than 50 Lb.:** Placing a small pig under 50 lb. in lateral recumbency can be done by reaching over its torso and grasping the front and hind leg on the side nearest the handler's body, picking it up and gently sliding it down the handler's body and onto its side.
        - **Medium-Sized Pigs, 50–80 Lb.:** See Procedural Steps 7.4.

Procedural Steps 7.4 Casting Medium-Sized Pigs for Lateral Restraint	
1.	The pig is first snubbed by its snout and then tied low to a post.
2.	Using a short rope with loops on each end, the loops are placed below the dewclaws on a front and hind leg on the same side.
3.	The handler stands on the side with the tied legs, and the mid part of the rope is pulled under the hog and upward causing the hog to lie on its side.
4.	The handler continues to hold the rope and places a knee just behind the hog's shoulder to maintain the restraint.

-
    -
        - **Hogs, More Than 100 Lb.:** For hogs more than 100 lb., a hock hobble can be used to lay a hog in lateral recumbency. A hock hobble is a snubbing rope applied around the upper jaw and then the standing end is run to a hind leg where a loop is applied above the hock. The snout is then pulled toward the hind leg forcing the hog to lie on its side.
        - **Large Hogs, More Than 300 Lb.:** Large hogs, more than 300 lb., are caught by the mouth with a snubbing rope and then cast with a rope at

least 15 ft long. After placing the rope around the hog's neck and tying with a bowline knot, the standing end of the rope is placed around the chest and flank with a couple of half hitches. Steady pulling on the end of the rope will cause the hog to lie down on its side in the same manner used to cast cattle with half hitches.

- **Restraint of the Head:** Restrain of the head with the use of halters or stanchions is not possible with swine. Hog snares or snubbing ropes restrain the head as much as is possible without chemical restraint.
- **Restraint of Asian Pot-Bellied Pigs:**
  - **Exotic Pets:** Asian (miniature) pot-bellied pigs are pigs from Vietnam with fat rolls over their eyes, a pot belly, and a swayback. Pot-bellied pigs became a fad pet in the United States during the 1980s. Although less popular now, they are still occasionally kept as pets and not treated like livestock.
  - **Behavior:** Pot-bellied pigs are uneasy about being picked up. They will struggle and can easily be dropped and injured. Dogs and pot-bellied pigs in the same household can cause problems because of competition for food and toys.
  - **Housing:**
    - **Tolerates Only Moderate Climates:** The preferred temperature range is 65 to 75°F.
    - **Outside Space for Rooting:** Outdoor housing should provide at least 50 square feet for each pig. Hay or straw should be provided for rooting and chewing.
    - **Moveable Shelter:** A shelter (three-sided shed or large dog house) from severe weather and sunlight should be provided. The pen and enclosure should be movable and relocated as soon as the pen's dirt has been rooted throughout the pen. If the pig is housed on concrete, the pen should be cleaned daily and fresh hay or straw added 3 to 4 times per week.
  - **Handling and Restraint:**
    - **General Handling:** General handling and restraint are more like the techniques used for dogs than for swine raised for meat production. Support slings can be useful in physical restraint of pet pigs.
    - **Hoof Trims:** Pot-bellied pigs need to have regular hoof trims about every 6 months if confined in pens with dirt and no abrasive surfaces (rocks, concrete, etc.).
  - **Routine Medical Procedures:**
    - **Castration:** Males should be castrated at 2 to 3 months of age. If they are not, boars more than 2 years of age can be more than 100 lb., aggressive, and dangerous.
    - **Trimming of Tusks:** Permanent canine teeth (tusks) should be trimmed at 1 year of age and annually thereafter. This requires chemical restraint.

INJECTIONS AND VENIPUNCTURE
- **Access to Veins:**
  - **Jugular Vein or Cranial Vena Cava:**
    - **Right Jugular Vein Preferred for Large Pigs or Hogs:** The blood vessel used for venipuncture in hogs is usually the right jugular or cranial vena cava (but not in miniature pigs). The left jugular is less desirable because it lies close to the phrenic nerve which can be inadvertently injured and cause paralysis of the diaphragm. The hog is usually caught with a snout snare and remains standing during the venipuncture.

○ **Jugular Venipuncture in Pigs:** Pigs less than 30 lb. are laid in ventrodorsal recumbency on a handler's lap or in a V-trough. The pig's head is tilted down and the front legs pulled back by an assistant. The phlebotomist holds the head extended with the non-dominant hand while performing jugular venipuncture.

● **Lateral Saphenous and Ear Veins:** The lateral saphenous veins in the hind legs, or central or lateral ear veins, are used less commonly. Restraint depends on the size of the pig or hog and usually involves a snare, single file alleyway, or crate.

● **Coccygeal Vein:** The coccygeal vein of the tail may be accessible in large hogs that have not been docked or in adult miniature pigs.

● **Injections:**

  ● **Intramuscular:** Intramuscular injections are given to hogs in the side of the neck, 2 to 3 inches behind and below the ear (Figure 7.10). Physical restraint is often not necessary. Due to the lack of muscle elsewhere, piglets are given IM injections in the semitendinosus and semimembranosus of the hind leg.

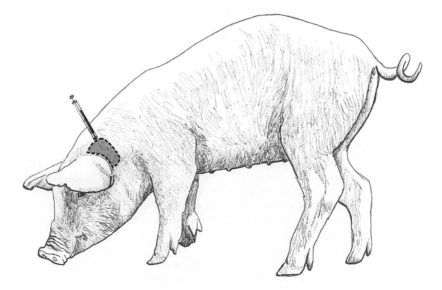

Figure 7.10 Intramuscular injection site in hogs.

  ● **Subcutaneous:** Pigs are given subcutaneous injections under the loose skin of the axilla behind a front leg or the flank fold while restrained by the inverted standing leg hold (Figure 7.11). Hogs are injected at the base of the ear often without restraint.

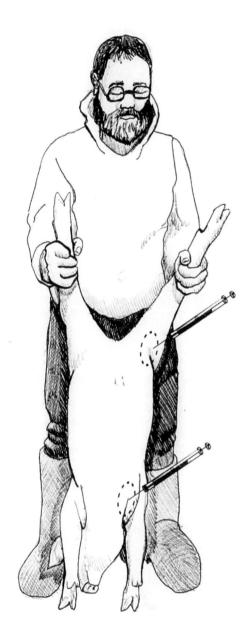

Figure 7.11   Subcutaneous injection sites in pigs.

ADMINISTRATION OF ORAL MEDICATIONS

Oral administration of medications to swine is done by the addition of the medication to their feed or water. Although oral examinations can be performed with a hand paddle oral speculum, this is not practical for repeated administration of oral medications. Piglets or small pet pigs may be able to be medicated by holding them vertically with their head up, while an assistant administers liquid medication with an oral syringe.

TRANSPORTING SWINE

RAMPS

- **Eliminate or Minimize Ramps:** When possible, swine should be loaded into transport vehicles from a level surface (a loading platform) rather than up a ramp into a transport vehicle. If a loading ramp is necessary, the incline should be less than 20 degrees with cleats.
- **Cleats on Ramps:** Cleats on ramps for adult pigs should be 8 inches apart and closer for smaller pigs.
- **Solid Ramp:** Swine will move up solid ramps better than slatted ramps with gaps.
- **Cover with Bedding:** The ramp should be covered with bedding used in the transport vehicle.

CHUTES

- **Size and Construction:** Loading chutes for hogs should have solid outside walls to prevent seeing handlers. Chute divisions should be 22 to 30 inches wide to prevent hogs from being able to turn around in the chute but wide enough to allow a handler to walk behind them. Center partitions in the chute should be see-through for hogs to see other hogs moving forward.
- **Group Size:** Small groups (three to six pigs) should be loaded at a time.

TRANSPORT VEHICLE

- **Clean and Disinfect:** The transport vehicle should be cleaned and disinfected after each use.
- **Create Small Groups with Partitions:** Transport vehicle partitions should be used to pen up to 20 to 25 hogs together.
- **Segregate Disagreeable Groups:**
  - **Hogs from Different Origins:** Mature hogs from different origins should not be mixed together due to fighting that will result.
  - **Mature Boars:** Mature boars should be penned individually.
- **Adverse Weather:**
  - **Hot Weather:** In hot weather, transported swine should be in a covered vehicle, bedded with moist sand, have openings in the trailer sides for ventilation, and hauled in the coolest part of the day. Extra space for each hog should be allowed and the vents adjusted to promote ventilation during travel.
  - **Cold Weather:** In cold weather, the top and most side openings should be closed and straw or wood shavings bedding should be provided.

BIBLIOGRAPHY

1. Kilbride AL, Mendi M, Statham P, et al. A cohort study of preweaning piglet mortality and farrowing accommodation on 112 commercial pig farms in England. Prev Vet Med 2012;104:281–291.
2. Klober K. Storey's Guide to Raising Pigs. 3rd edition. Storey Publishing, North Adams, MA, 2009.
3. Parsons TD, Deen J. How complexity of animal welfare issues can foster differences within the veterinary profession. J Am Vet Med Assoc 2015;247:240–241.
4. Stephens DB, Perry GC. The effects of restraint, handling, simulated and real transport in the pig (with reference to man and other species). Appl Anim Behav Sci 1990;28:41–55.

8

POULTRY

DOI: 10.1201/9781003110910-8

The chicken was the first domesticated poultry about 8,000 years ago in India and Southeast Asia. Today's poultry are raised for meat, eggs, feathers, and leather. Some are used for insect control and as property sentinels. The U.S. is the world's largest producer of poultry meat and is second to China in the world's production of eggs.

Domesticated poultry include chickens, turkeys, ducks, geese, guineafowl, and ratites (ostriches, emus, and rheas). Common terms used for poultry are provided in Table 8.1.

Table 8.1   Age and Gender Terminology for Poultry

•	**Hen**—Adult female poultry, although a female goose may be called a *goose*
•	**Pullet**—A female chicken under 1 year old
•	**Cock**—Adult male poultry; more specifically a male chicken is a **rooster**, a male turkey is a **tom**, a male duck is a **drake**, a male goose is a **gander**
•	**Capon**—A castrated male chicken
•	**Cockerel**—A young male chicken, under a year of age
•	**Broiler**—6- to 8-week-old chicken raised for meat
•	**Fryer**—7- to 10-week-old chicken raised for meat
•	**Roaster**—3- to 5-month-old chicken raised for meat
•	**Layer**—Adult hen raised for egg production
•	**Poult**—A young poultry, of either gender
•	**Jake**—A young male turkey
•	**Gosling**—Young goose
•	**Duckling**—Young duck.

NATURAL BEHAVIOR OF POULTRY

HIGHLY SOCIAL BUT TERRITORIAL
All poultry are highly social and disturbed by isolation. Strange birds of the same species added suddenly to an established group will be attacked and either injured or killed.

DAILY ACTIVITIES
Normal behavior of unstressed adult poultry with sufficient room for exercise includes wing-flapping, feather ruffling, leg stretching, and dust bathing.

- **Foraging:** In their natural environments, poultry spend nearly all their waking time foraging for food by pecking seeds, leaves, berries, worms, larvae, and insects to eat, picking up sand and gravel for their gizzards, or investigating their surroundings.
- **Dust Bathing:** Dust bathing occurs in the middle of the day several times per week.

ROOSTING
Areas with trees are preferred by small poultry to be used for roosting at night.

DEFENSES

- **Multiple Options:** The primary means of defense for most poultry is hiding in brush. Flying, vocalizing, pecking, clawing, and beating of wings are secondary defenses. Due to the danger from predators, females prefer to hide to lay eggs, and young birds are closely bound to wherever their mother goes.
- **Ability to Fly Is Variable:** Young poultry with prominent keel bones and large pectoral muscles such as some domestic chickens, turkeys, and ducks are capable of flying short distances and will perch or climb onto elevated resting spots. Ratites have small pectoral muscles, no keel bone, and cannot fly.

BEHAVIOR CAUSED BY CLOSE CONFINEMENT

- **Affected Species:** Most chickens and turkeys are raised commercially in high-density confinement.
- **Aggression:** Aggressiveness is enhanced by overcrowding. In these environments, birds do not have the opportunity to forage and receive the mental stimulation it provides.
  - **Head Pecking:** Head pecking of submissive or injured birds can be brutal and eventually kill the new member of the flock.
  - **Feather Pecking:** Feather pecking is also common in poultry confined on metal or concrete surfaces.

BEHAVIORS OF LESS COMMON POULTRY

- **Guineafowl:** Guineafowl stay in close groups and are ravenous foragers as they eat flying and crawling insects, ticks, worms, grubs, and snails. They will surround and attack small rodents, marauding birds, and snakes. They sleep in trees at night.
- **Shorebirds:** Ducks and geese get natural exercise by paddling through water. It is important for them to have sufficient water to immerse their bill and eyes to clean their face.
- **Ratites:** Ratite refers to a flat raft-like sternum in a type of birds with small pectoral muscles that cannot fly. Ratites, especially ostriches, have muscular legs and elongated toenails and are capable of swift running and lethal kicks. Ratites are not domesticated and can only become marginally tame.

SAFETY FIRST

HANDLER SAFETY

- **Defensive and Territorial Attacks by Poultry:** Most poultry protect themselves with escape by running or short flights. If escape is not possible, they will peck, scratch, and bat their wings. Chickens and turkeys may attack a handler perceived to be weak, particularly small children.
  - **Batting with Wings:** Injuries can occur from poultry wings during panic flying within an enclosure or being improperly held.
  - **Species Variations:**
    - **Chickens:** Aggressive chickens will peck and scratch, and roosters with spurs will use them to poke and scratch.

- Turkeys: Turkeys can inflict severe blows with their wings, but geese are more likely to use battery with their wings as a defense or offense mechanism.
- Geese: In addition to batting with their wings, geese will also peck with their beak, and rake with their toes.
- Ducks: Ducks are less prone to resist handling with defensive pecking and scratching.
- **Auditory and Respiratory Protection in Indoor Confinements:**
  - **Noise Risks:** Indoor confinement of poultry can expose handlers to excessive noise, and ear protection must be considered.
  - **Respiratory Risks:** Respiratory problems are also common in poultry handlers if the poultry are confined indoors. The primary causes of respiratory problems are organic dust composed of feathers, bacteria, and fungi, and ammonia from excrement containing urea. Appropriately rated respiratory masks should be worn, and poultry houses need to be frequently cleaned and well ventilated.
- **Ratites:**
  - **Unpredictable and Potentially Dangerous:**
    - **Adult Male Ostriches:** Adult male ostriches during breeding seasons are especially dangerous. They have a powerful forward and downward strike with a leg and sharp claws on two toes that can rip a handler's abdomen open or tear a femoral artery.
    - **Smaller Ratites:** Emus and rheas also strike forward with their feet. They both have three toes with a sharp claw on each toe.
    - **Never Stand in Front:** A handler should never stand directly in front of a ratite.
  - **Signs of Agitation:** An agitated male will stand tall and bump its chest against objects, hiss, gape its mouth, and flap its wings. A handler should never go into an ostrich pen without an assistant nearby.
  - **Run Faster Than Humans:** Humans cannot outrun an ostrich. If a handler is charged in the open by a male ostrich, it is recommended to lay flat on the ground to avoid a forward kick. They cannot kick low at an object on or near the ground.
  - **Peck at Shiny Objects:** Ratites will peck at any shiny object. Handlers should not wear sunglasses or jewelry when around ratites.

POULTRY SAFETY

- **Handling Can Impair Respirations:** Poultry, as with all birds, do not have a diaphragm between their thorax and abdomen. Therefore, they must be able to move their rib cage to breathe. Restraint methods involving their thorax must be loose enough to allow the bird to inhale.
- **Beak Trims:** Chicken pullets and turkey poults in close confinement have their beaks trimmed because of territorial aggression and risk of feather picking and cannibalism (Figure 8.1).
  - **Age of Trimming:** Hatcheries trim chick beaks using a beak-trimming machine at 6 to 8 days of age, but it can be performed up to 16 weeks of age. Turkey poults are trimmed at 2 to 5 weeks of age.
  - **Method:** It is done by cutting approximately one-half of the upper beak and blunting the lower beak. Beak-trimming machines cauterize the cut as it is made and prevents beak regrowth. If manual nippers are used, the beak will regrow.

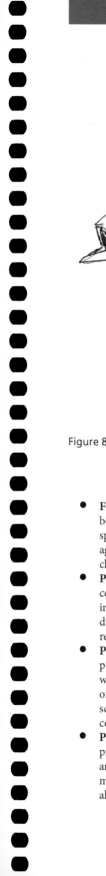

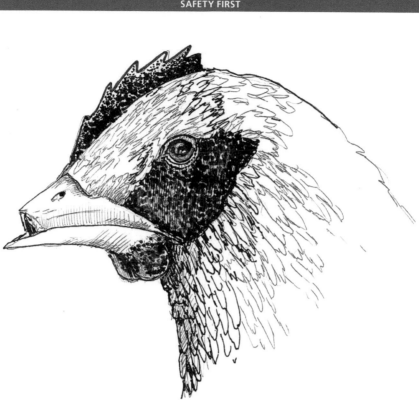

Figure 8.1 Debeaked chicken.

- **Feather Picking and Cannibalism:** The cause for feather picking and cannibalism can be varied, but overcrowding and boredom are factors. Providing at least 4 square feet of space for each chicken in a coop and 10 square feet in runs with an opportunity to forage (i.e., investigate and search for food), often prevents or eliminates feather picking in chickens.
- **Protecting Rooster Combs:** Chickens in close confinement will also peck at rooster combs, and roosters can cause injuries with their toes that lead to cannibalism of the injured bird. Preventive procedures used in large poultry confinement operations are dubbing of the comb, removal of the comb of young roosters, and toe dubbing, the removal of toes of breeding roosters.
- **Protecting Turkey Snoods:** The snood of turkeys is particularly vulnerable to being pecked by other turkeys in close confinement. The snood may be excised up to 3 weeks of age in situations where fighting or pecking has been a problem. Clipping of the two inside toes to remove the nails may be done at hatcheries to prevent scratches and skin tears to other turkeys when the turkeys are older and kept in close confinement.
- **Proposed Rules for Organic Production:** Proposed rules to the USDA to permit organic production of poultry labeling would prohibit beak trimming, desnooding, dewattling, and removal of combs. Poultry would have to be allowed sufficient room for freedom of movement and ability to engage in natural behaviors. The incidence of lameness would also have to be monitored.

Table 8.2 Diseases Transmitted from Healthy-Appearing Poultry to Healthy Adult Humans

Disease	Agent	Means of Transmission	Signs and Symptoms in Humans	Frequency in Animals	Risk Group*
Bites and Clawing	—	Direct injury	Bite wounds to face, arms, and legs	All poultry are capable of inflicting bite or claw wounds, or both	2
Salmonellosis	*Salmonella enteritidis* and other spp.	Direct, handling poultry and indirect from fomites (cages, bowls)	Diarrhea, systemic disease and abscesses	Common	3
Campylobacteriosis	*Campylobacter jejuni*, *C. coli*	Direct, fecal-oral	Diarrhea	Common, but transmission primarily by eating under-cooked poultry	2
Avian Influenza	Influenza A, H5N1 virus	Direct, poultry respiratory secretions	Influenza signs and symptoms (respiratory)	Possible if exposed to wild birds; outbreaks devastating to poultry flocks	3
Ornithosis	*Chlamydiophila psittaci*	Direct, respiratory secretions or fecal matter	Pneumonia	Rare	3
Newcastle Disease	Avian paramyxovirus	Direct	Conjunctivitis	Rare in U.S. due to vaccine	2
Poultry Mites	*Dermanyssus gallinae*	Direct and indirect from fomites	Itchy skin with red bumps	Common	2

*Risk Groups (National Institutes of Health and World Health Organization criteria. Centers for Disease Control and Prevention, Biosafety in Microbiological and Biomedical Laboratories, 5th edition, 2009.)
1. Agent not associated with disease in healthy adult humans.
2. Agent rarely causes serious disease and preventions or therapy possible.
3. Agent can cause serious or lethal disease and preventions or therapy possible.
4. Agent can cause serious or lethal disease and preventions or therapy are not usually available.

- **Risks of Foraging:**
  - **Predators:**
    - **Raptors and Canids:** Although providing poultry room to forage outdoors can eliminate common aggression injuries, poultry with access to the outdoors are endangered by a wide variety of predators such as hawks, owls, foxes, coyotes, and roaming dogs, among others.
    - **Rats:** Rodent control is important indoor and outdoors. In addition to eating grain and spreading disease, rats will kill chicks and poults.
  - **Duck Defenses:** Ducks are able to escape from predators in the wild more effectively than other poultry. Although most species of ducks sleep on the ground and are more vulnerable to predators, they can sleep literally with one eye open and escape by water or air.
- **Calm Announcement of Presence:** Signaling handler presence near poultry by speaking in a normal tone and moving smoothly, rather than erratically, reduces the risk of small poultry piling up from being startled, which could result in smothering.

KEY ZOONOSES

(NOTE: Apparently ill animals should be handled by veterinary professionals or under their supervision. Precautionary measures against zoonoses from sick animals are more involved than those required when handling apparently healthy animals and vary widely. The discussion here is directed primarily at handling apparently healthy animals.)

Apparently healthy poultry pose little risk of transmitting disease to healthy adult handlers who practice conventional personal hygiene. The risks of physical injury are greater than the risks of acquiring an infectious disease. However, most poultry are not routinely handled and feathers can hide signs of many illnesses (Table 8.2).

SANITARY PRACTICES

- **Appropriate Dress:** A handler of poultry should wear appropriate dress to protect against skin contamination with feathers and skin scales or urine, and other body secretions.
- **Basic Sanitary Practices:** Basic sanitary practices should be practiced, such as keeping hands away from eyes, nose, and mouth when handling poultry and washing hands after handling them. Eating and drinking in poultry containment or handling areas should be prohibited. Cleaning of food and water bowls and handling equipment should be done outside of human living quarters.
- **Precautions with Sick Poultry:** Special precautions are needed if sick poultry are handled, and sick poultry should be isolated from apparently normal poultry. New flock members should be quarantined for at least 2 weeks to reduce the risk of transmitting a disease that new birds could be incubating before introducing them to the rest of the flock.
- **Prevent Exposure to Migrating Waterfowl:** Ducks and geese are asymptomatic reservoirs for avian influenza which could mutate to become infectious to humans. Poultry should be prevented from contact with migrating waterfowl.

APPROACHING, CATCHING, AND ROUTINE HANDLING

CHICKENS

- **Gently Handle Individual Chickens Early in Their Life:** Chickens that are handled early in life and frequently as adults will offer no resistance nor appear distressed when gently handled. Those in large groups and having little to no experience being handled in the past will pile on top of each other in a corner resulting in injuries and death. If caught, they will flap their wings and scratch while trying to free themselves.

- **Use Food Rewards:** Chickens that are handled on a regular basis will come eat grain from a handler's hand and can be easily picked up by grasping them on both sides of their body and restraining their wings next to their body. The wings should not be held tightly enough to impair the chicken's respirations.
- **Capturing Untrained Chickens:**
  - **Trap in a Corner with a Panel:** Untrained chickens may be captured by hand while in a small enclosure or after a small group is herded to a corner of their enclosure using a folding mesh wire panel. Each panel unit should be 2 ft wide and 3 to 4 ft high for adult chickens. The handler should pin the group close enough together that they have just enough room to stand.
  - **Nets:** If a small enclosure is not available or the bird is on free range, a capture net can be used. Nets can be used on other poultry too, but the net should be the appropriate size for the bird, have a useful handle length, and possess a padded rim.
- **Reactivity Is Altered by Light:** If the time of day is not important for the capture, all poultry that are diurnal feeders can be caught more easily in an environment of subdued or blue light. Waiting until evening when they are roosting may be the least stressful time to capture chickens. Placing a cloth over a restrained chicken's head can simulate night-time and calm the bird.
- **Immobilize Wings without Impairing Respiration:**
  - **Capture Wings and Body with Quiet, Smooth, Rapid Movement:** When capturing a chicken, the handler approaches from behind and grasps the wings and body with both hands at the same time to immobilize the wings (Figure 8.2). The grip should be firm enough to provide restraint, but care must be taken not to impede the respiratory movements of the chest. Capture should be as quiet and smooth as possible to avoid upsetting the rest of the flock.
  - **Expect Continued Efforts to Escape:** The chicken must be held firmly since, if untrained, there will be repeated attempts to escape after periods of rest.
  - **Do Not Carry by the Legs:** The body should always be supported during restraint and chickens should not be carried only by the legs due to risk of injury to the bird.
  - **Careful Release:** During a release, the handler should return the bird to the ground or floor gently. The bird should not be dropped to the floor.
- **Poult Restraint:**
  - **Young Poults:** Restraint of a poult can be done with one hand over its back and making a ring around its neck with the thumb and forefinger. The bird's body should be supported by loosely wrapping the other three fingers around its body and trapping the legs between the ring and small fingers.
  - **Poults over 13 Weeks of Age:** Birds older than 13 weeks should be carried while restraining both wings and both legs.
- **Partial Restraint Causes Injuries:**
  - **Restraint Must Immobilize the Bird:** Chickens and all other poultry should never be held by the head, one wing, or one leg. Grabbing chickens by the leg and holding them upside down increases the risk of injury. Being returned to a flock with an injury could result in being attacked by other members of the flock.
  - **Demineralized Bones Are Fragile:** Chickens from battery cages are more likely to have demineralized bone from the lack of exercise. Fractures may result from being restrained by the legs.
- **Moving in and out of Cages:** See Procedural Steps 8.1.

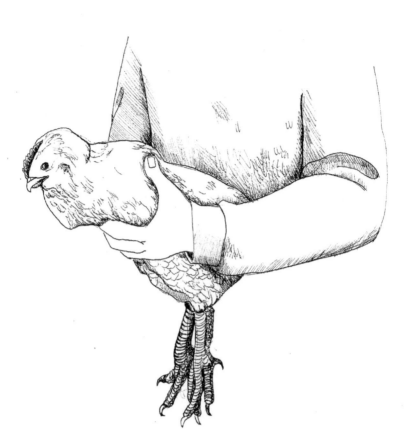

Figure 8.2   Restraint of a chicken.

Procedural Steps 8.1	Moving Chickens in and out of a Cage
1.	To remove a chicken from a cage, the handler should reach in and pin the chicken's body down and then turn its head toward the cage door.
2.	While keeping the hand on top of the bird, the handler should then slide the other hand underneath the bird to grasp the legs, with the index finger between the legs and the thumb just above the hock on one side, and the other fingers above the hock on the other side.
3.	The leg tendons are squeezed to extend the legs backward.
4.	Using both hands, the bird is removed from the cage headfirst.
5.	The chicken can be carried in the same position with its head between the handler's arm and body.
6.	To return the bird to a cage, it is rotated in the handler's hands and placed in the cage head first and placed on its feet.

GUINEAFOWL

Guineafowl are approached, captured, and handled in the same manner as chickens.

TURKEYS

- **Capturing Turkeys:** See Procedural Steps 8.2.

Procedural Steps 8.2	Capturing Turkeys
1.	The handler should herd 10 or fewer turkeys into a catch pen with a sorting panel in the same manner as chickens.
2.	The turkey to be captured is approached from behind.
3.	The handler kneels and grasps a wing where it joins the body and the legs between the hocks and the feet, holding the hocks straight and then place the turkey's breast on a platform, such as a bale of straw.
4.	If no platform is present, the breast can be rested on the handler's knee.
5.	A mature bird, which may weigh more than 50 lb., should be lifted from a kneeling position by the handler using their legs and keeping the back straight to reduce the risk of back injury.

- **Carrying Turkeys:** Turkeys can be carried by a handler with one arm, holding the legs with one hand and wrapping the arm around the bird's body with the head directed behind the handler.
- **Caution Needed with Tom Turkeys:** Domestic turkey hens are generally docile, but toms can be aggressive and should be watched more closely when a handler is in a pen with one. Male turkeys normally have a pale or blue-colored head. Aggressiveness may be signaled by the fleshy parts of the head becoming engorged with blood and red-colored.

WATERFOWL

The trachea of birds has complete cartilaginous rings and can withstand more compression than the trachea of mammals. Waterfowl, geese and ducks, have long necks and can be safely captured for restraint by grasping their necks and then their wings and feet (Figure 8.3). Compression on their chest must be mild to avoid inhibiting their breathing.

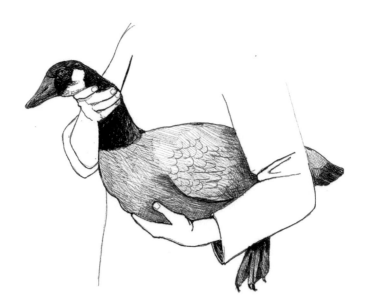

Figure 8.3 Restraint of a goose.

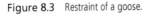

- **Ducks:**
  - **Capture and Carry:**
    - **Common Method:** The handler grasps the duck's neck from behind without firmly pressing on the trachea and esophagus in front. While pulling the duck upward, the wings are grasped near the attachment with the body with the other hand. The hand on the neck is then moved beneath the body to support the duck's body weight and the chest, abdomen, and legs are not restrained (Figure 8.4).

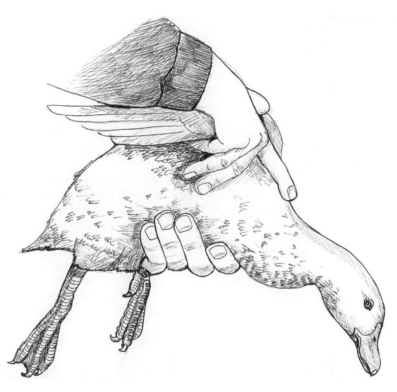

Figure 8.4 Restraint of a duck by its wings.

    - **Alternative Method:** A second method is to grasp the neck and then tuck the body under the other arm and against the handler's side with the duck's head pointed behind the handler.
  - **Use Sliding Release:** The release from being held should be with a sliding movement near the ground as if the duck is landing on water so that it will extend its feet to support its body.
  - **Dim Light Is Ineffective for Ducks:** Ducks are nocturnal feeders and have excellent night vision. Dimming lights in a handling room is not effective in reducing their reactivity.
- **Geese:**
  - **Pen Captures:**
    - **Catch Pens:** Geese walk slowly and should not be hurried or they will become panicked and stressed. Catch pens should not be overcrowded. Too many geese in the enclosure at one time can cause piling and suffocation might result.

- o **Manual Capture:** To capture a goose in a pen, a handler grasps its neck and then the base of the wings. Both wings can be held with one hand. The goose is picked up while the handler maintains a grasp on the neck, just below the goose's head, or the goose may peck at the handler's face.
- **Neck Crooks:** If a catch pen is not available, a neck crook can be used or an appropriate size and constructed net may be used. A handler should remain mindful that geese can cause painful blows with their wings and deep scratches with their feet.

RATITES

- **Ostrich Capture:**
  - **Chick Capture:** If a chick weighs less than 12 lb., the handler should support the whole body. If it weighs 12 to 30 lb., the handler should put a hand around the bird's body, pick it up, and allow the legs to dangle.
  - **Juvenile Capture:** Juveniles are 4 to 12 months old. They should be moved to a small collection pen with solid walls to be caught or caught with portable panels that have been covered with plastic or plywood. Juveniles may be moved by being held loosely in front of their chest with one arm and the other arm behind its rump while walking beside it.
  - **Adult Capture and Moving:**
    - o **Approach from Behind:** An approach to an adult ratite, especially ostriches, should always be from behind because ratites strike forward with their toes. T-shaped or V-shaped long-handled push poles are helpful in directing and sorting adult ratites. High-topped leather boots and leather chaps can provide some protection against a forward kick.
    - o **Panels/Shields:** Plywood or plastic shields can be used in a manner similar to hog sorting panels to move ratites, but an adult ostrich can still knock a handler with a shield down with a forward kick.
    - o **Moveable Squeeze Panels:** Moveable squeeze chutes can be constructed that are designed like a large notebook binder to capture and restrain a ratite.
- **Hoods:** Putting a hood over an ostrich's head will generally make them more manageable.
  - **Commercial and Improvised Hoods:** Commercial ratite hoods can be used, or a lightweight sleeve or sock with the toe cut out will suffice. Hoods should cover the eyes and extend about one-third down the neck, but it should not cover the nostrils.
  - **Application to a Non-Aggressive Ostrich:** Non-aggressive ostriches can be lured by grain in a bucket and hooded by grasping its beak with a hood everted over the hand. The hood is rolled off the hand and over the ostrich's head.
  - **Application to a Resistant Ostrich:**
    - o **Neck Crook:** Eight-foot long neck crooks can be used on ostriches just below the head to get their head down below the level of their back, preventing them from striking forward.
    - o **Prevent Backing Up:** The ostrich will pull back when its head is restrained. So, an assistant is needed to keep the bird from backing up while its head is being held down. The first handler, while keeping the crook on the bird's neck, must move forward to place a hood.
  - **Moving Hooded:** If an ostrich tolerates a hood, it may be able to be led without incident. Large ostriches should be led by three handlers, one on each wing, and one to gently push the bird forward and guide it.

- **Emu and Rhea Capture and Moving:**
  - **Avoid Hoods and Grasping the Neck:** An emu's or rhea's head or neck should not be grasped nor hooded because they do not tolerate handling of their head as well as ostriches. Emus have thin, fragile skin. Plus, their head and neck have little muscle or soft tissue protection from injury and their trachea can be easily collapsed.
  - **Capture and Restraint:** Emus and rheas are approached from behind and grasped around their wings, lifted up, and tipped back slightly, or they can be slowly pushed toward the ground and straddled while holding their neck.
- **Transport of Ratites:** Level loading bays to transport vehicles are recommended because ratites are reluctant to walk up inclines. Transport vehicles should provide enough room for the bird's head when it is standing.

HANDLING FOR COMMON MEDICAL PROCEDURES

INJECTIONS AND VENIPUNCTURE
- **Access to Veins:**
  - **Small Poultry:** Small poultry are held on their side on a table for venipuncture. The handler uses one hand to hold the legs with one finger between the bird's legs while the other hand elevates the uppermost wing over the bird's back. The phlebotomist accesses the wing (brachial) vein (Figure 8.5).

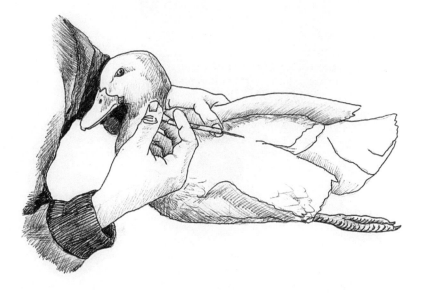

Figure 8.5   Venipuncture of a brachial vein in the wing of a goose.

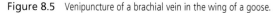

- **Ratites:**
  - ○ **Ostriches:** A wing vein (brachial vein) is used for venipuncture in adult ostriches. The neck cannot be adequately restrained to safely access the jugular vein. The ostrich is hooded and restrained with its head below the level of its back with an assistant to keep it from backing up while the wing vein is accessed.
  - ○ **Emus and Rheas:** Rheas or emus are grasped around the wings from behind and picked up slightly and tilted back. Venipuncture is done from a jugular vein or medial metatarsal leg vein.
- **Injections:**
  - **Intramuscular:**
    - ○ **Small Poultry:** To administer an intramuscular injection, a handler holds small poultry by both legs with one hand positioning an index finger between the legs, while the other hand holds both wings at their base. The injection is given by another person into the pectoral muscle of the chest (Figure 8.6).

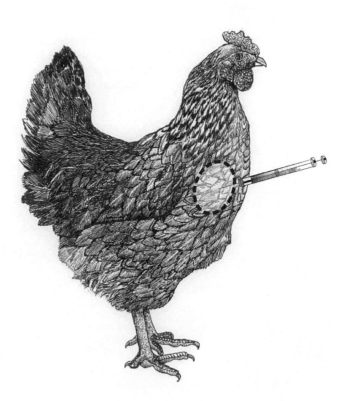

Figure 8.6   Intramuscular injection site in poultry.

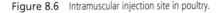

- ○ **Ratites:** Ratites are held in the same manner as for venipuncture to administer an IM injection into the pectoral muscles or thigh muscles.
- **Subcutaneous:** Subcutaneous injections are given to poultry in the wing web at the base of the wings. The same restraint needed for IM injections is used.

ADMINISTRATION OF ORAL MEDICATIONS

Most vaccines and medications for flocks are administered in the drinking water or by aerosol and do not involve handling or restraint.

BIBLIOGRAPHY

1. Damerow, G. Storey's Guide to Raising Poultry. 3rd edition. Storey Publishing, North Adams, MA, 2010.
2. Drowns, G. Storey's Guide to Raising Poultry. 4th edition. Chickens, Turkey, Ducks, Geese, Guineas, Game Birds. Storey Publishing, North Adams, MA, 2012.
3. Gauthier J, Ludlow R. Chicken Health for Dummies. Wiley, Somerset NJ, 2013.
4. Greenacre CB, Morishita TY. Backyard Poultry Medicine and Surgery: A Guide for Veterinary Practitioners. Wiley-Blackwell, Ames, IA, 2014.

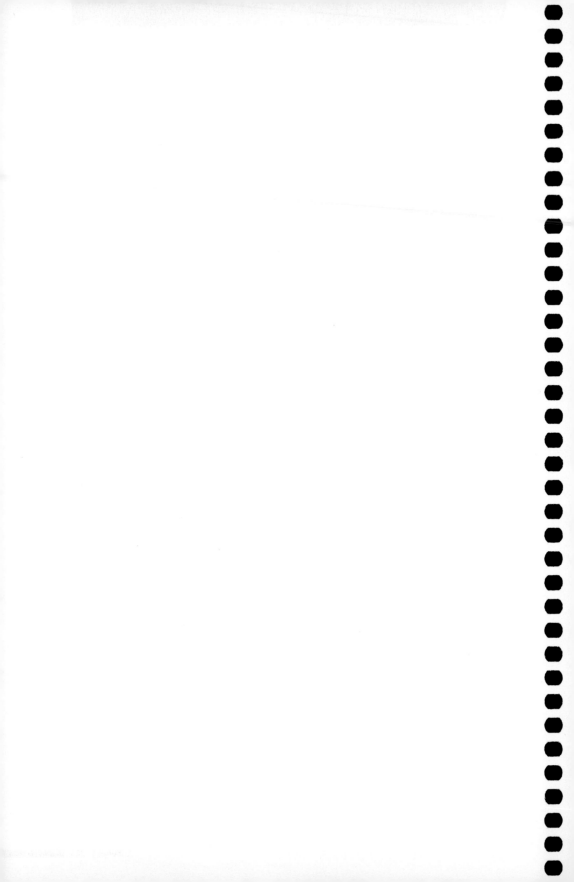

APPENDIX

SUPPLY SOURCES OF LARGE ANIMAL HANDLING AND RESTRAINT EQUIPMENT

Behlen Mfg. Co.
P.O. Box 569
Columbus, NE 68602
402-564-3111
behlencountry.com
Horse and Beef Cattle Equipment

D-S Livestock
18059 National Pike
Frostburg, MD 21532
800-949-9997
dslivequip@gmail.com
Cattle, Sheep, and Goat Equipment

Nasco
901 Janesville Ave.
P.O. Box 901
Fort Atkinson, WI 53538
800-558-9595
enasco.com
Alpaca, Dairy Cattle, Beef Cattle, Goat, Hog, Horse, Poultry,
and Sheep Supplies and Equipment

National Ropers Supply
4650 S. U.S. Hwy
287, Decatur, TX 76234
940-310-8363
nrsworld.com
Horse equipment and supplies

Priefert Ranch Equipment
2630 S. Jefferson
P.O. Box 1540
Mt. Pleasant, TX 75456
800-527-8616
priefert.com
Horse and Beef Cattle Equipment

Valley Vet Supply
1118 Pony Express Hwy.
Marysville, Kansas 66508
800-419-9524
valleyvet.com
Horse, cattle, goats, sheep, swine, and poultry equipment and supplies

MULTI-SPECIES BIBLIOGRAPHY AND RECOMMENDED READINGS

1. Ackerman N, Aspinall, V. Aspinall's Complete Textbook of Veterinary Nursing. 3rd edition. Elsevier, Orlando, FL, 2016.
2. Anderson RS, Edney ATB. Practical Animal Handling. Pergamon Press, Oxford, 1991.
3. Angulo FJ, Glaser CA, Juranek DD, et al. Caring for pets of immuno compromised persons. J Am Vet Med Assoc 1994;205:1711–1718.
4. Ballard B, Rockett J. Restraint and Handling for Veterinary Technicians and Assistants. Delmar, Clifton Park, NY, 2009.
5. Ballard B, Cheek R. Exotic Animal Medicine for the Veterinary Technician. 3rd edition. Wiley-Blackwell, Hoboken, NJ, 2017.
6. Baker WS, Gray GC. A review of published reports regarding zoonotic pathogen infection in veterinarians. J Am Vet Med Assoc 2009;234:1271–1278.
7. Bassett JM, Thomas J. McCurnin's Clinical Textbook for Veterinary Technicians. 9th edition. Elsevier, Orlando, FL, 2017.
8. Broom DM, Fraser AF. Chapter 21. Handling, Transport and Humane Control of Domestic Animals. In Domestic Animal Behaviour and Welfare. 4th edition. Oxford University Press, Oxford, 2007:199–215.
9. Campbell KL, Campbell JR. Companion Animals. 2nd edition. Pearson Education, Inc. Upper Saddle River, NJ, 2009.
10. Centers for Disease Control and Prevention: Injury Prevention & Control. www.cdc.gov/injury.
11. Colville JL, Berryhill DL. Handbook of Zoonoses: Identification and Prevention. Mosby Inc, St. Louis, MO, 2007.
12. Crow SE, Walshaw SO, Boyle JE. Manual of Clinical Procedures in Dogs, Cats, Rabbits, & Rodents. 3rd edition. Wiley-Blackwell, Ames, IA, 2009.
13. Fowler ME. Restraint and Handling of Wild and Domestic Animals. 3rd edition. Wiley-Blackwell, Ames, IA, 2008.
14. French D, Tully T. Restraint and Handling of Animals. In McCurnin DM, Bassert JM. Clinical Textbook for Veterinary Technicians. 6th edition. W.B. Saunders, Philadelphia, PA, 2005.
15. Grandin T. Improving Animal Welfare: A Practical Approach. CAB International, Cambridge, MA, 2010.
16. Grandin T, Johnson C. Animals in Translation: Using the Mysteries of Autism to Decode Animal Behavior. Scribner, New York, 2005.
17. Grandin, T, Johnson C. Animals Make Us Human: Creating the Best Life for Animals. First Mariner Books, New York, 2010.
18. Herron ME, Shreyer T. The pet-friendly veterinary practice: A guide for practitioners. Vet Clin Small Anim 2014;44:451–481.
19. Holtgrew-Bohling, K. Large Animal Clinical Procedures for Veterinary Technicians. 4th edition. Elsevier, St. Louis, MO, 2019.
20. Leahy JR, Barrow P. Restraint of Animals. 2nd edition. Cornell Campus Book Store, Ithaca, NY, 1953.
21. National Association of State Public Health Veterinarians Animal Contact Compendium Committee 2013. Compendium of measures to prevent disease associated with animals in public settings. J Am Vet Med Assoc 2013;243:1270–1288.
22. National Association of State Public Health Veterinarians. Compendium of standard precautions for zoonotic disease prevention in veterinary personnel. www.nasphv.org/Documents/VeterinaryStandardPrecautions.pdf, 2015.

23. National Center for Infectious Diseases. Healthy pets healthy people. www.cdc.gov/healthypets/child.htm, October 2016.
24. Pickering LK, Marano N, Bocchini JA, et al. Exposure to nontraditional pets at home and to animals in public settings: Risks to children. Pediatrics 2008;122:876–886.
25. Romich JA. Understanding Zoonotic Diseases. Thompson Delmar Learning, Clifton Park, NY, 2008.
26. Sheldon CC, Sonsthagen T, Topel JA. Animal Restraint for Veterinary Professionals. Mosby, St. Louis, MO, 2006.
27. Vanhorn B, Clark RW. Veterinary Assisting: Fundamentals & Applications. Delmar Cengage Learning, Clifton Park, NY, 2010.
28. Warren DM. Small Animal Care & Management. 4th edition. Delmar, Cengage Learning, New York, NY, 2015.

INDEX

Note: **Boldface** page references indicate tables. *Italic* references indicate figures.

gender, 59–60, 79, 245–246
goats, 210–211
habituation training methods and, 42
handler safety, 5, 26–27
health assessment and, 43, **43**
herd, 78–79, 156–157
hierarchy of animals, 27–28
inherent species, 5
instincts, 26
leaders, 28
manifestations of, 44
mules, 153
point of balance, 29
poultry, 268–269
predator, 26–27, 36
prey, 26–27, 36, 43
reinforcements of, 42
resistance, 38–40
respect for handler, 6
ruminants, 209
sheep, 210
socialization with humans, 28–29
stereotypic, 43–44, **44**
swine, 244–246
varied, 5
bends, **58**, 59
benzodiazepines, 20
best interest of animals, 22
bezerk male syndrome, 214
bib, 125
bird deterrence, 15, 88
bird handling, 34, *see also* poultry
blanketing horses, 119–121
blindfolds, 34, 107, 239
blocker tie ring, *104*
boars, 246, *see also* swine
body language, *see also specific type*
  of animals, 26, 80, 83, 210–211
  care/management handling of animals and, 4
  of handler, 4, 27
bolusing animals, 231
boss mare, 78
Brahman cattle, 159
breakaway cross ties, 106
breed behavior, 80
breeding stallion halters, 116
bucks (male goats), 213–214, 233, *see also* goats
bud's box, 172, **173**, *174*, 189, 250
bulls, 39, 156, 159, **159–160**, 186–187, *see also* cattle
Burley method, 195, *196*
butt bars, 177

C

calf tilt table, 179–180, *179*
California-style horseback roping, 72
calves, 158, 160, 166–169, *168*, **168**, 179–180, *179*, 204, *see also* cattle

camelids
  aggression in male, 214
  alleyways for, 237
  approaching, 237–238
  auditory communication by, 32
  behavior of, 211, *212*
  bezerk male syndrome, 214
  breeds of, 208, 237, **237**
  catching, 237–238
  characteristics of, 208, *209*
  chukkering, 240
  communication by, 32, 211
  defense tactics of, 211
  equipment for handling, 238–240, *238, 239*
  halters for, 239–240, *239*
  handler safety with, 214, **214**
  injections/venipuncture and, 240
  kicking by, 214
  kushing, 212, *213*, 240
  medical procedures and, 240
  mobile rope corral method and, 239
  moving, 239
  neck hug and, 237
  pens for, 238–239
  restraining, 237–240, *239*
  separating, 239
  social bonding of, 211
  spitting by, 214
  stocks for, 238, *238*
  temperature and, adversity to extreme, 212
  terminology, **237**
  territory and, protectiveness of, 211, 214
  transporting, 241
cannabidiol, 46
canvas slings for restraining swine, 260
care/management handling of animals, *see also specific animal*
  adaptation to special circumstances and, 6–7
  affection and, 3
  animal abuse regulations and, 19
  aromatherapy, 31–32
  attitude for, proper, 3
  best interest of animals and, 22
  body language and, 4
  clothing of handler and, 7–8, *7*, **7**, *8*, 17
  conditions for, 9–10
  dangerous animals, 19
  drugs for, 20–21
  duration of, 11
  early, risks of, 29
  effects on animals, 10, **10**
  elderly animals, 7
  ethical concerns, 17–18, **17**
  examples of good, 2, **2**
  facilitating, 26
  flexibility and, 22
  force and, use of, 18
  freedoms of domesticated animals, 2, **2**
  handlers seen as predators and, 27

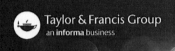

Concise Textbook of Large Animal Handling

A Practical Handbook

This concise instructional guide condenses the most important aspects of large animal handling. It provides a portable, durable, beside-the-animal means of learning, as well as a convenient way to refresh on how to strive for safety and efficacy in animal handling techniques. It is ideal for use during veterinary placements in all settings from farm to laboratory, to riding school. The text covers:

- Handler safety
- Animal safety
- Sanitation
- Approach and capture
- Routine handling and release procedures
- Handling for medical procedures
- Use and supply sources of restraint equipment

A Companion Website provides additional self-assessment questions and answers to aid learning.

Important reading for undergraduate veterinary students on EMS rotations, as well as practicing veterinarians, technicians, and assistants, the book covers species encountered in farm, equine, and laboratory settings.

FREE
INSTRUCTOR & STUDENT RESOURCES

Please visit the Companion Website at
www. routledgetextbooks.com/textbooks/9780367628093

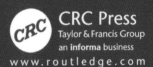

CRC Press
Taylor & Francis Group
an **informa** business

www.routledge.com

CRC Press titles are available as eBook editions in a range of digital formats

VETERINARY MEDICINE

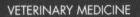
978-0-367-62809-3

9 780367 628093